Comprehensive Healthcare Simulation

Series Editors:

Adam I. Levine
Samuel DeMaria Jr.

This new series focuses on the use of simulation in healthcare education, one of the most exciting and significant innovations in healthcare teaching since Halsted put forth the paradigm of "see one, do one, teach one." Each volume focuses either on the use of simulation in teaching in a specific specialty or on a cross-cutting topic of broad interest, such as the development of a simulation center. The volumes stand alone and are also designed to complement Levine, DeMaria, Schwartz, and Sim, eds., THE COMPREHENSIVE TEXTBOOK OF HEALTHCARE SIMULATION by providing detailed and practical guidance beyond the scope of the larger book and presenting the most up-to-date information available. Series Editors Drs. Adam I. Levine and Samuel DeMaria Jr. are affiliated with the Icahn School of Medicine at Mount Sinai, New York, New York, USA, home to one of the foremost simulation centers in healthcare education. Dr. Levine is widely regarded as a pioneer in the use of simulation in healthcare education. Editors of individual series volumes and their contributors are all recognized leaders in simulation-based healthcare education.

More information about this series at http://www.springer.com/series/13029

Shad Deering • Tamika C. Auguste
Dena Goffman

Editors

Comprehensive Healthcare Simulation: Obstetrics and Gynecology

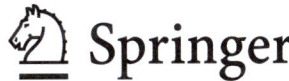 Springer

Editors
Shad Deering
Department of Obstetrics and
Gynecology
Uniformed Services University
of the Health Sciences
Bethesda, MD, USA

Tamika C. Auguste
Department of Obstetrics and
Gynecology
MedStar Washington Hospital Center
Washington, DC, USA

Dena Goffman
Department of Obstetrics and
Gynecology
Columbia University Irving Medical
Center
New York, NY, USA

ISSN 2366-4479   ISSN 2366-4487   (electronic)
Comprehensive Healthcare Simulation
ISBN 978-3-319-98994-5   ISBN 978-3-319-98995-2   (eBook)
https://doi.org/10.1007/978-3-319-98995-2

Library of Congress Control Number: 2018966143

This Springer imprint is published by the registered company Springer Nature Switzerland AG
The registered company address is: Gewerbestrasse 11, 6330 Cham, Switzerland

We dedicate this book to Sterling B. Williams, MS, MD, PhD, with our deepest respect and gratitude. As a result of his leadership and foresight, the ACOG Simulation Working Group (formerly Consortium) was launched in 2008. This group that he advocated to create has made tremendous contributions and continues to work to establish simulation as a pillar in education for women's health through collaboration, advocacy, research, and the development and implementation of multidisciplinary simulations-based educational resources and opportunities for obstetricians and gynecologists. We are most appreciative for his vision, passion, and tireless efforts mentoring the future leaders in OBGYN education.

Foreword

Simulation in obstetrics and gynecology permeates all levels of education and is recognized as key component of patient safety and quality improvement initiatives. Although J. Whitridge Williams recognized simulation as an important element in teaching in the 1890s, its use in our field did not explode until the end of the twentieth century. The requirement for simulation in our training programs and the recognition of simulation in our certification process drive innovation today.

In the 1990s, I served as a military physician. Impressed by the aviation and military applications of simulation, the Department of Defense invested in medical simulations. Shad Deering was a resident in the Uniformed Services University program. His passion for harnessing simulation to improve education and care delivery sparked the beginning of an extraordinary career. The Society of Maternal-Fetal Medicine and the American College of Obstetricians and Gynecologists supported adding young physicians as faculty to our continuing education courses at our annual meetings. Shad Deering, Dena Goffman, and Tamika C. Auguste were part of that team. Today they are the recognized leaders in simulation in our specialty and subspecialties.

Every month our journals and online publications describe simulations applied to education, training, and safety initiatives. Trying to decipher the best ways to implement and reap the benefits of simulation may be analogous to trying to drink from a fire hose. Drs. Deering, Goffman, and Auguste and their team of authors assembled a resource to allow readers to access useful information in one place. *Simulation in Obstetrics and Gynecology* provides a roadmap for implementation of simulation in obstetrics and gynecology. It fills a necessary and important niche in this exciting and relevant field. Whether you are a learner, educator, clinician, or simply interested in improving care to patients and their families, you will benefit from their efforts.

Andrew J. Satin, MD, FACOG
Johns Hopkins Medicine
Baltimore, MD, USA

Preface

In our specialty, we have moved from the time when a select few providers started using simulation because they felt it had the potential to improve outcomes to where it is now recommended by national organizations and almost universally used in training programs for all levels of providers. As more evidence continues to be published supporting its effectiveness in improving actual patient outcomes, its use will only continue to increase. But, even though simulation is now widely accepted as a necessary step in training, there remains a gap in practical advice and instruction on how to implement this training. Motivated providers and educators have to start from scratch and create programs at their own institutions. They learn by trial and error and expend a significant amount of time and resources in the process. Since most of us started this way, we applaud the efforts of everyone who has done this, but felt there needed to be a single place where anyone can go to find what they need to set up a program to fit their institution based on their specific needs.

What the editors have worked to provide you in this book is a clear path to success in whatever area of simulation you are interested in within the specialty of obstetrics and gynecology. To this end, we have assembled a team of leading experts in the field who use simulation every day at their local institutions and bring their wealth of experience to share. One thing you will find if you are around these people is that they are passionate about making a difference. They constantly strive to both improve training and outcomes while at the same time critically examine their methods and the evidence to make sure what they are doing is effective.

You will also see that they love to share what they have developed and do not want others to have to reinvent the same things and waste time when they could be training others! We have worked hard to focus the chapters and make sure this translates in the book to deliver both a solid background and concrete examples to get you up and running in as little time as necessary.

So, going forward, we recommend that you remember a few simple things about simulation in general and also as they apply to OB/GYN:

1. Think of your audience first and the simulator last: Since starting to do medical simulation, one of the most common questions we hear is "which type of simulator should I buy?" It is a fair thing to ask and one that definitely has to be answered, but it is also not the first thing to do. The first

question should always be, "who am I training and what do I need them to learn."

2. Be ready to learn and change with every training event: I often tell people who are starting to run simulations that after they write and prepare for the training, it is important to practice them prior to using them with actual learners. No matter how clear you think you have been in writing out your instructions, and even if you are certain about what the learners actions/ reactions will be, you will be surprised every time. I have yet to run a course or event where a provider did not ask a question or do something I had not anticipated or there was some kind of issue with a simulator or script that came up. Being prepared to adjust in the middle is part of what makes simulation training effective, because it is just like real life. So, when this happens, do not get frustrated. Embrace the unexpected and use it to improve the next simulation and the overall experience.

3. Do not ever stop being curious: Being curious when you run and debrief simulation training events is critical. When you use simulation, it is inevitable that people will make mistakes during the training sessions. Always remember that they had a reason for making the error. It may be a lack of knowledge or something they were previously taught. They may not have known what to do and decided to "just do something" to try and save face or possibly had a rough night on call and are too tired to think straight. Remember that no one gets up in the morning and decides they want to make a mistake. There is a reason for everything people do. Ask questions and be genuinely curious, always focusing on understanding why the decision was made and then helping to reframe the discussion to allow them to improve for the next time they have an actual case with a real patient.

4. Always remember why: Finally and most importantly, always remember why you are doing the training. The end result of everything that we do with simulation is to improve the care provided to the patient. This translates directly to a better quality of life for the patients and their families, and it also affects the stress levels of the providers because every bad outcome weighs on them as well. While we have endeavored to explain the objective evidence that demonstrates simulation training makes a difference in our specialty in this book, it is the individual stories that your learners will tell you about how your training made a difference that brings the true importance into focus.

You have taken the first step in your journey to better and more effective training by reading this far. Simulation training takes more effort and resources than traditional lectures, but the return is more than worth it. So, embrace the quest, and thank you for working to make a difference.

Bethesda, MD, USA   Shad Deering, MD

Acknowledgments

We would like to acknowledge all of the hard work and contributions of every author and publishing staff member who was part of the creation and final delivery of this book. It has truly been a labor of love inspired by the impact we see every day that simulation can make in our patient's lives. Without the time and efforts of the entire team, it would not have been possible.

Contents

Contributors

Arnold Patrick Advincula, MD Columbia University Medical Center/New York-Presbyterian Hospital, Department of Obstetrics and Gynecology, New York, NY, USA

Mary & Michael Jaharis Simulation Center, New York, NY, USA

Chetna Arora, MD Columbia University Medical Center/New York-Presbyterian Hospital, Department of Obstetrics and Gynecology, New York, NY, USA

Tamika C. Auguste, MD Department of Obstetrics and Gynecology, MedStar Washington Hospital Center, Washington, DC, USA

Komal Bajaj, MD, MS-HPEd NYC Health + Hospitals Simulation Center, Bronx, NY, USA

Albert Einstein College of Medicine, Bronx, NY, USA

Les R. Becker, PhD, MS.MEdL, NRP, CHSE MedStar Health, Simulation Training and Education Lab (SiTEL), Washington, DC, USA

Department of Emergency Medicine, Georgetown University School of Medicine, Washington, DC, USA

Brian C. Brost, MD Wake Forest School of Medicine, Department of Obstetrics and Gynecology, Division of Maternal-Fetal Medicine, Winston-Salem, NC, USA

E. Britton Chahine, MD Department of Gynecology and Obstetrics, Emory University School of Medicine, Atlanta, GA, USA

Angela Chaudhari, MD Division of Minimally Invasive Gynecology, Fellowship in Minimally Invasive Gynecologic Surgery, Department of Obstetrics and Gynecology, Northwestern University, Feinberg School of Medicine, Chicago, IL, USA

Chi Chiung Grace Chen, MD MHS Department of Gynecology and Obstetrics, Division of Female Pelvic Medicine and Reconstructive Surgery, Johns Hopkins University School of Medicine, Baltimore, MD, USA

Meleen Chuang, MD, FACOG Albert Einstein College of Medicine/
Montefiore Medical Center, Bronx, NY, USA

Lou Clark, MFA, PhD Uniformed Services University of the Health
Sciences, Val G. Hemming Simulation Center, Silver Spring, MD, USA

Mary K. Collins, DO Walter Reed National Military Medical Center,
Bethesda, MD, USA

Kay Daniels, MD Department of Obstetrics and Gynecology, Stanford
Health Care, Palo Alto, CA, USA

Shad Deering, MD, FACOG Department of Obstetrics and Gynecology,
Uniformed Services University of the Health Sciences, Bethesda, MD, USA

Renee M. Dorsey, BS (Biology) Uniformed Services University of the
Health Sciences, Val G. Hemming Simulation Center, Silver Spring, MD,
USA

Etoi A. Garrison, MD, PhD Department of Obstetrics and Gynecology,
Vanderbilt University Medical Center, Nashville, TN, USA

Dena Goffman, MD Department of Obstetrics and Gynecology, Columbia
University Irving Medical Center, New York, NY, USA

Toni Huebscher Golen, MD Department of Obstetrics and Gynecology,
Beth Israel Deaconess Medical Center, Boston, MA, USA

Bethany Crandell Goodier, PhD Department of Communication, College
of Charleston, Charleston, SC, USA

Christopher G. Goodier, MD Department of Maternal Fetal Medicine,
Medical University of South Carolina, Charleston, SC, USA

Kimberly S. Harney, MD Stanford University School of Medicine,
Department of Obstetrics & Gynecology, Stanford, CA, USA

Belinda A. Hermosura, MSN, RN, CHSE MedStar Health, Simulation
Training & Education Lab (SiTEL), Washington, DC, USA

Erin Higgins, MD Department of Obstetrics and Gynecology, Cleveland
Clinic, Cleveland, OH, USA

Jin Hee Jeannie Kim, MD Columbia University Medical Center/New York-
Presbyterian Hospital, Department of Obstetrics and Gynecology, New York,
NY, USA

Colleen A. Lee, MS, RN Department of Quality and Patient Safety, New York
Presbyterian/Weill Cornell Medical Center, New York, NY, USA

Emily K. Marko, MD, FACOG, CHSE Department of Obstetrics and
Gynecology, Inova Health System, Falls Church, VA, USA

David Marzano, MD Department of Obstetrics and Gynecology, University
of Michigan, Ann Arbor, MI, USA

Shirley McAdam, CHSE Clinical Simulation Laboratory at the University of Vermont, Burlington, VT, USA

Michael Meguerdichian, MD, MHP-Ed NYC Health + Hospitals Simulation Center, Bronx, NY, USA

Harlem Hospital Center, Emergency Department/H+H Simulation Center, New York, NY, USA

Emily Nicole Bernice Myer, MD Department of Gynecology and Obstetrics, Division of Female Pelvic Medicine and Reconstructive Surgery, Johns Hopkins University School of Medicine, Baltimore, MD, USA

Joshua F. Nitsche, MD, PhD Wake Forest School of Medicine, Department of Obstetrics and Gynecology, Division of Maternal-Fetal Medicine, Winston-Salem, NC, USA

Jessica L. Pippen, MD Department of Obstetrics and Gynecology, The Ohio State University Wexner Medical Center, Columbus, OH, USA

Jean-Ju Sheen, MD Department of Obstetrics and Gynecology, New York Presbyterian/Columbia University Irving Medical Center, New York, NY, USA

Vanessa Strickland Uniformed Services University of the Health Sciences, Val G. Hemming Simulation Center, Silver Spring, MD, USA

Chelsea Weaks, M.Ed. Gynecological Teaching Associate Program, School – Eastern Virginia Medical School, Sentara Center for Simulation and Immersive Learning, Norfolk, VA, USA

Part I

Introduction to Simulation for Obstetrics and Gynecology

The History of Simulation in Obstetrics and Gynecology

David Marzano

Introduction

Simulation use in medicine is not a new concept. Many teaching and training techniques over the centuries have utilized "models" to allow learners to develop, practice, and demonstrate skills related to the practice of medicine. For the purposes of this overview, "simulation" will be defined according to the Society for Simulation in Healthcare: "an educational technique that replaces or amplifies real experiences with guided experiences that evoke or replicate substantial aspects of the real world in a fully interactive manner" [1]. Most medical students' first induction to simulation is learning human anatomy. Anatomic dissection using human cadavers, a very high-fidelity simulator, is a rite of passage for most medical students. Cadaveric dissection allows learners to touch, feel, and experience body systems in their natural state. Modern medical educators, like their earlier counterparts, recognize the drawbacks of using human cadavers for demonstration of techniques beyond identification and familiarity with anatomy. There are limitations of using preserved (and in very early medical education less well preserved) cadavers: limited availability, need for facilities, expense, and less than ideal practice for specific skills and techniques [2]. Those same limitations were present for early medical educators [3]. The need for models that were reusable, stable, and representative of the skills to be taught became apparent. This led to the development of some of the early simulators allowing students to practice, repetitively, and hone skills prior to practice on patients.

Simulators have evolved over the centuries. A simulator, as defined by the Society for Simulation in Healthcare, is "any object or representation used during training or assessment that behaves or operates like a given system and responds to the user's actions" [1]. From very early models used in ancient China, developed to train in the field of acupuncture, to glass and wooden models to replicate the female pelvis, to CPR trainers (Resusci-Annie), and to the complex full-body human simulators and virtual-reality (VR) trainers in use today, advances in computer technology and moulaging techniques have led to the most cutting-edge simulators in use in OB/GYN today [4]. More importantly, the history of simulation must also include a discussion of the development of curricula to make use of these simulators. Simulators, or the physical object or representation of full or part task to be replicated [5], are the tools or means for instruction in specific skills or techniques. The simulator is a device used during an educational encounter informed by a curriculum with specific goals, objectives, and measurable outcomes. Unfortunately, while there exist brief descriptions of simulators used in centuries

D. Marzano (✉)
Department of Obstetrics and Gynecology, University of Michigan, Ann Arbor, MI, USA
e-mail: damarz@umich.edu

past, very little specifics of curricula survive. With the advancement in simulation and development of simulators, there has also been an explosion of medical curricula used in modern medical training, which will serve as one of the most important contributions to future medical training.

From its nascent beginnings to modern times, along with development of simulation as a teaching pedagogy, the study and implementation of simulation has evolved as well. National organizations, such as the Society of Simulation in Healthcare, have been created to define, create, study, and disseminate simulation-based research. Medical and nursing schools now have simulation centers to provide resources and materials as well as curricula and educational faculty, for the education of future practitioners, and to conduct research into future uses of medical simulation. Medical specialty societies have developed simulation sections, including the American College of Obstetricians and Gynecologists, to define, design, and implement educational programs to advance the safe delivery of healthcare to patients.

> **Key Learning Points**
> - Simulation has been used in obstetrics and gynecology for many years and is a critical part of training.
> - Training for procedures as well as communication and teamwork can be done in obstetrics and gynecology.
> - Research into simulation and its use in the specialty continues to build.
> - Simulation use in the specialty will continue to increase and is likely to be incorporated into both certification and licensure.

The History of Simulation in Obstetrics

Dating as far back as the 1700s, the need for simulation in obstetrics was recognized. For most of recorded history, women were delivered by other women, which evolved into the practice of midwifery. In 1543, *de conceptu et generatione hominis* was published by Jacob Rueff, a surgeon, in which the method of delivery of the obstructed fetus was described. The publication of this book is thought to have made it possible for men to become educated in the practice of obstetrics and thus began the contentious relationship between physicians and midwives [6]. The view that midwives were not well trained sparked the development of some of the early simulation models. The need to educate midwives in the practice of obstetrics was recognized by Giovanni Antonio Galli, who designed one of the first "high-fidelity" simulators, creating a uterus comprised of glass with a flexible baby [4]. Prior to this point, most simulators were made of wood or clay. Galli, as an early simulation educator, recognized not only the need for a model to teach but the necessity to assess performance. He is reported to have had his students perform the simulation blindfolded, demonstrating the ability to demonstrate their skills [7]. This early form of an assessment was a key development in simulation training that remains today.

The use of obstetrics simulation continued to became more popular, with institutions in Europe utilizing various models for learners to practice and develop skills. Marie-Catherine Biheron, an anatomist, was known for her creation of wax replications of female anatomy that were considered very realistic. Her models were used in teaching institutions for over 50 years [8]. Angelique Marguerite Le Boursier du Coudray advanced both the practice of simulation as well as the development of the need to incorporate education and practice for skills development. King Louis XV, in an attempt to reduce the falling live birth rate in France, called upon du Coudray to educate midwives in the practice of obstetrics. She developed life-size simulators that would still be considered high fidelity today. Her simulators had interchangeable cervices, the ability to change cervical dilation, and different-sized fetuses. She could replicate rupture of membranes and hemorrhage as well. Perhaps equally as important, she developed an instructional course that was comprised of 40 hours of practice, representing a very early forerunner of modern-day medical simulation education [9].

Throughout the 1800s, simulation was being used throughout Europe, with various models, some with descriptions, others only mentioning the use of mannequins. At the same time, medical schools in the United States were using simulation as a means of compensating for the lack of hospital-based births [10]. During this same time period, organizations were developed to shape the structure of medical education in the United States. In 1876, the first meeting of what was to become the Association of American Medical Colleges occurred, defining their purpose as "the object of the convention is to consider all matters relating to reform in medical college work" [11]. In 1910, Abraham Flexner presented his report on medical education in the United States and Canada to the Carnegie Foundation for the advancement of teaching. As part of this significant report that would shape medical training throughout the twenty-first century, he commented on the poor state of medical education in North America. He made a specific reference on the importance of the use of simulation as a medical educational tool. He was particularly critical of the training in obstetrics, stating, "the very worst showing is made in the matter of obstetrics" [12]. He suggested that students should practice on a mannequin first, followed by graduated responsibility to direct patient care. He also pointed that didactic lectures were not useful for the teaching of obstetrics and yet the use of "mannequin" was of limited value, as clinical teaching and experience is necessary. Unfortunately at that time, there were limited deliveries because most women delivered outside of the hospital and in some cases no formal departments of obstetrics and gynecology existed [12].

With technological advances, the introduction of computers and electronics propelled simulation use in many other fields, including the fields of business, military, and aviation. In 1968, there was the introduction of Harvey, a mannequin that incorporated computer technology to allow for learners to assess vital signs and heart sounds and perform procedures. Harvey was the first modern-day high-fidelity simulator [13]. This set the wheels in motion for the development of the many commercially available obstetric simulators used today. These include high-fidelity full-body mannequins with computer control of vital signs, control of the descent of the fetal presenting part, ability to bleed, replication of cesarean sections, and the ability to provide a very realistic environment to allow the learner of obstetrics to practice. High-fidelity simulators today utilize wireless technology, radio-frequency recognition, and even allow for verbal interaction. There are also numerous obstetric partial task trainers, such as pelvises to visualize the fetus moving through the birth canal and those that allow the provider to place forceps and practice shoulder dystocia maneuvers. Low-fidelity models continue to be in regular use with many educators creating models to fulfill the specific goal they are trying to achieve.

Interestingly a 1978 airplane crash provided obstetric simulation its next giant step forward in terms of team training. The FAA investigation into the cause of the crash, which identified a malfunctioning light which then distracted the pilot from recognizing and listening to his crew warning him of the lack of engine fuel, led to the development of the program known as crew resource management (CRM). The key elements of this program identify that responsibilities of all members of the team are important and focus on safety. This included flight attendants, ground crews, and air traffic control. Pilot training was already making use of simulation, but the addition of CRM changed training from merely how to operate to how to interact with the crew, respond to changes, and identify problems [14]. In 1999, the Institute of Medicine published *To Err is Human: Building a Safer Health System*, identified team training as a need in the delivery of healthcare and cited CRM as one successful model [15]. In a similar fashion, the American College of Obstetrics and Gynecology (ACOG) released a joint statement calling for the use of simulation as a means of improving patient care through improved teamwork [16]. This added the current level of advancement in obstetric simulation present in modern day. In conjunction with the Department of Defense, the Agency for

Healthcare Research and Quality (AHQR) set out to apply the key elements of CRM to medical teams; several programs were created. The earliest advances were made with anesthesia crew resources management. Since then additional programs have been developed including MedTeams, the Medical Team Management program, and currently the Team Strategies and Tools to Enhance Performance and Patient Safety (TeamSTEPPS). These are a several examples of such programs that were applied to train medical teams including obstetrics teams [17].

Obstetric simulation, a part of medical education in training for centuries has evolved into a stepwise fashion to include (1) individual development of specific skills (e.g., placement of forceps), (2) individual development and practice of skills in an environment with a clinical scenario present (e.g., forceps delivery for arrest of descent in a patient with a bradycardia), and finally (3) development and practice of skills in a team, with all members of the labor and delivery, including additional disciplines (pediatrics and anesthesia), nursing, certified nurse midwives, medical aides, and clerical staff during a clinical scenario (e.g., arrest of descent with bradycardia, forceps delivery, postpartum hemorrhage).

The History of Simulation in Gynecology

The field of obstetrics and gynecology is unique in that it combines almost all aspects of healthcare delivery to women. An exploration of the history of gynecologic simulation first starts in examining the beginnings of surgical simulation. While the use of simulation in obstetrics has a rich history, that history is less well documented for gynecology and even surgery as a whole. One of the oldest surgical "textbooks," the Sushruta Samhita, survives from around 600 BC [18]. Sushruta, who pre-dates Hippocrates by about 150 years, was an Indian surgeon who documented his experience in surgery. While commonly referred to as the father of plastic surgery for his description of procedures such as rhinoplasty and cleft lip repairs, he also described the

use of simulation in his manual. Specifically, he used fruits and vegetables, as well as rotted wood as models for teaching his students [18].

In 1909, describing his experience with litholapaxy, the destruction of a stone in the bladder, the use of a "phantom" bladder for practice is referenced. During a discussion at the American Urological Association, Dr. Krotoszyner described his practice at litholapaxy on a phantom bladder, stating, "By these means I have acquired so much practice that my results with litholapaxy has been of late very satisfactory." [19]. Not only does this demonstrate the use of simulation early in the twentieth century but acknowledges its usefulness in practicing a surgical procedure and improving performance.

While laparoscopy is frequently considered a modern-day procedure, the history of laparoscopy and the implementation of its routine use was a major driver of advancement in the use of simulation for gynecologic procedures. The first laparoscopic procedure was performed in 1901 by George Kelling, who initially performed his procedure on dogs [20]. Kurt Semm, sometimes referred to as the father of modern laparoscopy, was instrumental in the development of the use of laparoscopy. In addition to his development of techniques, instruments, and critically an insufflator, he also developed a pelvic trainer to be used in practicing laparoscopic skills. It was transparent to allow for visualization of techniques [21]. Modifications of this concept, now known as box trainers, are present in simulation centers throughout the world.

As the use of laparoscopy became more frequently employed, the complexity of intraoperative procedures increased, including oocyte retrieval, tubal ligation, adhesiolysis, salpingostomy, and eventually in 1988, Harry Reich performed the first laparoscopic hysterectomy [22]. By the beginning of the twenty-first century, minimally invasive procedures were becoming the mainstay of gynecologic surgery. The next big step forward for minimally invasive surgery came shortly thereafter with the introduction of robotic surgery. Though there were many early versions, in 2005 the DaVinci surgical system (Intuitive Surgical, Inc.) was FDA approved for the use of gynecologic surgery [23]. This ushered in a new era for minimally invasive surgery.

With the advancement of laparoscopy, the need for a platform for education also emerged. The use of training platforms began with Semm's development of his laparoscopic trainer. This has led to use of box trainers, which can be used for development of multiple skills, including eye-hand coordination, economy of movement, and proper visualization. Other simulation platforms have included live animals and cadavers, as these provide a true high-fidelity experience, replicating actual tissue planes, and in the case of cadavers true human anatomy. Unfortunately, several barriers to this type of training exist: cost, availability, need for facilities to maintain and procure specimens, and, in the case of animals, recent ethical considerations [24].

Further technologic advances have led to the development of virtual-reality (VR) surgical trainers, with the ability not only to allow learners to practice basic skills but actual procedures that will be performed in practice. Many of these VR trainers also allow for a more formative evaluation, as computer programs are able to score performances based upon programmed objectives [24]. The current state of medical education and training now has many simulation tools at its disposal for teaching future gynecologist in a safe environment without putting the patient at increased risk.

Despite the explosion in simulation opportunities, needs in laparoscopic training and evaluation still exist. As is evident by a recent call to action, "…there is no standardized evidence-based laparoscopy program to teach gynecology residents laparoscopic surgery…" [25]. The authors suggest three steps forward: (1) simulation education should be implemented in all training programs, (2) training programs should adopt a standardized curriculum, and (3) a standardized assessment should be conducted to ensure competency [25]. While there are many publications detailing individual methods used for training, no formal curriculum exists in the field of gynecology. The surgical discipline has made this step forward in the adoption of the fundamentals of laparoscopic surgery, a simulation-training program. The fundamentals of laparoscopic surgery are an example of a validated curriculum currently utilized by the American Board of Surgery (ABS). The ABS has required that all applicants graduating after 2010 be certified in FLS [26]. No such requirement is currently required of graduating obstetrics and gynecology residents. Likely simulation will provide a role in the future.

The use of minimally invasive gynecologic surgery has now become the mainstay of practice in modern gynecology. As outlined, this has significantly driven the need for simulators and simulation curricula to train future physicians. Just as Flexner noted in his 1901 report about lack of opportunities for deliveries for obstetrics students, modern-day educators have seen a new gap in gynecology resident training: the infrequent performance of abdominal hysterectomies. As a result of the success of minimally invasive techniques, fewer and fewer abdominal hysterectomies are performed in teaching hospitals in the United States. As a result, there is a paucity of learning experiences for what was once an abundant, common procedure. Because of this lack of training, perhaps the next wave of advancement for gynecologic surgical simulation will be the development of abdominal hysterectomy models.

Pelvic models have also been used for introduction of medical learners to the pelvic exam, pelvic anatomy, and office-based procedures such as IUD placement and endometrial biopsy [27].

The History of Simulation Education and Research

While education and training have always been at the root of the development of simulation, the modern age has seen the development of simulation education as a field of research. The full gamut of simulators is currently being used for medical education, including high- and low-fidelity models, partial task trainers, homegrown models, simulated patient instructors, and VR trainers. Simulation centers, partnered with educational experts have been established to optimize simulation curricula and research into the use of simulation. Yet, this research is still working on the answer to the big question: Does it improve outcomes? The evolution of simulation as field of study is based on this question. Numerous publications have addressed the development, realism, acceptance, and finally validation of curricula to use simulation as a means of education. While previously described presentations on medical training mention simulation, the first major conference to provide a means for dissemination of simulation research was held in 1991. In 2001, the first International Meeting on Medical Simulation met as part of an anesthesiology technology conference [28]. The year 2004 saw the creation of the Society for Simulation in Healthcare (SSH), with the goal to provide an organization dedicated to educators and researchers in the field of medical simulation, acknowledging that simulation bridges specialties and disciplines. In 2006, the journal *Simulation in Healthcare* was created to provide a means for dissemination of research in the "science of simulation" [29]. In addition to SSH, individual specialties have devoted resources to the development of simulation, including the American College of Obstetrics and Gynecology (ACOG). The ACOG Simulations Consortium (now Working Group) was established in 2009 with the mission of "establishing [simulation] as a pillar in education for women's health through collaboration, advocacy, research, and the development and implementation of multidisciplinary simulation-based educational resources and opportunities for Obstetrics and Gynecology" [30].

Conclusion

Medical simulation is not new to medical training, having evidence of its use as a means of teaching and evaluation dating back as far as 600 BC. The field of obstetrics and gynecology has been part of this endeavor from the beginning and has grown from vague descriptions to very detailed published research dealing with all aspects of simulation: (1) design of simulators,

(2) development of curricula, (3) development and validation of assessment tools, and (4) evaluation of these tools. Obstetrics and gynecology, being unique among medical fields in its breadth and depth of types of care, has seen the use of simulation for teaching for individual skills training, practice, and evaluation. With the most recent focus on patient safety and the need for team training, this field, operating in a realm of complex teams, has seen the expansion of the use of simulation in team training. More recently simulation has begun to be used for maintenance of certification. The American Board of Medical Specialties (ABMS) states in its 2014 Standards for the ABMS Program for Maintenance of Certification (MOC) that in addition to other requirements "…other commonly used evaluations include oral examinations and simulation exercises…" can be used for assessment of skills [31]. The future of simulation in obstetrics and gynecology will likely see the use of simulation for residency assessment, board examinations, and credentialing.

References

1. Lopreiato JO (Ed.), Downing D, Gammon W, Lioce L, Sittner B, Slot V, Spain AE (Associate Eds.), the Terminology & Concepts Working Group. Healthcare simulation dictionary; 2016. Retrieved from http://www.ssih.org/dictionary.
2. Badash I, Burtt K, Solorzano CA, Cary JN. Innovations in surgery simulation: a review of past, current and future techniques. Ann Transl Med. 2016;4(23):453. https://doi.org/10.21037/atm.2016.12.24.
3. Elizondo-Omaña RE, Guzmán-López S, De Los Angeles García-Rodríguez M. Dissection as a teaching tool: past, present, and future. Anat Rec. 2005;285B:11–5. https://doi.org/10.1002/ar.b.20070.
4. Owen H. Early use of simulation in healthcare. Simul Healthc. 2012;7(2):102–16. https://doi.org/10.1097/SIH.0b013e3182415a91.
5. Cooper JB, Taqueti VR. A brief history of the development of mannequin simulators for clinical education and training. Qual Saf Health Care. 2004;13(Suppl 1):i11–8. https://doi.org/10.1136/qshc.2004.009886.
6. Drife J. The start of life: a history of obstetrics. Postgrad Med J. 2002;78:311–5.
7. Acton R. The evolving role of simulation in teaching in undergraduate medical education. In: Brown KM, Paige JT, editors. Simulation in surgical training and Practice. Phildeplhia: Elsevier; 2015. p. 740–1.

8. Haines CM. International women in science: a biographical dictionary to 1950. Santa Barbara: ABC-CLO, Inc; 2001. p. 32.

9. Clark V, Van de Velde M, Fernando R. Oxford textbook of obstetric anaesthesia. Oxford: Oxford University Press; 2016. p. 853.

10. Owen H, Pelosi M. A historical examination of the Budin-Pinard Phantom: what can contemporary obstetrics education learn from simulators of the past? Acad Med. 2013;88(5):652–6.

11. Association of American Medical Colleges [Interent] AAMC History. Available at: https://www.aamc.org/about/history/. Last accessed Feb 2017.

12. Flexner A. Medical education in the United States and Canada: a report to the Carnegie Foundation for the advancement of teaching. New York; 1910:117. [Internet] Available from: http://archive.carnegiefoundation.org/pdfs/elibrary/Carnegie_Flexner_Report.pdf. Last accessed Feb 2017.

13. Gordon MS, Ewy GA, DeLeon AC Jr, Waugh RA, Felner JM, Forker AD, et al. "Harvey," the cardiology patient simulator: pilot studies on teaching effcctiveness. Am J Cariol. 1980;45(4):791–6.

14. Helmreich RL. Managing human error in aviation. Sci Am. 1997;276(5):52–7.

15. Committee on Quality of health Care in America; Institute of Medicine. In: Kohn LT, Corrigan JM, Donaldson MS, editors. To Err is human: building a safer health system. Washington, DC: National Academies Press; 2000.

16. Lawrence HC III, Copel JA, O'Keeffe DF, Bradford WC, Scarrow PK, Kennedy HP, et al. Quality patient care in labor and delivery: a call to action. Am J Obstet Gynecol. 2012;207(3):147–8. https://doi.org/10.1016/j.ajog.2012.07.018.

17. Chapter 4. Medical team training: medical teamwork and patient safety: the evidence-based relation. Agency for Healthcare Research and Quality, Rockville; 2005. Available from: http://archive.ahrq.gov/research/findings/final-reports/medteam/chapter4.html. Last accessed Feb 2017.

18. Saraf S, Parihar R. Sushruta: the first plastic surgeon in 600 BC. Int J Plast Surg. 2006;4(2):1–7.

19. Cumston CG, editor. 7th Suprapubic operation for stone with immediate closure of wound. Transactions of the American Urological Association. Brookline: Riverdale Press; 1909. p. 98.

20. Spner SJ, Warnock GL. A brief history of endocopy, laparoscoy, and laparoscopic surgery. J Laparoendosc Adv Surg Tech A. 1997;7(6):369–73.

21. Moll FH, Marx FJ. A pioneer in laparoscopy and pelviscopy: Kurt Semm (1927–2003). J Endurology. 2005;19(3):269–71.

22. Lau WY, Leow CK, Li AKC. History of endoscopic and laparoscopic surgery. World J Surg. 1997;21(4):444–53.

23. Advincula AP, Wang K. Evolving role and current state of robotics in minimally invasive gynecologic surgery. J Minim Invasive Gynecol. 2009;16(3):291–301.

24. Badash I, Burtt K, Solorzano CA, Carey JN. Innovations in surgery simulation: a review of past, current and future techniques. Am Transl Med. 2016;4(23):453.

25. Shore EM, Lefebvre GG, Grantcharov TP. Gynecology resident laparoscopy training: present and future. Am J Obstet Gynecol. 2015;212(3):298–301, 298. e1. https://doi.org/10.1016/j.ajog.2014.07.039. Epub 2014 Jul 25.

26. Buyske J. The role of simulation in certification. Surg Clin North Am. 2010;90(3):619–21. https://doi.org/10.1016/j.suc.2010.02.013.

27. Nitschmann C, Bartz D, Johnson NR. Gynecologic simulation training increases medical student confidence and interest in women's health. Teach Learn Med. 2014;26(2):160–3. https://doi.org/10.1080/10401334.2014.883984.

28. Rosen KR. The history of medical simulation. J Crit Care. 2008;23(2):157–66. https://doi.org/10.1016/j.jcrc.2007.12.004. https://www.ncbi.nlm.nih.gov/pubmed/18538206.

29. Gaba DM. The future's here. We are it. Simul Healthc. 2006;1:1–2.

30. American Congress of Obstetrics and Gynecology [Internet] working group goals and objectives. Available from: http://www.acog.org/About-ACOG/ACOG-Departments/Simulations-Consortium/Consortium-Goals-and-Objectives. Last accessed Feb 2017.

31. American Board of Medical Specialties [Internet] Standards for the ABMS program for maintenance of certification (MOC). January 15, 2014. Available from: www.abms.org/media/1109/standards-for-the-abms-program-for-moc-final.pdf. Last accessed Feb 2017.

Simulation Education Theory

2

Les R. Becker and Belinda A. Hermosura

Introduction

Simulation-based educational methods are recognized as an established component of medical training for medical students, residents, and fellows [1]; have been shown to be low-cost and cost-effective [2]; and most recently have been linked to convincingly improved training outcomes for high-risk, low-frequency obstetrical emergencies [3]. This chapter offers an overview of educational theory supporting simulation-based education (SBE) methods.

Experiential learning theory (ELT) serves as the endoskeleton of simulation-based education. David Kolb and colleagues have devoted a lifetime to the examination of the underpinnings of experiential learning [4–6]}. In this chapter, we provide an overview of their approach to SBE and weave related constructs into a useful primer.

L. R. Becker, Ph.D., MS.MEdL, NRP, CHSE (✉)
MedStar Health, Simulation Training and Education Lab (SiTEL), Washington, DC, USA

Department of Emergency Medicine, Georgetown University School of Medicine,
Washington, DC, USA
e-mail: les.becker@email.sitel.org

B. A. Hermosura, MSN, RN, CHSE
MedStar Health, Simulation Training & Education Lab (SiTEL), Washington, DC, USA
e-mail: belinda.hermosura@email.sitel.org

> **Key Learning Points**
> - Simulation-based education is built on experiential learning theory and permits significant activation of the learner.
> - Understanding of the underlying learning theories behind simulation education help educators in the development of new simulation programs.
> - It is important to consider fidelity of the simulator and to choose the one that best fits the educational learning objectives.

The Origins of ELT

Though Kolb [4] is commonly cited in the simulation literature, a more recent edition of the historic work was published several years [6] ago and has largely escaped the attention of the simulation community. In this 2014 volume, Kolb revisits his early work and also integrates key refinements. This discussion begins with a summary of one of Kolb's earliest descriptions of experiential learning theory and the model.

Kolb [7] and thereafter [4, 6] characterize learning as a four-stage cycle (Fig. 2.1). A learner engages in a "concrete experience," in our context, a simulated medical procedure or patient encounter, and the components of that

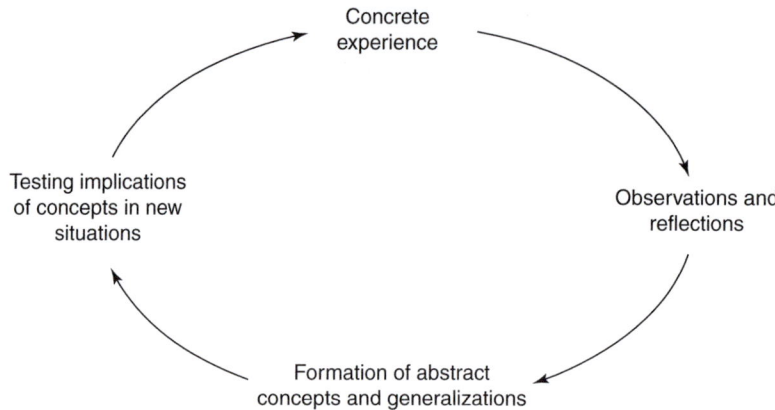

Fig. 2.1 The experiential learning model [7]. (Reprinted with permission)

experience form the basis for the second step of the cycle, "observation and reflection." As a result of this second step, learners develop their internalized operational model for working through a procedure or encounter. In the third step, learners test their operational model in a new situation (another simulation or actual clinical encounter), resulting in additional concrete experience, and the cycle repeats itself, until if and when a learner achieves mastery [8–10]. Even in his earliest works, Kolb [7, 11] emphasized the importance of four essential learner traits essential to achieving success via the cycle. These included concrete experience, reflective observation, abstract conceptualization and active experimentation (Fig. 2.1). During engagement the learner must be fully involved and open to new experiences without bias, willing to integrate observations into logical theories and then use those to make decisions and apply them to solve problems [7].

The ELT model appears deceptively simple, but in both his 1984 and 2015 publications, Kolb acknowledges the foundational contributions of Piaget, Lewin, and Dewey to ELT by referring to this trio as the "foremost intellectual ancestors of experiential learning theory [6]." Though Piaget's lifelong studies focused upon children, Kolb drew upon Piaget's descriptions of cognitive-development processes and their role in learning and education. Kolb [4] summarized Piaget by writing that "Piaget's theory describes how intelligence is shaped by experience. Intelligence

is not an innate internal characteristic of the individual but arises as a product of the interaction between the person and his or her environment." Piaget [12] characterized this process as the "effects of the physical environment on the structure of intelligence" and further that "Experience of objects, of physical reality, is obviously a basic factor in the development of cognitive structure." Analogously, specific knowledge of new procedures and approaches to patient and colleague interaction arise through experiencing them in the simulation lab.

Dr. Kurt Lewin is recognized as the founder of the field of American social psychology [13]. Lewin [14] wrote that "to understand or to predict behaviour, the person and his environment have to be considered as one constellation of interdependent factors." T-groups were an early form of reflective learning [15], "a cyclic process in which learning recurs in increasing depth [16]. The experiences surrounding Lewin's T-groups influenced Kolb as he developed ELT. Daily evening discussion periods, at first only open to staff, led to dynamic discussions involving the learners as well. Kolb [6] summarizes Lewin's contributions to ELT in a global context:

> ...the discovery was made that learning is best facilitated in an environment where there is dialectic tension and conflict between immediate, concrete experience and analytic detachment. By bringing together the immediate experiences of the trainees and the conceptual models of the staff in an open atmosphere

where inputs from each perspective could challenge and stimulate the other, a learning environment occurred with remarkable vitality and creativity.

Lastly, Kolb [6] characterizes John Dewey as "the most influential educational theorist of the twentieth century." The educational approaches that were ultimately spawned by Dewey's [17] volume and his legacy we take for granted today. Apprenticeships, internships, work/study programs, cooperative education, and other experiential forms were all at one time viewed to be evolutionary, if not revolutionary. Though Dewey [17] was focused globally, in his Chap. 3, "Criteria of Experience," aspects of his writing resonate strongly in our modern era of simulation-based education, whether in the lab or in situ. He wrote, "A primary responsibility of educators is that not only be aware of the general principle of the shaping of actual experience by environing conditions, but that they also recognize in the concrete what surroundings are conducive to having experiences that lead to growth [6]."

Learning Styles and Learning Spaces

In Kolb and Kolb's discussion [5] and review [18] of ELT in higher education, the authors expanded Kolb's earlier discussion [4] of learning styles and learning spaces. They expanded upon his earlier [4] statement that "knowledge results from the culmination of grasping and transforming experience" and also his descriptions of the four basic learning styles: diverging, assimilating, converging, and accommodating. Grasping experience can occur through concrete experience (CE) or its counterpart abstract conceptualization (AC); transforming experience can occur through reflective observation (RO) or its counterpart active experimentation (AE). Kolb and Kolb [5] described how each of the four learning styles is derived from an admixture of balanced tendencies or strengths in grasping and transforming experience combined with an individual's dominant predisposition towards one or more learning approach.

Kolb and Kolb [18] presented a rich but compact description of ELT built on six propositions:

1. Learning is best conceived as a process, not in terms of outcome.
2. All learning is relearning … as beliefs and ideas are examined, tested and integrated with new, more refined ideas.
3. Learning requires alternate bouts of reflection and action and feeling and thinking.
4. Learning is holistic process … involves the integrated functioning of the total person – thinking, feeling, perceiving and behaving.
5. Learning results from … transactions between the person and the environment … assimilating new experiences.
6. Learning is the process of creating knowledge.

Equipped with an understanding of these fundamentals, we can now move on to a discussion of the "learning space [18]." Note that each of the six propositions is active and dynamic. These activities occur in the "learning space [6, 18]." Kolb and Kolb [18] further note that "In ELT the experiential learning space is defined by the attracting and repelling forces (positive and negative valences) of the two poles of the dual dialectics of action/reflection and experiencing/conceptualizing, creating a two dimensional map of the regions of the learning space."

Each of the six propositions above could just as easily describe participation in a high-fidelity medical simulation scenario, whether mannequin- or computer-based, and the congruence is enhanced by the essential component of debriefing. The learning style model is plausibly related to simulation education and even more directly to OB/GYN simulation education.

Proposing the "Simulation Space"

The term "simulation space" has been typically used in the medical simulation context to describe the physical space associated with simulation activities (e.g., [19]) and even to describe the testbeds for molecular-level biochemical simulations [20]. Kolb [6] includes the physical, cultural, institutional, social, and psychological dimensions in his updated definition of the learning space.

In this chapter, we define the simulation space to be "The learning environment of the simulation activity in concert with the experiential learning process inherent to such a space and process." Our definition meshes smoothly with Kolb and Kolb's [18] description of ELT as "a process of locomotion through the learning regions that is influenced by a person's position in the learning space" and his multidimensional [6] learning space that includes the physical, cultural, institutional social, and psychological dimensions of learning. Furthermore, these concepts are included in Kolb's experiential learning theory (Fig. 2.2) as he talks about contemporary applications of ELT and links them to the foundational trio of Lewin, Dewey, and Piaget (Fig. 2.3).

Kolb's Revised Model

Having provided an overview of the foundational influences of Kolb's experiential learning theory, we can now view the ELT model in its current form (Fig. 2.2).

Key elements of the model are paired, gaining new knowledge through actual concrete experience (CE), and abstract conceptualization (AC) and then transforming experience through reflective observation (RO) and active experimentation (AE) [6].

From Cycle to Spiral

Less well known than the learning cycle is the "learning spiral" discussed in Kolb [6]. Kolb's learning spiral is derived from art, philosophy,

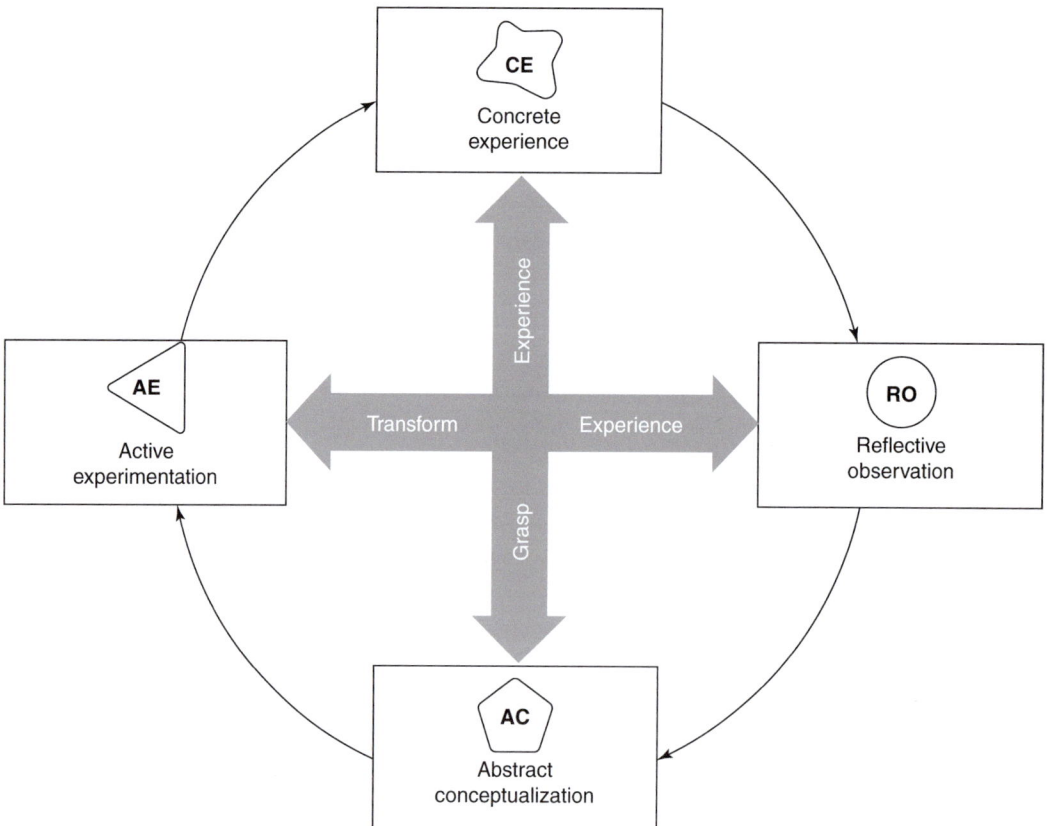

Fig. 2.2 Kolb's [6] experiential learning model. (©2015. Reprinted by permission of Pearson Education, Inc., New York, New York)

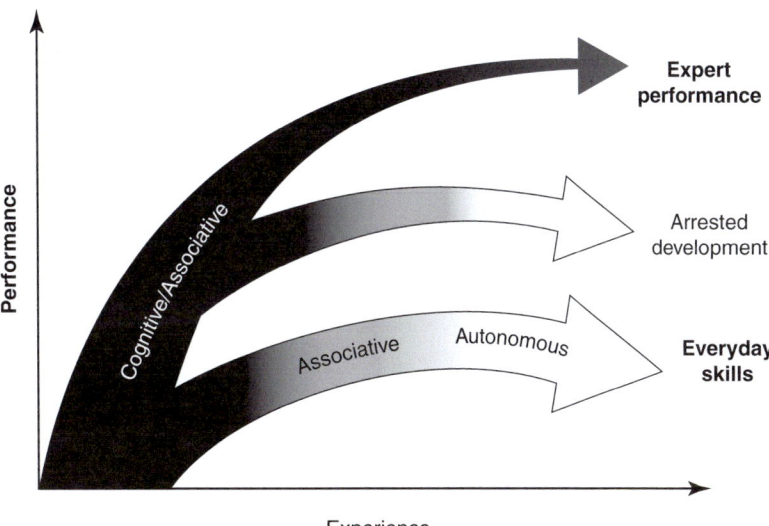

Fig. 2.3 Ericsson's [74] figure explains the divergence between learners that develop expert performance and those that remain at everyday levels or experience arrested development. (Reprinted with permission)

nature, and even the physical sciences. The most concise description of the learning spiral is drawn from Kolb's appreciation of the work of Sir Thomas Cook, an early twentieth-century scholar, art historian, and journalist [21].

> One of the chief beauties of the spiral as an imaginative conception is that it is always growing, yet never covering the same ground, so that it is not merely an explanation of the past, but is also a prophesy of the future; and while it defines and illuminates what has already happened, it is also leading constantly to new discoveries (423).
> Cook [21] quoted in Kolb [6]

Not only does the spiral perfectly characterize the learning cycle as Kolb remarks, but it also perfectly characterizes simulation-based learning where each experience contributes to the next. He also has incorporated the spiral into his discussion of knowledge creation. We further propose the learning spiral as the fundamental basis of reflective practice in lifelong learning. Mann and colleagues [22] provide evidence for reflective practice among practicing healthcare professionals. Further, reflection seems to be triggered by complex clinical encounters. So, by accelerating the trip along the spiral via simulated encounters, we can trigger reflective practice and contribute to lifelong learning.

Supporting Bodies of Theory

By necessity, our review of ELT merely scratches the surface. Nevertheless, we must visit several other theoretical domains to address some of the "how" of simulation education. In the next section, we discuss cognitive scaffolding, Vygotsky's theory on the zone of proximal development, and a general discussion of the role of fidelity in simulation education.

Fidelity

Though early discussions of simulation fidelity date back to the 1950s, more recent definitions of simulation fidelity arose from work in the 1980s and 1990s performed for the US Army [23, 24], the Federal Aviation Administration [25], and academic discussions focusing upon aviation simulators [26, 27]. From that era, Hays and Singer [28] defined simulation fidelity as:

> The degree of similarity between the training situation and the operational situation which is simulated. It is a two dimensional measurement of this similarity in terms of: the physical characteristics, for example, visual, spatial, kinesthetic, etc.; and the functional characteristics, for example, the informational, and stimulus and response options of the training situation.

Table 2.1 Typologies of simulation and simulator fidelity

Author(s)	Fidelity typology type	Elements
Rehmann et al. [25]	Simulation	Environmental fidelity – degree to which the simulator duplicates motion, visual, and sensory clues Equipment fidelity – degree to which the simulator duplicates appearance and feel of the real system Psychological fidelity – degree to which the trainee believes the simulation to be a surrogate for the task
Seropian [99]	Simulation	Plausible environment Plausible responses Plausible interactions Familiar equipment Realistic simulation equipment

Maran and Glavin [30]	Simulators	Part task trainers
		Computer-based systems
		Virtual reality and haptic systems
		Simulated environments
		Integrated simulators
		  Instructor-driven simulators
		  Model-driven simulators

Commercialization of full-body patient simulators beginning in the 1990s [29] and thereafter led to competition, a growing array of simulator features and much ongoing discussion of high- vs. mid-fidelity simulators. The discussion of fidelity continued in a flight-simulator context [25] and expanded to include typologies of simulation fidelity [30, 31], summarized in Table 2.1.

Liu and colleagues [32] published a comprehensive typology of fidelity types. In Table 2.2, we have included more recent published definitions and suggest that the typology presented in [25] remains the most useful overall classification scheme for fidelity.

A review of Tables 2.1 and 2.2 leads one to conclude that a potentially dizzying array of decisions enter into the choice of a simulation modality for a given learning situation and/or group of learners. Norman et al. [34] published a watershed study in the simulation fidelity realm.

They specifically identified studies that compared performance outcomes associated with low- and high-fidelity simulators vs. no-intervention controls in three clinical domains: (1) auscultation skills and use of heart-sound simulators, (2) basic motor skills, and (3) complex crisis management skills. Their analysis confirmed conventional wisdom that in nearly all cases, both high- and low-fidelity simulation (HFS and LFS, respectively) activities resulted in "consistent improvements in performance in comparison with no-intervention control groups. However, nearly all the studies showed no significant advantage of HFS over LFS, with average difference ranging from 1% to 2% [34]." Lee et al.'s [35] pilot study in intensive care paramedic training, Bredmose et al.'s [36] study of training London Helicopter Emergency Medical Service physicians and paramedics, and studies by Levett-Jones and colleagues in nursing education [37, 38] are consistent with Norman et al.'s [34] findings. Before exploring the instructional implications of their findings, let us review a small number of more recent studies.

Three additional reviews serve to summarize the current state of the art regarding fidelity and the diverging viewpoints [33, 39, 40]. Paige and Morin [39] have proposed a multidimensional model of simulation fidelity incorporating (1) physical fidelity of equipment and the environment, (2) task fidelity (reflecting real situations), (3) functional fidelity (realism of simulation responses), (4) psychological fidelity and (5) conceptual fidelity as well as two broad classes of cueing ..conceptual- and reality-cueing. They emphasize that "all aspects of fidelity significantly hinge on the learner's perceived realism of the context of the learning episode as compared to any particular feature of the learning environment." Their model arrays the realism, stimuli, and cues among the dimensions of the patient (or confederate), the clinical scenario, and the healthcare facilities (including equipment). Hamstra et al. [40] promote an alternative viewpoint, calling for the abandonment altogether of the term "fidelity" and replacing it with terminology focusing upon "physical resemblance and functional task alignment" and focus instead upon more operationally and consensus-based approaches

Table 2.2 Classification of fidelity types based upon an overview of the refereed literature

Terminology	References	Definition
Environmental		
Physical fidelity	Allen [100]	Degree to which device looks, sounds, and feels like actual environment
Environmental fidelity	Rehmann et al. [25] Paige and Morin [39]	Degree to which the simulator duplicates motion, visual, and sensory clues
Visual–audio fidelity	Rinalducci [101]	Replication of visual and auditory stimulus
Simulation fidelity	Gross et al. [102]; Alessi [26]	Degree to which device can replicate actual environment, or how "real" the simulation appears and feels
Motion fidelity	Kaiser and Schroeder [103]	Replication of motion cues felt in actual environment
Physical (engineering)	Dahl et al. [104]	Degree to which device looks, sounds, and feels like actual environment
Patient fidelity	Tun et al. [33]	Representations of interactions with all or part of the patient
Equipment		
Functional fidelity	Allen [100] Dahl et al. [104]	How device functions, works, and provided actual stimuli as actual environment
Equipment fidelity	Zhang [105] Rehmann et al. [25]	Replication of actual equipment hardware and software
Task fidelity	Zhang [105] Roza [106] Hughes and Rolek [107] Dahl et al. [104]	Replication of tasks and maneuvers executed by user
Healthcare simulation fidelity	Tun et al. [33]	Representations of the clinical equipment and environment
Psychological		
Psychological fidelity	Rehmann et al. [25]	Degree to which the trainee believes the simulation to be a surrogate for the task
Psychological/psychological–cognitive fidelity	Kaiser and Schroeder [103] Beaubien and Baker [108] Dahl et al. [104]	Degree to which device replicates psychological and cognitive factors (i.e., communication, situational awareness)
Psychological Task attributes Conceptual attributes	Paige and Morin [39] Dieckmann et al. [109] Paige and Morin [39]	Extent to which events and scenario plots reflect real situations
Clinical scenario fidelity	Tun et al. [33]	Representations relating to the script and progression of a scenario

such as "transfer of learning, learner engagement and suspension of disbelief."

How Can We Utilize Fidelity?

Given the capital investment in simulators in healthcare education and the limited likelihood that the term fidelity will be abandoned, how can medical educators make best use of their equipment inventories with regard to potential educational outcomes? Alessi's [26] foundational paper addressed not whether high fidelity is a critical, but whether for particular levels or categories of learners or instructional goals, different levels of fidelity might be more or less appropriate and beneficial. He wrote:

> it appears we are faced with a dilemma in simulation design. Increasing fidelity, which theoretically should increase transfer, may inhibit initial learning which in turn will inhibit transfer. On the other hand, decreasing fidelity may increase initial

learning, but what is learned may not transfer to the application situation if too dissimilar.. Simulations meant for initial presentations or guidance would be simplified and have lower fidelity while those intended for independent practice would have higher fidelity [26].

Thus, the solution to the dilemma lies in "ascertaining the correct level of fidelity based on the student's current instructional level. As a student progresses, the appropriate level of fidelity should increase." Then, as now, this guidance is derived from cognitive-load theory [41, 42]. Early learning should occur in relatively low-fidelity environments to reduce cognitive load [42]. Later learning can involve increased fidelity and resultant load, while approaching clinical practice.

Returning to Paige and Morin's [39] model, they suggest that simulation design should be driven by careful, separate, consideration of the fidelity levels of the physical, psychological, and conceptual fidelity dimensions. In their example, learning a new skill might be associated with high physical, low psychological, and medium conceptual fidelity. Hysteroscopic resection simulation as described by Burchard et al. [43] serves as an excellent example of this approach.

In summary, how can we logically and effectively vary fidelity in an effort to optimize training outcomes? We suggest that lower fidelity simulation approaches might be employed in the training of novices, initial training of a skill regardless of learner level, and in performance improvement settings for any level of learner. Higher fidelity approaches may best be utilized with advanced learners, training where the emphasis is upon transfer to the real-world setting and in high-stakes assessment.

Scaffolding

Cognitive Scaffolding

Holton and Clarke [44] have said that just as a construction scaffold allows workers to construct or repair buildings, so does a "cognitive scaffold" support the learning of new actions. More importantly, scaffolding allows "learners to reach places that are otherwise inaccessible [44]." Finally, when the learning or construction task is complete, "the scaffolding is removed...and not seen in the final product [44]."

Simulation-based education clearly draws upon the principles of cognitive scaffolding. Jerome Bruner, a cognitive psychologist who devoted a lifetime to the study of child development (e.g., [45]), is widely recognized for his foundational work that ultimately led to the development of the concept of "cognitive scaffolding." He described skill acquisition in children as "goal-directed skilled action … conceived as the construction of serially ordered constituent acts whose performance is modified towards less variability, more anticipation and greater economy by benefit of feed-forward, feedback and knowledge of results [45]."

Scaffolding draws upon Vygotsky's [46] "zone of proximal development" originally defined for children as "the distance between the actual development as determined by independent problem solving and the level of potential development as determined through problem solving under adult guidance or in collaboration with more capable peers." Wood et al. emphasized the social context of learning and noted that problem solving or skill acquisition "involves a scaffolding process that enable a child or a novice to solve a problem, carry out a task or a achieve a goal which would be beyond his unassisted efforts [47]."

Clinical problems in medicine are ill structured [48]. In ill-structured environments, novices are unlikely to develop the expertise necessary for independent problem solving [49]. Saye and Brush [50] conceptualized two categories of scaffolding to aid the novice in an ill-structured environment. The authors define "hard scaffolds" as "static supports that can be anticipated and planned in advance based on typical student difficulties with a task [50]." In the simulation context, examples of hard scaffolding include procedural videos ("technical scaffolds" described by Yelland and colleagues [51]) and formative task checklists. In contrast, soft scaffolds are "dynamic and situational [50]" and might include the availability of dedicated simulation station proctors or roving faculty [52]. Thus, faculty and learners have availed opportunities for questioning and feedback, respectively. A further value of scaffolding is not only that it "supports the immediate construction of knowledge by the learner … [it] provides the basis for future independent learning of the individual [44]." Thus scaffolding by mentors and even peers, "reciprocal scaffolding" [44] early and throughout one's career can form the basis for lifelong learning. Both Sibley and Parolee [53] and Paramalee and Hudes [54] acknowledge the importance of scaffolding in team-based learning. We suggest that the reciprocal scaffolding of Holton and Clarke [44] is the substrate of team-based or group learning's contributions to lifelong learning; Tolsgaard et al.'s [55] review acknowledges the value of scaffolding in the earlier stages of learning in health professions education. Simulation-based education in medicine also relies upon expert scaffolding [44, 56–59], where a faculty member dynamically evaluates a learner's level of expertise and guides the learner through their zone of proximal development, facilitating mastery of needed knowledge [60]. Van Lier [61] has characterized this type of scaffolding as "contingent scaffolding."

In earlier works, Jonassen [62] emphasized the importance of scaffolding in computer-driven case-based learning environments,[1] and Hmelo and Day [63] pioneered the practice of embedding contextualized questions in problem-based learning [64] simulations focusing upon basic clinical sciences education. Choules's [65] review of learning in medical education identified strategies of scaffolding for use with self-directed learners in virtual patient scenarios designed to teach and strengthen skills in diagnostic reasoning and patient management through interactivity. Wu et al. [66] have recently demonstrated the value of scaffolding via cognitive representation in a clinical reasoning instructional tool. The importance of scaffolding, both cognitive and through auditory, visual, and haptic clues

is well established in the virtual world. Lemheney and colleagues [67] mention scaffolding in their recent virtual reality (VR) simulation for office-based medical emergencies as do Kizakevich et al. [68] in a VR simulation for multicasualty triage training.

Moving to more traditional simulation topics and approaches, Rawson et al. [69] highlighted the importance of scaffolding in their basic and clinical science fluid therapy simulation. Nel [70] emphasized a dual theoretical underpinning of his clinical simulation activities for psychology trainees incorporating both scaffolding and the concept of the zone of proximal development [46]. In a simulation-based curriculum introducing key teamwork principles, Banerjee et al. [71] identified scaffolding of desired knowledge, skills, and abilities as an important lesson learned. Finally from the lesser known field of telesimulation; Papanagnou [72] identifies inherent barriers to scaffolding and suggests that telesimulation is perhaps a modality better suited to the advanced learner.

We conclude that scaffolding is more than just a construct for pedagogical inquiry, but rather that it constitutes an important component of health professions simulation and education. Depending upon the particular simulation topic and type, the scaffold may in fact be the simulator itself, but more often than not, the scaffold is the faculty member, proctor, or peer working alongside or serving as a co-learner.

Deliberate Practice

Expert Performance and Deliberate Practice

In this section, we briefly introduce expert performance and the path whereby to become an expert …deliberate practice. Subsequently, we introduce the concept of mastery learning in medicine and close by describing the interrelationship of mastery learning and deliberate in modern medical education.

K. Anders Ericsson has devoted a lifetime to the study of expert performance and its

---

[1]Categorized as a Level 2 simulation in Alinier's 35. Alinier [35]. Typology.

underpinnings, and a comprehensive review of his contributions is beyond the scope of this chapter. Much of his work since the early 1990s has focused upon deliberate practice, and in the past decade he expanded his work to integrate these concepts with learning and, more recently, simulation. Studying pianists, Ericsson et al. [73] "identified a set of conditions where practice had been uniformly associated with improved performance. Significant improvements in performance were realized when individuals were (1) given a task with a well-defined goal, (2) motivated to improve, (3) provided with feedback, and (4) provided with ample opportunities for repetition and gradual refinements of their performance [74]." Ericsson and his colleagues further established that "deliberate efforts to improve one's performance beyond its current level demands full concentration and often requires problem-solving and better methods of performing the task [74]" and that these models often required development of new approaches to mental modeling of the task themselves, described as "mental representations that allow them [expert performers] to plan and reason about potential courses of action and these representations also allow experts to monitor their performance, thus providing critical feedback for continued complex learning [75]." Ericsson's [73] study is also well known for its finding that by age 20, the best musicians had spent over 10,000 h of practice, anywhere from two for times more than musicians of lesser caliber. This study and others (e.g., [76]) achieved clear description of the qualitative difference between everyday activities and sustained improvement of expert performance. Figure 2.3 from Ericsson [74], shows that everyday skills are honed to a level where they stable and autonomous, Fitts and Posner's [76] third stage of performance where little cognitive effort is required, ultimately leading to arrested development. In contrast, experts remain in the cognitive and associative phases of learning and develop increasingly complex mental representations as described previously. As described below, simulation provides a means to engage in deliberate practice and serves as a pathway to expert performance [77].

Deliberate Practice, Mastery Learning, and General Medical Education (GME)

McGaghie [78] succinctly describes mastery learning's central tenets as: "1) educational excellence is expected and can be achieved by all learners, and 2) little or no variation in measured outcomes will be seen among learners in a mastery environment." In addition, mastery learning intends that trainees' acquisition of knowledge, skills, and affect time, and professional attributes are measured rigorously and compared with fixed achievement standards. All learners are offered sufficient time to reach mastery learning results that are uniform among learners, consistent with the principles of competency-based medical education, its forebear [79], the time invested by learners may vary. Deliberate practice is a pathway to mastery learning.

Simulationists in the GME community have embraced the deliberate practice and mastery learning paradigms. The ground-breaking work in this area includes that of Diane Wayne at Northwestern University where she applied these concepts to advanced cardiac life support skills [80] and thoracentesis [81]. Dr. Wayne's colleague Jeffrey Barsuk's team has firmly established the value of the triumvirate of simulation, mastery learning, and deliberate practice in various skill areas including hemodialysis catheter insertion [82], adult lumbar puncture [83], paracentesis [84], and most recently maintenance of central lines [85]. Other studies have demonstrated gains in various training domains including infant lumbar puncture [86], neonatal resuscitation [87–89], neurosurgical practice and care [90], operating room surgical performance [91], and video laryngoscopy [92]. Deliberate practice by residents has been demonstrated to produce superior training outcomes in hysteroscopic technique [93, 94]. Lastly, deliberate practice-based mastery learning is associated with higher-level health outcomes at the patient and population level [95–98].

In closing, this chapter, intended as a primer in experiential simulation-based medical education theory, has provided an overview of the roots of this field, reviewed recent concepts in simulation fidelity, discussed the functional importance of cognitive scaffolding, and has closed with an overview of the closely related endeavors of deliberate practice and mastery learning.

References

1. Deering S, Auguste T, Lockrow E. Obstetric simulation for medical student, resident, and fellow education. YSPER. 2013;37(3):143–5.
2. Bruno CJ, Glass KM. Cost-effective and low-technology options for simulation and training in neonatology. YSPER. 2016;40(7):473–9.
3. Fisher N, Bernstein PS, Satin A, Pardanani S, Heo H, Merkatz IR, et al. Resident training for eclampsia and magnesium toxicity management: simulation or traditional lecture? Am J Obstet Gynecol. 2017;203(4):1–5.
4. Kolb DA. Experiential learning. Englewood Cliffs: Prentice-Hall; 1984.
5. Kolb AY, Kolb DA. Learning styles and learning spaces: enhancing experiential learning in higher education. Acad Manag Learn Edu. 2005;4(2):193–212.
6. Kolb DA. Experiential learning: experience as the source of learning and development. 2nd ed. Pearson Education: Saddle River; 2015.
7. Kolb DA. Management and the learning process. Calif Manag Rev. 1976;XVIII(3):21–31.
8. Dreyfus SE, Dreyfus HL. A five-stage model of the mental activities involved in directed skill acquisition. DTIC Document: Berkeley; 1980.
9. Dreyfus SE. The five-stage model of adult skill acquisition. Bull Sci Technol Soc. 2004;24(3):177–81.
10. Ericsson KA. The influence of experience and deliberate practice on the development of superior expert performance. In: Ericsson KA, Charness N, Feltovich PJ, Hoffman RR, editors. The Cambridge handbook of expertise and expert performance. Cambridge: Cambridge University Press; 2006. p. 683–704.
11. Kolb DA. On management and the learning process. Cambridge, MA: Massachusetts Institute of Technology; 1973.
12. Piaget J. Development and learning. In: Gauvain M, Cole M, editors. Readings on the development of children, vol. 1997. New York: Scientific American Books; 1964. p. 19–28.
13. Marrow AJ. The practical theorist: the life and work of Kurt Lewin, vol. 1969. New York: Basic Books; 1969.
14. Lewin K. Resolving social conflicts & field theory in social science. Washington, DC: American Psychological Association; 2008 [1946].
15. Hampden-Turner CM. An existential "learning theory" and the integration of T-group research. J Appl Behav Sci. 1966;2(4):367–86.
16. Bradford L, Gibb J, Benne K, editors. T-group theory and laboratory method: innovation in re-education. New York: Wiley; 1964.
17. Dewey J. Education and experience. New York: Simon and Schuster; 1938.
18. Kolb AY, Kolb DA. Learning styles and learning spaces: a review of the multidisciplinary application of experiential learning theory in higher education. In: Sims RR, Sims SJ, editors. Learning styles and learning. New York: Nova Science Publishers, Inc.; 2006. p. 45–91.
19. Arafeh JMR. Simulation-based training: the future of competency? J Perinat Neonatal Nurs. 2011;25(2):171–4.
20. Toofanny RD, Simms AM, Beck DA, Daggett V. Implementation of 3D spatial indexing and compression in a large-scale molecular dynamics simulation database for rapid atomic contact detection. BMC bioinformatics. 2011;12:234.
21. Cook T. The curves of life. London: Constable and Company; 1914.
22. Mann K, Gordon J, MacLeod A. Reflection and reflective practice in health professions education: a systematic review. Adv Health Sci Educ. 2009;14(4):595.
23. Hays RT. Simulator fidelity: a concept paper. DTIC Document; 1980.
24. Hays RT. Research issues in the determination of simulator fidelity: proceedings of the ARI sponsored workshop 23–24 July, 1981.
25. Rehmann AJ, Mitman RD, Reynolds MC. Federal aviation administration technical C. A handbook of flight simulation fidelity requirements for human factors research; 1995. 25 p.
26. Alessi SM. Fidelity in the design of instructional simulations. J Comput-Based Ins. 1988;15:40–7.
27. Alessi SM. Simulation design for training and assessment. Aircrew Train Assess. 2000;
28. Hays RT, Singer MJ. Simulation fidelity in training system design: bridging the gap between reality and training. New York: Springer; 1989.
29. Bradley P. The history of simulation in medical education and possible future directions. Med Educ. 2006;40(3):254–62.
30. Maran NJ, Glavin RJ. Low-to high-fidelity simulation–a continuum of medical education? Med Educ. 2003;37(s1):22–8.
31. Alinier G. A typology of educationally focused medical simulation tools. Med Teach. 2007;29(8):e243–50.
32. Liu D, Macchiarella N, Vincenzi D. Simulation fidelity. Boca Raton: CRC Press; 2008. p. 61–73.
33. Tun JK, Alinier G, Tang J. Redefining simulation fidelity for healthcare education. Simul Gaming. 2015;46(2):159–74.
34. Norman G, Dore K, Grierson L. The minimal relationship between simulation fidelity and transfer of learning. Med Educ. 2012;46(7):636–47.
35. Lee KHK, Grantham H, Boyd R. Comparison of high- and low-fidelity mannequins for clinical

performance assessment. Emerg Med Australas. 2008;20(6):508–14.

36. Bredmose PP, Habig K, Davies G, Grier G, Lockey DJ. Scenario based outdoor simulation in pre-hospital trauma care using a simple mannequin model. Scandinavian. Journal of Trauma, Resuscitation and Emergency Medicine. 2010;18(1):13.

37. Lapkin S, Levett-Jones T. A cost-utility analysis of medium vs. high-fidelity human patient simulation manikins in nursing education. J Clin Nurs. 2011;20(23–24):3543–52.

38. Levett-Jones T, Lapkin S, Hoffman K, Arthur C, Roche J. Examining the impact of high and medium fidelity simulation experiences on nursing students' knowledge acquisition. Nurse Educ Pract. 2011;11(6):380–3.

39. Paige JB, Morin KH. Simulation Fidelity and cueing: a systematic review of the literature. Clin Simul Nurs. 2013;9(11):e481–e9.

40. Hamstra SJ, Brydges R, Hatala R, Zendejas B, Cook D. Reconsidering fidelity in simulation-based training. Acad Med. 2014;89(3):387–92.

41. van Merrienboer JJG, Sweller J. Cognitive load theory and complex learning: recent developments and future directions. Educ Psychol Rev. 2005;17(2):147–77.

42. Reedy GB. Using cognitive load theory to inform simulation design and practice. Clin Simul Nurs. 2015;11(8):355–60.

43. Burchard ER, Lockrow EG, Zahn CM, Dunlow SG, Satin AJ. Simulation training improves resident performance in operative hysteroscopic resection techniques. Am J Obstet Gynecol. 2007;197(5):542–e4.

44. Holton D, Clarke D. Scaffolding and metacognition. Int J Math Educ Sci Technol. 2006;37(2):127–43.

45. Bruner JS. Organization of early skilled action. Child Dev. 1973;44(1):1–11.

46. Vygotsky L. Mind in society: the development of higher psychological processes. Oxford: Harvard University Press; 1978.

47. Wood D, Bruner JS, Ross G. The role of tutoring in problem solving. J Child Psychol Psychiatry. 1976;17(2):89–100.

48. Barrows HS, Feltovich PJ. The clinical reasoning process. Med Educ. 1987;21(2):86–91.

49. Land SM, Hannafin MJ. Patterns of understanding with open-ended learning environments: a qualitative study. Educ Technol Res Dev. 1997;45(2):47–73.

50. Saye JW, Brush T. Scaffolding critical reasoning about history and social issues in multimedia-supported learning environments. Educ Technol Res Dev. 2002;50(3):77–96.

51. Yelland N, Masters J. Rethinking scaffolding in the information age. Comput Educ. 2007;48(3):362–82.

52. Simons KD, Klein JD. The impact of scaffolding and student achievement levels in a problem-based learning environment. Instr Sci. 2007;35(1):41–72.

53. Sibley J, Parmelee DX. Knowledge is no longer enough: enhancing professional education with team-based learning. New Dir Teach Learn. 2008;2008(116):41–53.

54. Parmelee DX, Hudes P. Team-based learning: a relevant strategy in health professionals' education. Med Teach. 2012;34(5):411–3.

55. Tolsgaard MG, Kulasegaram KM, Ringsted CV. Collaborative learning of clinical skills in health professions education: the why, how, when and for whom. Med Educ. 2015;50(1):69–78.

56. Borders LD, Eubanks S, Callanan N. Supervision of psychosocial skills in genetic counseling. J Genet Couns. 2006;15(4):211–23.

57. Hess A. Growth in supervision: stages of supervisee and supervisor development. In: Kaslow F, editor. Supervision and training: models, dilemnsa, and challenges. New York: The Hawoth, Inc.; 1986. p. 51–67.

58. Middelton LA, Peters KF, Helmbold EA. Programmed instruction: genetics and gene therapy: genes and inheritance. Cancer Nurs. 1997;20(2):129–51.

59. Read A, Donnai D. New clinical genetics. 3rd ed. Oxfordshire: Scion; 2015.

60. Venne VL, Coleman D. Training the Millennial learner through experiential evolutionary scaffolding: implications for clinical supervision in graduate education programs. J Genet Couns. 2010;19(6):554–69.

61. Van Lier L. Interaction in the language curriculum: awareness, autonomy, and authenticity. London: Longman; 1996.

62. Jonassen DH. Scaffolding diagnostic reasoning in case-based-learning environments. J Comput High Educ. 1996;8(1):48–68.

63. Hmelo C, Day R. Contextualized questioning to scaffold learning from simulations. Comput Educ. 1999;32(2):151–64.

64. Barrows HS. How to design a problem-based curriculum for the preclinical years. New York: Springer Pub Co; 1985.

65. Choules AP. The use of elearning in medical education: a review of the current situation. Postgrad Med J. 2007;83(978):212–6.

66. Wu B, Wang M, Johnson JM, Grotzer TA. Improving the learning of clinical reasoning through computer-based cognitive representation. Med Educ Online. 2014;19:25940.

67. Lemheney AJ, Bond WF, Padon JC. Developing virtual reality simulations for office-based medical emergencies. J Virtual Worlds Res. 2016;9:1–18.

68. Kizakevich P, Furberg R, Hubal R, editors. Virtual reality simulation for multicasualty triage training. Proceedings of the 2006 I/ …; 2006/01/01.

69. Rawson RE, Dispensa ME, Goldstein RE, Nicholson KW, Vidal NK. A simulation for teaching the basic and clinical science of fluid therapy. Adv Physiol Educ. 2009;33(3):202–8.

70. Nel PW. The use of an advanced simulation training facility to enhance clinical psychology trainees' learning experiences. Psychol Learn Teach. 2010;9(2):65.

71. Banerjee A, Slagle JM, Mercaldo ND, Booker R, Miller A, France DJ, et al. A simulation-based

curriculum to introduce key teamwork principles to entering medical students. BMC Med Educ. 2016;16(1):295.

72. Papanagnou D. Telesimulation: a paradigm shift for simulation education. AEM Educ Train. 2017; 1:137.

73. Ericsson KA, Krampe RT, Tesch-Römer C. The role of deliberate practice in the acquisition of expert performance. Psychol Rev. 1993;100(3):363–406.

74. Ericsson KA. Deliberate practice and acquisition of expert performance: a general overview. Acad Emerg Med. 2008;15(11):988–94.

75. Ericsson KA. The scientific study of expert levels of performance: general implications for optimal learning and creativity1. High Abil Stud. 1998;9(1):75–100.

76. Fitts PM, Posner MI. Human performance. 1967.

77. Ericsson KA. Deliberate practice and the acquisition and maintenance of expert performance in medicine and related domains. Acad Med. 2004;79(10 Suppl):S70–81.

78. McGaghie WC. Mastery learning. Acad Med. 2015;90(11):1438–41.

79. McGaghie WC, Miller G, Sajid A, Tedler T. Competency-based curriculum development in medical education. An introduction. Public health papers no. 68. Geneva: World Health Organization; 1978. 96 p.

80. Wayne DB, Butter J, Siddall VJ, Fudala MJ, Wade LD, Feinglass J, et al. Mastery learning of advanced cardiac life support skills by internal medicine residents using simulation technology and deliberate practice. J Gen Intern Med. 2006;21(3):251–6.

81. Wayne DB, Barsuk JH, O'Leary KJ, Fudala MJ, McGaghie WC. Mastery learning of thoracentesis skills by internal medicine residents using simulation technology and deliberate practice. J Hosp Med. 2008;3(1):48–54.

82. Barsuk JH, Ahya SN, Cohen ER, McGaghie WC, Wayne DB. Mastery learning of temporary hemodialysis catheter insertion by nephrology fellows using simulation technology and deliberate practice. Am J Kidney Dis. 2009;54(1):70–6.

83. Barsuk JH, Cohen ER, Caprio T, McGaghie WC, Simuni T, Wayne DB. Simulation-based education with mastery learning improves residents' lumbar puncture skills. Neurology. 2012;79(2):132–7.

84. Barsuk JH, Cohen ER, Vozenilek JA, O'Connor LM, McGaghie WC, Wayne DB. Simulation-based education with mastery learning improves paracentesis skills. J Grad Med Educ. 2012;4(1):23–7.

85. Barsuk JH, Cohen ER, Mikolajczak A, Seburn S, Slade M, Wayne DB. Simulation-based mastery learning improves central line maintenance skills of ICU nurses. J Nurs Adm. 2015;45(10):511–7.

86. Kessler DO, Auerbach M, Pusic M, Tunik MG, Foltin JC. A randomized trial of simulation-based deliberate practice for infant lumbar puncture skills. Simul Healthc. 2011;6(4):197–203.

87. Sawyer T, Sierocka-Castaneda A, Chan D, Berg B, Lustik M, Thompson M. Deliberate practice using

simulation improves neonatal resuscitation performance. Simul Healthc. 2011;6(6):327–36.

88. Barry JS, Gibbs MD, Rosenberg AA. A delivery room-focused education and deliberate practice can improve pediatric resident resuscitation training. J Perinatol. 2012;32(12):920–6.

89. Cordero L, Hart BJ, Hardin R, Mahan JD, Nankervis CA. Deliberate practice improves pediatric residents' skills and team behaviors during simulated neonatal resuscitation. Clin Pediatr. 2013;52(8): 747–52.

90. Marcus H, Vakharia V, Kirkman MA, Murphy M, Nandi D. Practice makes perfect? The role of simulation-based deliberate practice and script-based mental rehearsal in the acquisition and maintenance of operative neurosurgical skills. Neurosurgery. 2013;72(Suppl 1):124–30.

91. Palter VN, Grantcharov TP. Individualized deliberate practice on a virtual reality simulator improves technical performance of surgical novices in the operating room: a randomized controlled trial. Ann Surg. 2014;259(3):443–8.

92. Ahn J, Yashar MD, Novack J, Davidson J, Lapin B, Ocampo J, et al. Mastery learning of video laryngoscopy using the Glidescope in the Emergency Department. Simul Healthc. 2016;11(5):309–15.

93. Chudnoff SG, Liu CS, Levie MD, Bernstein P, Banks EH. Efficacy of a novel educational curriculum using a simulation laboratory on resident performance of hysteroscopic sterilization. Fertil Steril. 2010;94(4):1521–4.

94. Rackow BW, Solnik MJ, Tu FF, Senapati S, Pozolo KE, Du H. Deliberate practice improves obstetrics and gynecology residents' hysteroscopy skills. J Grad Med Educ. 2012;4(3):329–34.

95. Barsuk JH, Cohen ER, Potts S, Demo H, Gupta S, Feinglass J, et al. Dissemination of a simulation-based mastery learning intervention reduces central line-associated bloodstream infections. Qual Saf Health Care. 2014;23(9):749–56.

96. Griswold S, Ponnuru S, Nishisaki A, Szyld D, Davenport M, Deutsch ES, et al. The emerging role of simulation education to achieve patient safety: translating deliberate practice and debriefing to save lives. Pediatr Clin N Am. 2012;59(6): 1329–40.

97. McGaghie WC, Issenberg SB, Cohen ER, Barsuk JH, Wayne DB. Medical education featuring mastery learning with deliberate practice can lead to better health for individuals and populations. Acad Med. 2011;86(11):e8–9.

98. McGaghie WC, Issenberg SB, Barsuk JH, Wayne DB. A critical review of simulation-based mastery learning with translational outcomes. Med Educ. 2014;48(4):375–85.

99. Seropian MA. General concepts in full scale simulation: getting started. Anesth Analg. 2003;97(6): 1695–705.

100. Allen J. Maintenance training simulator fidelity and individual difference in transfer of training. Hum Factors. 1986;28(5):497–509.

101. Rinalducci E. Characteristics of visual fidelity in the virtual environment. Presence Teleop Virt. 1996;5(3):330–45.
102. Gross D, Freemann R, editors. Measuring fidelity differentials in HLA simulations. Fall 1997 Simulation Interoperability Workshop; 1997.
103. Kaiser M, Schroeder J. Flights of fancy: the art and sceince of flight simulation. In: Vidulich M, Tsang P, editors. Principles and practices of aviation psychology. Mahwah: Lawrence Erlbaum Associates; 2003. p. 435–71.
104. Dahl Y, Alsos OA, Svanæs D. Fidelity considerations for simulation-based usability assessments of mobile ICT for hospitals. Int J Hum Comput Interact. 2010;26(5):445–76.
105. Zhang B. How to consider simulation fidelity and validity for an engineering simulator. Flight simulation and technologies. Guidance, navigation, and control and co-located conferences. American Institute of Aeronautics and Astronautics; 1993.
106. Roza M, Voogd J, Jense H, editors. Defining, specifying and developing fidelity referents. 2001 European simulation interooperability workshop. London; 2001.
107. Hughes T, Rolek E, editors. Fidelity and validity: issues of human behavioral representation requirements development. 2003 Winter simulation conference. New Orleans; 2003.
108. Beaubien JM, Baker DP. The use of simulation for training teamwork skills in health care: how low can you go? Qual Saf Health Care. 2004;13(suppl 1):i51–i6.
109. Dieckmann P, Gaba D, Rall M. Deepening the theoretical foundations of patient simulation as social practice. Simul Healthc. 2007;2(3):183–93.

Essentials of Scenario Building

Toni Huebscher Golen

Introduction and Background

There are many driving forces for creating simulation content: a recent adverse event, new regulatory pressure, developing technology, or moving educational goalposts. Simulation scenarios are designed to be formative or summative; they may assess a learner's capability or teach something new. Simulation scenarios aim to improve communication or technical skill, or both. All simulation scenarios share a common goal, though: to enhance practice.

There is strong temptation to imagine a fancy scenario that includes all of the details, nuances, and what-ifs of actual care – or else, the educator worries, it may not be realistic. Steven Spielberg, the great filmmaker, has said, "Audiences are harder to please if you're just giving them effects, but they're easy to please if it's a good *story*." A similar principle applies to writing simulation scenarios – worry less about the effects and focus on telling the right *story*. The story, in medical simulation, should embody the teaching points. All else is window dressing. This chapter will provide a step-by-step guide to writing scenarios that effectively tell the story and captivate the learner, using established teaching principles and

avoiding unnecessary details. See the Scenario building template at the end of this chapter (Fig. 3.1).

> **Key Learning Points**
> - Limit the use of simulation scenarios to clinical challenges that cannot be taught as effectively using conventional methods.
> - Begin the scenario by establishing the desired outcome.
> - Choose the setting that most naturally fits with the clinical problem.
> - Fully developed roles for characters in the scenario create realism.
> - Thoughtful learning objectives easily become a facilitator's checklist.
> - Debriefing, or reflection, marks the conclusion of successful simulation scenarios

Theory and Evidence

Sound educational practice is the starting point of all good simulation. Simulation scenario design has been exhaustively considered by Jeffries et al. [1] and the National League for Nursing, [2] who have identified several key educational

T. H. Golen (✉)
Department of Obstetrics and Gynecology, Beth Israel Deaconess Medical Center, Boston, MA, USA
e-mail: tgolen@bidmc.harvard.edu

© Springer International Publishing AG, part of Springer Nature 2019
S. Deering et al. (eds.), *Comprehensive Healthcare Simulation: Obstetrics and Gynecology*,
Comprehensive Healthcare Simulation, https://doi.org/10.1007/978-3-319-98995-2_3

practices – active learning [3], feedback [4], attention to diverse learning styles, and having high expectations for success [5] – that increase the likelihood of greater learning in simulation.

Beyond foundational education principles, certain design features of simulation scenarios lead to success. Attention to objectives, fidelity, problem-solving, learner support, and opportunity for debriefing should be addressed when writing a scenario. Each feature may be included more or less in a particular scenario depending on the purpose and setting, as well as the intended outcome of the exercise.

In many simulation exercises, learners listen to or are provided with a standardized description of the scenario before beginning. This can clarify the setting and the players and take away unnecessary surprises that do not contribute to the learning environment [6].

Fidelity describes the degree to which a simulation is true to reality. A scenario may call for either high- or low-fidelity simulation. The objective of the simulation dictates the type of fidelity that is required, for example, mastering the skills of laparoscopic lymph node dissection may require high fidelity, whereas a low-fidelity simulation may be extremely effective for teaching the repair of a second-degree vaginal laceration or for practicing teamwork and communication [7].

Every simulation scenario should present an opportunity for the learner to solve a problem. The number and difficulty of problems to be solved are related to the knowledge and skill level of the learner. The scenario should present a challenge, but not a challenge that is insurmountable unattainable. There should be an expectation of success. It is important to avoid giving the learner too much information just because it is possible to do so. The learner, faced with a problem, should be expected to assess, provide care, and then reflect on their performance [8]. As the learner exits the simulation experience, she should feel confident, challenged, and motivated.

The simulation scenario should be constructed so that it is clear how and when the learner may need help, support, cues, or additional information. There are a variety of ways to blend this type of information into a scenario script – a facilitator may provide it ahead of time or in real time, it may be provided by another individual involved in the simulation, or it can be communicated with a properly timed phone call, an ultrasound report, or other way of delivering information that fits naturally into the scenario. For example, when building a scenario aimed at learning how to manage eclampsia, a learner may be so narrowly focused on treating blood pressure that she does not notice the mannequin has begun to seize. A well-delivered alarmed exclamation from a nurse may help to shift the focus and move the simulation forward.

Reflective thinking, or debriefing, should be built into every simulation scenario, no matter how simple. Debriefing takes place once the simulation is complete. Participants are told the simulation has ended and the debriefing will follow. Specifics of the debriefing procedure are described elsewhere in this text. In writing scenarios, many authors cite debriefing as the most critical part of simulation; without it, learning just does not take place in an effective way. Essential characteristics of good debriefing include obtaining feedback from the facilitator, the opportunity for the learner to speak about her feelings and impressions, a review of the timeline of the scenario as it played out, and a conversation that involves mutual sharing of learners' experiences [9–13].

Building a great simulation scenario demands careful planning ahead of time that incorporates principles of educational theory, knowledge, and experience with simulation and best clinical practice, as well as an outlook of continuous improvement [14].

Choosing Clinical Topics

Not every opportunity for learning requires simulation. Given the resources required to carry out effective simulation events, it is wise to select topics that present a critical thinking challenge, a new or rarely used technical skill, or opportunities to improve inter-professional communication.

Specific examples in obstetrics and gynecology include:

- High acuity, low-frequency diagnoses
  - Pulmonary embolism
  - Amniotic fluid embolism
  - Sepsis
  - Diabetic ketoacidosis
  - Eclampsia
  - Cardiac arrest
- Challenging communication
  - Maternal death
  - Miscarriage
  - Peer-to-peer conflict
  - Impaired physician/provider
  - Poor leadership
- Protocol compliance
  - Safety checklist compliance
  - Interruptions
  - Handoffs
  - Massive hemorrhage
  - Established practice outside of typical space (e.g., a delivery in the emergency department)
- Medical-legal challenges
  - Documentation/EMR compliance
  - Clinical discord
  - Physician-patient relationship
  - Fatigue
- Technical proficiency
  - Laparoscopy
  - Cesarean hysterectomy
  - Uterine compression sutures (B-Lynch)
  - Shoulder dystocia
  - Forceps delivery
  - Vaginal breech delivery
  - Circumcision
  - Third- and fourth-degree laceration repair

Establishing Outcomes

The outcome of the scenario is the knowledge, skill, or behavior that the facilitator or instructor is expecting to see in the learner as a result of participation in the simulation. The story that is created must allow for the learner to have a key role in creating the outcome of the story. In other words, it must be an interactive and student-centered experience [15, 16].

The outcome must suit the learner. From a practical standpoint, all learners involved in a scenario may not be at the same level, so scenarios must be flexible enough to meet different levels of expertise. Effective scenarios address the pertinent domains of learning (e.g., knowledge, communication, technique) and ensure that the goals correspond to the level of the learner, are properly matched with the overall outcomes, are evidence-based, reflect a holistic view of the patient, and are achievable in the given time frame [17].

Is there a particularly difficult communication challenge that the learner should demonstrate proficiency with? Is there a need to show competency with patient handoffs? Is there a new protocol that needs practice? Is there a technique that needs development? Why is the scenario being created? These questions should be addressed and answered in the outcome.

If the simulation involves a laparoscopic ovarian cystectomy, is the facilitator expecting to see proper placement of trocars or only the technical aspects of the cystectomy itself? If simulating a shoulder dystocia, is the learner expected to demonstrate technical proficiency for all shoulder dystocia maneuvers or just one or two? Or the simulation may involve a communication challenge after a maternal death. Is the learner expected to provide emotional support only or be able to explain the medical details?

The desired outcomes will depend on the proficiency of the learner, the time, personnel, space available for the simulation, and the course director or facilitator's assessment of the most pressing educational need.

The Setting

The setting for the story provides realism – the story contains the learning points, and the setting should be familiar enough to the learner that the next time the learner encounters a similar story, she recalls what she learned, in part because the setting evokes a memory.

The scenario might unfold in a fully equipped simulation center, on an unused clinical unit, or in an empty labor room or operating suite. Along with these considerations, a list of needed equipment, supplies, and people is created. It is important that this list reflects the desired outcomes. For example, simulation of an obstetric hemorrhage may be most valuable in the actual labor and delivery unit in order to meet the desired outcome that, for example, staff know where to find emergency medications or equipment in their native environment. If the desired outcome were different – for example, the demonstration of technical skills involved in cesarean hysterectomy – the best setting might be a simulation center with higher-fidelity mannequins.

Learning Objectives

Once the outcome and the setting for the simulation are determined, the learning objectives flow naturally. Keep Steven Spielberg's advice in mind – "Audiences are harder to please if you're just giving them effects, but they're easy to please if it's a good story." Focus on telling the right *story*. The story, in medical simulation, should shine a very bright light on the learning objectives. As the scenario is built, learning objectives easily give rise to a checklist for the simulation facilitator.

Limit learning objectives to no fewer than two, and no more than five, depending on the complexity of the clinical scenario and the proficiency of the learner. The learning objectives are the specific behaviors expected from the learner.

Consider the learning objectives for a few simulation scenarios in obstetrics and gynecology:

– Outcome: demonstrate ability to prioritize and delegate tasks while caring for a patient in cardiac arrest at 35-week gestation.
  • Setting: simulation center, high-fidelity mannequin, nursing/anesthesia/obstetrician teams participating
    – Learning objectives
      1. Identify pulseless state.
      2. Initiate CPR.
      3. Provide handoff to resuscitation team.
      4. Deliver fetus in timely fashion.

– Outcome: demonstrate ability to place laparoscopic trocars for surgical treatment of ectopic pregnancy.
  • Setting: simulation center, low-fidelity anterior abdominal wall model, learner and expert facilitator participating
    – Learning objectives
      1. Position patient correctly.
      2. Test laparoscopic equipment prior to placement.
      3. Identify anatomic landmarks.
      4. Grasp and position trocars correctly for safe placement.
– Outcome: demonstrate ability to move patient quickly to the operating room for emergency cesarean delivery for umbilical cord prolapse.
  • Setting: labor and delivery unit, nursing/anesthesia/obstetrician staff participating
    – Learning objectives
      1. Identify prolapsed cord on physical exam.
      2. Elevate fetal head.
      3. Communicate situation and plan with team.
      4. Move patient to operating room without delay.

Organizing the Scenario

The building blocks of the scenario story include the clinical topic, the outcomes, setting, and the learning objectives; these inform how the scenario flows. It may be helpful to think of the simulation in three phases: beginning, middle, and end. Each phase should contain an outline of the patient assessment findings, the environment, and the expected learner actions. The triggers that cause movement to the next phase should also be identified (this may be a change in the patient's status or a passage of time) [14].

Setting the Scene: The Beginning Phase

The learner enters your story at the beginning phase. Anything that has occurred up to the moment the learner enters the scenario and begins to provide care, communicating and solving problems should be accounted for in the beginning phase. Any equipment needed should be identified at the beginning phase as well.

Think of this phase as setting the scene. What does the learner need to know and have access to in order to play her part? A bedside handoff from a colleague may provide the learner with vital signs (hypoxia, hypertension), an initial assessment (pain, confusion), or other complicating factors (the patient has no support person, the surgeon has not answered an urgent page). During this phase, the learner begins to immerse herself in make-believe, acclimates to the environment, and begins to solve problems. This phase often lasts no more than 5 min, depending on the complexity of the situation and level of proficiency of the learner, and it is crucial. Skipping this phase may deprive the learner of the opportunity to fully understand where she is and what is expected of her, causing the learner to feel unprepared, unsuccessful, or unfairly judged. To fully appreciate this, imagine the challenge of a real-life crisis where providers were forced to solve problems without any accompanying history whatsoever.

Imagine the beginning phase of a simple scenario involving a ruptured ectopic pregnancy.

– Outcome: demonstrate ability to move unstable patient quickly to operating room for treatment of ruptured ectopic pregnancy.
  • Setting: emergency department
    – Learning objectives
      1. Assess vital signs.
      2. Perform physical exam.
      3. Confirm patient is pregnant.
      4. Communicate need to move patient to operating room.

The beginning phase of this scenario should include a way for the learner to understand the setting (e.g., a sign that says "Emergency Department"), the initial vital signs (e.g., a monitor display), the identity of the patient (e.g., an ID band), and some description of other characters in the scenario.

Characters that will have roles in the story should be presented and described in the beginning phase. They should be described in enough detail so that they become real people and so that actions may be anticipated or explained by their backstory. The patient is often the principal character, but others may play an important role in achieving the outcome as well. Description of characters can sometimes be woven into a script, but it does not need to be. A nurse, for example, may introduce herself to the learner upon meeting and give a brief background of herself, or a learner can be handed a printed role description of all of the characters ahead of time.

"The nurse caring for the patient is named Susan. Susan is new to her role in the Emergency Department, but has 10 years of experience in the ICU. Her shift is ending in 20 minutes."

In this example, a learner would expect Susan to know how to clinically respond to critically ill patients, to possibly not know the location of equipment in the current setting (e.g., an ultrasound machine) or procedures for moving patients from the emergency department to the operating room, and to be tired or rushed because it is the end of her shift. These details allow the learner to acclimate and adjust expectations appropriately in order to solve clinical problems, achieve the desired outcome of the scenario, and meet learning objectives.

Using the ruptured ectopic scenario, and focusing on the last learning objective (expeditiously moving the patient to the operating room), the learner may encounter difficulty doing this in a timely fashion due to nursing inexperience in the emergency department. The beginning phase, in telling the story of Susan's character, creates realism and provides a sense of fairness for the learner. The fact that Susan does not know how to move a patient from the emergency department to operating room should not come as a great surprise because the learner has been told that this is a nurse who likely lacks specific experience with this.

Character background assists the learner in exploring how people will respond in a scenario. This information should be ready to be provided to the learner. All characters should be able to answer these questions: What is your background? Why are you here? What is your current emotional state? What do you expect to happen as a result of interacting with the learner? Enough information should be provided so that characters will respond appropriately as the learner interacts with them [18].

Returning to the ruptured ectopic example, another character may be the patient's partner. His role description may be provided to the learner on paper ahead of time, or may be worked in organically to the scenario. In either case, this character would be presented in the beginning phase and should be able to respond to key questions:

What is your background? I am the patient's husband.

Why are you here? I was at work, and I was called by my wife's co-worker to say she was being taken to the hospital by ambulance.

What is your current emotional state? Afraid.

What do you expect to happen as a result of interacting with the learner? The learner is going to explain the plan.

The role of the patient must be described well enough for the story to make sense. It should, similar to other roles, have details to create realism but be simple enough to avoid distractions and confusion. The desired outcome and learning objectives will inform the character of the patient. For example, if the outcome of the scenario is the demonstration of successful prioritization of tasks in a pregnant patient experiencing cardiac arrest, the role of the patient should account for possible risk factors for this complication while avoiding superfluous medical facts – it would be important, for example, that the patient had chronic hypertension but unnecessary and potentially confusing if the patient had recurrent urinary tract infections.

Aschenbrenner et al. [18] note that role descriptions should not be so elaborate that the learner is forced to stray away from the intended outcomes and learning objectives that are to be covered in the simulation. An example of a story line that may confuse a scenario is a patient or support person for whom English is not a preferred language. If cultural competence is a learning objective, then a role such as this is effective. If this has little to do with the objective, then a language barrier may actually get in the way of the learner's performance, cause frustration, and make it unnecessarily difficult to reach the objective of the scenario.

Moving the Story: The Middle Phase

The middle phase of the scenario presents the learner with the opportunity to solve problems; this part challenges the participant to use critical thinking and make course-altering decisions. This comes together once the clinical topic is chosen, the outcome of your story is decided, learning objectives are clear, the setting is agreed on, roles of characters are flushed out, and a story is laid out.

The transition from beginning to middle phase must be marked by a trigger that is obvious to the learner. This may take the form of a change in the patient's vital signs, a concern raised by another provider, an argument started by a peer or family member, and a phone call with new information – any signal that tells the learner that the scenario they entered at first, where they were given the opportunity to adjust, assimilate, and immerse themselves, has now altered course in a way that requires some action.

The middle phase is also marked by uncertainty. In order for the learner to solve problems, the correct answers must not be completely obvious. The degree of difficulty is always related to the experience level of the learner.

A time estimate for the middle phase should be determined in advance. This may be affected by room or personnel schedules, availability of equipment, or complexity of the clinical topic but usually lasts 10–15 min.

Attention to varying learning styles is part of a successful middle phase. As much as possible, the middle phase should account for those who learn best through tactile methods (palpation, manipulation), auditory cues (fetal heart tones, breath sounds, verbal explanations), or visual displays (a changed facial expression, a pregnant-appearing abdomen, a flashing alarm). Learners use all of these to incorporate data and formulate their decision-making. In the middle phase, as the learner is confronted with a situation that requires action and decision-making, there is ideally a collection of consistent information presented that sends a unifying message about the problem to be solved [15].

Consider this scenario:

– Outcome: demonstrate ability to prioritize and delegate tasks while caring for a patient in cardiac arrest at 35-week gestation.

- Setting: simulation center, high-fidelity mannequin, nursing/anesthesia/obstetrician teams participating

    – Learning objectives

        1. Identify pulseless state.
        2. Initiate CPR.
        3. Provide handoff to resuscitation team.
        4. Deliver fetus in timely fashion.

→ Beginning phase (5 min)

Roles

Learner: resident physician

Patient: 28-year-old para 1 at 35-week gestation. History of chronic hypertension

Patient's partner: at bedside, called in from work by patient, has had distressing experiences in hospitals before

Nurse: 15 years of experience working on L and D

Rapid response team: available as needed. Includes another nurse, anesthesiologist, and respiratory therapist

Equipment

Vital signs monitor

Fetal monitor

Code cart

Patient Assessment

Temp: 98.6 F.

HR = 110 bpm.

RR = 24 per minute.

BP = 160/95.

Oxygen saturation: 97% on 2 L/min by nasal cannula.

Patient comments: "My stomach hurts. I'm bleeding a little. My baby isn't due for 5 more weeks."

Setting/Environment

Labor and delivery triage room (sign on wall)

Patient on stretcher with pillow under right hip

Patient's partner at bedside, curious, anxious

"What's wrong with her?"

"Is the baby okay?"

"Our 3-year-old needs to be picked up from daycare soon."

Expectations of Learner from Beginning Phase

___ Introduces self to nurse, patient, and partner

___ Asks for handoff from nurse

___ Confirms fetal viability/well-being

___ Reassures patient and partner

___ Advises alternative childcare plan when asked about their 3-year-old child

___ Informs patient and partner of abnormal blood pressure without alarming them

→ Trigger to move to middle phase: patient states, "I can't breathe. I can't breathe."
→ Middle phase

Patient Assessment
    Patient is unresponsive.
    No palpable pulse.

Setting/Environment
    Support person begins shouting and shaking the patient to wake up.
    Nurse asks resident what to do.
    Monitor alarm sounding.

Expectations of Learner from Middle Phase
    ___ Verbalizes that the patient is pulseless
    ___ Initiates chest compressions
    ___ Calls for help
    ___ Positions patient for effective chest compressions (firm board, left lateral tilt)
    ___ Provides SBAR handoff when rapid response team arrives
        ___ Situation: Patient became pulseless 1 min ago.
        ___ Background: 35-week pregnant, chronic hypertension.
        ___ Assessment: possible amniotic fluid embolism, pulmonary embolism, stroke.
        ___ Recommendation: rapid response team takes over CPR and ACLS, and obstetrician will need to perform cesarean delivery at approximately 4 min.
    ___ Instructs someone to inform patient's partner
    ___ Instructs someone to keep time
    ___ Relinquishes chest compression duty when rapid response team indicates ability to take over
    ___ Verbalizes need for scalpel and cesarean delivery by 4 min
    ___ Does not take time to move patient to another location
    ___ Performs cesarean delivery at approximately 4 min following beginning of pulseless state

That Is a Wrap: The Ending Phase

The ending phase happens once the learner has met, or demonstrated her inability to meet, the learning objectives. Learners should be given enough time and supportive cues from the facilitator in order to meet the objectives; rarely, scenarios simply must be terminated if the learner demonstrates she is not well suited to the scenario. Scenarios that are planned carefully, with attention to appropriate clinical problems, realistic outcomes, familiar settings, flushed-out roles, and achievable learning objectives, should not end with the learner sensing failure. Remember that failure to accomplish the objectives of the simulation is a reflection of ineffective planning more often than inadequate learner knowledge or skills.

The ending phase is marked by a clear announcement from a facilitator that the simulation scenario has ended and that the individuals involved in the simulation will now debrief, or discuss, the experience. The goal is to give the learner an opportunity to consider the consequences of her actions.

Debriefing, or reflection, takes place in a room separate from where the simulation action has occurred, in order to facilitate a psychological transition from pretending to reality. A debrief should be part of every simulation scenario; it is the opportunity for the leader or facilitator to make connections between the decisions and actions undertaken in the scenario and the predetermined outcomes of the script. The styles and strategies for the content of debriefs are beyond the scope of this chapter.

Summary

Impactful simulation builds on appropriate clinical topics. These may spring from new evidence, changing regulations, advancing technology, revised documentation requirements, or a recent adverse event. In developing a simulation scenario, the learner should be considered the centerpiece of the story, and the content must be both timely and specific for that learner's level of experience. The setting and role descriptions should reflect the reality most familiar to the learner. The principal outcome of the scenario will determine the learning objectives, which are action-oriented. The learning objectives create the basis for a facilitator's checklist. Debriefing, or reflection, is necessary in order to have a successful simulation experience.

a

Scenario Building Template

Clinical topic (4 words or fewer): _____

Domain for Learning (check 1 or 2)
____ High acuity, low frequency diagnosis
____ Communication
____ Protocol compliance
____ Medical-legal challenges
____ Technical proficiency

Outcome of the Scenario (one sentence; the knowledge, skill or behavior the learner will demonstrate as a result of the scenario: e.g., *The learner will be able to compassionately communicate bad news to a patient.*)

Setting:
____ Simulation Center
____ Operating room (in situ)
____ Labor room (in situ)
____ Nursing station
____ Emergency department
____ other (describe):

Primary Learning Objectives (No fewer than 2, no more than 5 specific behaviors expected from the learner. Statements should contain no more than 8 words and always begin with a verb, e.g., *Perform directed physical exam, or Explain diagnosis to patient and family*).

1.
2.
3.
4.
5.

Role Descriptions:
  Learner(s) experience level and profession:

  Confederate staff:
  ____ Nurse(s)
  ____ Midwife(s)
  ____ Physician(s)
  ____ Rapid response team
  ____ Operating room personnel
  ____ Pharmacy:
  ____ Clergy
Information related to roles (fatigue, psychological state, novice level, distractions):

Fig. 3.1 (**a–d**) Scenario building template

b

Patient:
Name:

Age:

Gravidity, Parity:

Pregnant: Yes / No

Medical/surgical history:

Medications:

Allergies:

Social factors:

Psychological state:

Support Person(s)/Family
Name:

Relationship:

Reason for being present:

Expectations of learner (what does this person want the learner to do?):

Psychological state:

Equipment:
_____ Mannequin
_____ Task trainer
_____ IV pump
_____ IV fluids
_____ IV tubing
_____ Foley catheter
_____ Laparoscopic instruments
_____ Hysteroscopic instruments
_____ Vital sign monitor
_____ Fetal monitor
_____ Fluids
_____ Synthetic blood
_____ Medication prop
_____ Suture material
_____ Surgical instruments
_____ Code cart
_____ Images
_____ Audio of fetal heart rate, alarm
_____ Documentation forms, chart, EMR
_____ other:

Fig. 3.1 (continued)

c

Learner set-up checklist (what the learner needs to know to succeed):
____ Participant role description
____ Setting
____ Guidelines and expectations
         o   This is a safe environment
         o   Mistakes are expected and encouraged
         o   Act as naturally as possible
         o   Have fun while learning
____ Verify completion of pre-simulation requirements (e.g., reading, video)
____ Provide necessary data to begin problem-solving portion of simulation
(e.g., patient's name, age, initial lab results)

Scenario Timeline:
0 to 5 minutes
      Beginning phase
      Introduce learner to her role, roles of others, the patient, the setting, guidelines,
      expectations, provide necessary data to begin problem-solving
Trigger (e.g., change in vital signs):
      Role of person providing trigger:
5–15 minutes
      Middle phase
      Learner solves problems and performs tasks
15–25 minutes
      Ending phase
      Debrief, reflect

Checklist for Facilitators
The checklist for facilitators is a tool that holds the scenario designers accountable for the
learning objectives and once completed, helps to guide debriefing and reflection.
To create the checklist, begin with the primary learning objectives and determine the
actions that the learner must complete to satisfy each learning objective. These individual
actions make up the facilitator's checklist.

CHECKLIST:
1. LEARNING OBJECTIVE:
      a. Learner is expected to do X to fulfill learning objective
      b. _____
      c. _____
      d. _____
2. LEARNING OBJECTIVE:
      a. Learner is expected to do X to fulfill learning objective
      b. _____
      c. _____
      d. _____

Fig. 3.1 (continued)

d

3. LEARNING OBJECTIVE:

    a. Learner is expected to do X to fulfill learning objective.

    b. _____

    c. _____

    d. _____

Example checklist:

Learning objectives:

    1. Assess vital signs

    2. Perform physical exam

    3. Confirm patient is pregnant

    4. Communicate need to move patient to operating room

➙ Checklist for Facilitator

____ Learner determines temperature

____ Learner determines heart rate

____ Learner determines respiratory rate

____ Learner determines blood pressure

____ Learner communicates recognition of abnormal blood pressure

____ Learner determines oxygenation status

____ Learner auscultates heart

____ Learner auscultates breath sounds

____ Learner palpates abdomen

____ Learner orders pregnancy test

____ Learner communicates with nurse need to go to operating room

____ Learner or delegate calls operating room and communicates urgency

____ Learner communicates with patient need for urgent surgery

____ Learner consents patient for surgery

____ Patient moved to operating room

Debrief and Reflect:

____ Explain that the purpose of simulation is to learn, and mistakes are natural and expected.

____ How did the learner(s) and participants feel during the experience?

____ Describe the objectives that were achieved.

____ Did the learners feel that they had the appropriate knowledge and skills?

____ What went particularly well?

____ Where were the opportunities to improve?

____ What do the learner(s) think was the diagnosis?

____ How can we improve this simulation in the future?

Fig. 3.1 (continued)

References

1. Jeffries PR. A framework for designing, implementing, and evaluating simulations used as teaching strategies in nursing. Nurs Educ Perspect. 2005;26(2):28–35.
2. National League for Nursing (NLN). http://www.nln.org/professional-development-programs/simulation. Accessed 26 Mar 2017.
3. Reilly DE, Oermann M. Behavioral objectives: evaluation in nursing. 3rd ed. New York: National League for Nursing; 1990. (Health Sciences Library WY 18 R362b 1990)
4. Henneman EA, Cunningham H. Using clinical simulation to teach patient safety in an acute/critical nursing course. Nurse Educ. 2005;30(4):172–7.
5. Vandrey C, Whitman M. Simulator training for novice critical care nurses. Am J Nurs. 2001;101(9):24GG–LL.
6. Jeffries P, editor. Simulation in nursing education: from conceptualization to evaluation. 2nd ed. New York: National League for Nursing; 2012. p. 32–9.
7. Medley CF, Horne C. Using simulation technology for undergraduate nursing education. J Nurs Educ. 2005;44(1):31–4.
8. Rauen C. Using simulation to teach critical thinking skills. Crit Care Nurs Clin North Am. 2001;13(1):93–103.
9. Cantrell MA. The importance of debriefing in clinical simulations. Clin Simul Nursing. 2008;4(2):e19–23.
10. McDonnell LK, Jobe KK, Dismukes RK. Facilitating LOS debriefings: a training manual. NASA technical memorandum 112192. Moffett Field: Ames Research Center: North American Space Administration; 1997.
11. O'Donnell JM, Rodgers D, Lee W, et al. Structured and supported debriefing (interactive multimedia program software). Dallas: American Heart Association (AHA); 2009.
12. Decker S. Integrating guided reflection into simulated learning experiences. In: Jeffries PR, editor. Simulation in nursing education from conceptualization to evaluation. New York: National League for Nursing; 2007.
13. Phrampus P, O'Donnell J. Debriefing using a structured and supported approach. In: Levine A, DeMaria S, Schwartz A, Sim A, editors. The comprehensive textbook of healthcare simulation. New York: Springer Science + Business Media; 2013. p. 73–93.
14. Bambini D. Writing a simulation scenario: a step-by-step guide. AACN Adv Crit Care. 2016;27(1):62–70.
15. Clapper TC. Beyond knowles: what those conducting simulation need to know about adult learning theory. Clin Simul Nurs. 2010;6:e7–e14.
16. Jeffries P. Simulation in nursing education: from conceptualization to evaluation. 2nd ed. New York: National League for Nursing; 2012. p. 26–37.
17. Lioce L, Reed CC, Lemon D, et al. Standards of best practice: simulation standard III- participant objectives. Clin Simul Nurs. 2013;9(6s):S15–8.
18. Aschenbrenner D, Milgrom L, Settles J. Designing simulation scenarios to promote learning in simulation. In: Jeffries P, editor. Nursing education: from conceptualization to evaluation. 2nd ed. New York: National League for Nursing; 2012. p. 43–74.

Essentials of Debriefing and Feedback

4

Emily K. Marko

Introduction

Facilitating a debrief is one of the most difficult skills to acquire in simulation. It is the phase that occurs after a simulation when the facilitators and learners come together to discuss and reflect upon the simulation experience. We often say that this is where the magic of learning happens. Educational theory supports the fact that when learners are guided through reflection, their experience will be transformed into new knowledge ready for application in the next experience. In this chapter we will review learning theory and a learner-centered approach that is crucial to debriefing. There are many methods for facilitating a debrief and limited evidence-based research that would favor one method over another, and therefore several debriefing methodologies will be highlighted and key themes presented. The debriefing methods are driven by the objectives, the type of simulation experience, the level of the learner, the environment, equipment, and the experience of the facilitator. The skilled facilitator uses the debrief to help learners reflect on their actions, identify gaps in knowledge and skills, reframe their decision-making, and improve teamwork. When planning a simulation curriculum, the debriefing phase should allow for extra time, and a practical rule to follow is at least twice the time as the actual simulation. A practical, structured guide to debriefing will be described. Several tools for debriefing and evaluating the facilitator will be highlighted.

> **Key Learning Points**
> - Debriefing occurs after the simulation exercise and takes at least twice as long.
> - The premise of debriefing is experiential learning theory and reflective practice.
> - Simulation learning is solidified through reflection on action during the debrief.
> - Objectives must be clearly stated or visually presented.
> - There are many methodologies for simulation debriefing including advocacy-inquiry, plus-delta, rapid cycle deliberate practice, etc., but all involve structured feedback.
> - Psychological safety is essential for learning in a simulation debrief.
> - Diffusion of emotions is critical to allow for participants to partake in meaningful engagement in a debrief.
> - Checklists or protocols are useful tools to clinical debriefing.

E. K. Marko (✉)
Department of Obstetrics and Gynecology, Inova Health System, Falls Church, VA, USA
e-mail: Emily.marko@inova.org

© Springer International Publishing AG, part of Springer Nature 2019
S. Deering et al. (eds.), *Comprehensive Healthcare Simulation: Obstetrics and Gynecology*,
Comprehensive Healthcare Simulation, https://doi.org/10.1007/978-3-319-98995-2_4

- Feedback to learners needs to be specific and depersonalized.
- Teamwork debriefing is aided by TeamSTEPPS® concepts and tools.
- Challenges to facilitating a debrief may be addressed by multiple strategies such as "parking lot issues" and co-debriefing.
- Facilitating a debrief requires skill and practice.

Description/Background

Debriefing originates from the military and is used after a mission to collect, process, and disseminate information as well as to determine if members are ready to return to duty. Medical debriefing is commonly used after a major event such as a code, trauma, or patient death. The purpose is to review what went well and identify areas for improvement. It also provides healthcare workers an opportunity to talk about their emotions. Medical simulation is based on experiential learning theory, and the debriefing phase is where significant learning occurs through a process of guided reflection.

Experiential learning theory developed by Kolb states that "knowledge is created through the transformation of experience. Knowledge results from the combination of grasping and transforming experience." He designed a four-stage learning cycle including "Do, Observe, Think, Plan" which highlights reflection and analysis [1]. Schön's work on professional practice described two important concepts: "reflection in action" during an event and "reflection on action" after an event [2]. These educational theories lay the groundwork for adult learning through reflection during a simulation debrief.

Ericsson's work on deliberate practice provides the basis for providing learners with multiple opportunities to refine skills. The key is that timely and specific feedback is provided between repetitions so that the learner may develop skills [3]. This concept is most applicable to learners developing new skills or moving from novice to expert level of skills.

Simulation debriefing of medical teams involves reflecting on teamwork and communication. Team Strategies and Tools to Enhance Performance and Patient Safety (TeamSTEPPS®) is an evidence-based set of teamwork tools, aimed at optimizing patient outcomes by improving communication and teamwork skills among healthcare professionals [4]. It was developed by the Department of Defense and the Agency for Healthcare Research and Quality to integrate teamwork into practice. The tools and strategies as well as the entire curriculum are publically available and have been implemented widely through federal agencies and healthcare and academic institutions. The simulation debrief may be enhanced by reviewing examples of and opportunities for incorporating TeamSTEPPS® tools and strategies into clinical practice.

Evolving Evidence: Debriefing Methodologies

A significant work over two decades in the field of simulation debriefing has been done by Rudolf et al. [5] The focus of their work is on reflective practice and using good judgment when exercising a debrief. Rudolf's debriefing model involves three phases: determining the conceptual framework of the learner, providing respectful performance evaluation, and using advocacy and inquiry to help the learner improve. These methods help promote the psychological safety that is necessary for healthcare workers to participate in a simulation exercise. By using the advocacy and inquiry method, the skilled simulation debriefer identifies actions that are questionable, helps the learner find cognitive frames or beliefs that caused the actions, and illuminates unintended consequences of these actions.

Others have provided us with a blended approach to debriefing by promoting excellence and reflective learning in simulation (PEARLS) [6]. Facilitators are often hesitant to provide critical feedback because of perceived negative effects on the learner. Eppich and Cheng devised a scripted approach to debriefing divided into four phases: reactions, description, analysis, and summary phases [6]. The reactions phase allows for emotional decompression of all learners. The description phase is a brief summary of the events and key issues for objectives of the debrief so that everyone is on the same page. The analysis phase can be done through learner self-assessment of what went well and what did not (plus-delta method), directive feedback on specific behaviors, or focused facilitation using the advocacy-inquiry method. The summary phase reviews the objectives and summarizes key learning points. The PEARLS framework and debriefing script allow for a standardized structure for facilitators at varying levels of expertise.

The American Heart Association (AHA) and the Winter Institute for Simulation Education and Research (WISER) collaborated to develop the structured and supported debriefing that is a learner-centered process for debriefing in three phases: gather, analyze, and summarize (GAS) [7]. This method is commonly used by the AHA for advanced cardiac and pediatric advanced cardiac life support program debriefing. It involves active listening to participants as they narrate their perspective of the simulation. This is followed by facilitated reflection with the aid of the recording of events and reporting observations. A summary phase reviews lessons learned.

Debriefing for Meaningful Learning (DML) by Dreifuerst uses the Socratic method of questioning to uncover the thought process related to action. Probing the assumptions, rationale, and consequences helps learners to reflect in, on, and beyond the simulation [8].

Another structured debriefing hybrid tool called TeamGAINS was developed by Kolbe et al. [9] It integrates three approaches: guided team self-correction, advocacy-inquiry, and systemic-constructivist techniques. The latter involves circular questions and a view from outside by a "reflecting team" at the interactions of participants. This is useful when larger groups are involved in simulation events and some are able to observe and provide their input. The steps in TeamGAINS involve a reactions phase, clarifying clinical issues, transfer from simulation to reality,

reintroducing the expert model, and summarizing the learning experience. The authors were able to demonstrate improved psychological safety and inclusiveness using these methods.

The anesthetists nontechnical skills (ANTS) is a framework of four key skills categories: situation awareness, decision-making, task management, and teamwork/leadership [10]. It uses a four-point behavior rating scale for each category of the framework. The ANTS tool is used in simulation debriefing and in the workplace for providing constructive feedback. This tool has been disseminated worldwide for anesthetists.

"Rapid Cycle Deliberate Practice" is a debriefing and feedback methodology coined by Hunt et al. based on Ericsson's work on deliberate practice [11]. Facilitators rapidly cycle between deliberate practice and directed feedback until skill mastery is achieved. It was developed for resident learning and applies the coaching principles of directed feedback followed by repetitive practice in order to maximize muscle memory learning in a short period of time. Simulations are interrupted for deviations from the gold standard then repeated until done correctly. Psychological safety and expert coaching were essential. These techniques resulted in improved mastery of procedural and teamwork skills for novice learners.

In summary, the main themes for debriefing a simulation include ensuring psychological safety, allowing for emotional decompression so that learning can occur, providing opportunities for all learners to participate, using methodology of reflective practice, promoting clinical expertise through practice, and optimizing teamwork and communication.

How to Implement: A Practical Guide to Debriefing in Simulation

Incorporating the extensive work of others, a practical guide to simulation debriefing in a systematic manner is presented here. In obstetrics and gynecology simulation programs, specific skill expertise and teamwork and communication are essential components of learning. The nature of our specialty is one of the high emotions as well as rapid, coordinated team actions during emergencies. Therefore this practical guide addresses several key components of the obstetrics and gynecology simulation debrief. Table 4.1 summarizes the structure, and Table 4.2 lists best practices.

Address Learning Climate

Plan the location for the simulation debrief. Moving the group to another location may be beneficial when a simulation exercise involved significant action and emotion. This helps learners to decompress as they transition to a new environment. Address the learning climate by making sure that learners are all seated around a table or in a circle and at the same physical level. Limit distractions by silencing pagers and cell phones. The use of video debrief works well in this setting where everyone is able to view the simulation video.

If debriefing in the simulation room, have the learners move into a circle seated or standing so that everyone is on an equal physical level. The advantages of debriefing in the simulation room are that specific tasks may be demonstrated or repeated where the equipment is readily at hand. Co-debriefing works best if the facilitators are on opposite sides, so they can maintain eye contact and be part of the group.

It is very useful to have a board, tripod, or paper on a clipboard marked as "Parking Lot Issues." Prepare the group to write down concerns that are brought up during the debrief that have to do with systems or operations that cannot be adequately addressed during the debrief and need further attention from other leaders. The facilitator may defer issues that distract from the team debrief and return with recommendations from leadership at a later time.

Diffuse Emotions

As soon as possible, diffuse the emotions. Experiential learning involves an emotional response to the actions, and learners coming out of a simulation exercise often experience a range of emotions. In order for them to enter the reflective phase of debriefing, the emotions need to be settled down. One way to do this is to ask everyone how they are feeling. Some learners will immediately speak, and others may remain quiet. Each participant should be encouraged to contribute. It is important to validate feelings and provide reassurance that in simulation we expect mistakes to happen. Reinforce psychological safety and "Vegas rules." These are the rules of engaging in simulation and are usually discussed at the pre-brief. Participants are informed that the mistakes that inevitably happen in simulation exercises are not to be recorded or discussed outside of the simulation program. Set the agenda for the debrief by focusing on the objectives of the simulation.

Discuss Objectives of Debrief

Providing an outline and objectives of the debrief is important for learner participation and setting expectations. State that time will be allotted to reviewing any clinical issues followed by the majority of the debrief being spent reflecting on teamwork and discovering gaps in knowledge, skills, or attitudes. Engage learners by having them contribute to and agree upon the objectives of the debrief.

Clinical Debrief

Learners will often want to discuss clinical issues, and it is a good idea to address these early in the debrief. Using a clinical checklist helps to focus this part of the discussion. During the simulation, the facilitator may use the checklist or assign an observer to mark expected tasks based on standards of care. Clinical checklists and validated performance assessment tools are readily available through national organizations such as the American College of Obstetricians and Gynecologists patient safety checklists [12], patient safety bundles [13], and MedEdPortal [14]. The facilitator should also document spe-

Table 4.1 Structured debriefing guide for obstetrics and gynecology simulation faculty

Component	Description	Sample statements	Suggested time
Learning climate	Move to a debriefing area that is conducive to group discussion Bring checklists and/or video review Set up "parking lot issues" chart	Let's gather around this area and talk about the simulation; please silence your phones and pagers. If we come across issues that need to be taken to leadership or operations, then we will write them down here	1–2 minutes
Diffuse emotions	Allow everyone to express their emotions about the simulation exercise, validate emotions, and reinforce psychological safety and "Vegas rules"	Simulation often invokes a variety of emotions, how are you feeling at this time? Everyone is well trained and trying to do their best for their patient. It is common to feel emotion after an event such as this. Remember that simulation is a safe environment where we come together to learn as a group. What happened here in simulation stays here. We destroy any videos that were recorded unless you give us permission to keep them	3–5 minutes
Objectives	Provide an agenda for the debrief Review the objectives of the simulation that were stated in the brief Ask participants if there are any other objectives they would like to address	For the next 20–30 minutes, we are going to review our simulation exercise and everyone will be asked to provide their input. We will spend the first few minutes going over any clinical issues or skills and then spend the rest of our time reflecting on our teamwork and communication during this event. Let's review the objectives for the simulation…is there anything else anyone would like to add?	3–5 minutes
Clinical debrief	Use a validated checklist or protocol, and have the group review the steps to discover gaps in knowledge or skills Provide expert feedback with deliberate practice as needed for specific clinical tasks Review use and availability of medical equipment	Let's look at our checklist/protocol…was there anything we missed? What could have helped us remember? Does anyone want to review or practice a skill? (Or let's take a moment to review this skill…) Was there any equipment that was not available?	10–15 minutes
Teamwork debrief	Use open-ended questions to initiate reflection and dialogue on teamwork Request each member to reflect and communicate about their perspective of the scenario Use advocacy-inquiry to discover opportunities for improvement by reframing Use video debrief, facilitator notes, or a teamwork performance assessment	How was our teamwork and communication? What is your perception of the events in this simulation? Were you missing any information? What information would you have preferred to receive? When you did…I noticed…I'm curious …what were you thinking about at that time? Let's provide examples of TeamSTEPPS® concepts and tools that were used today and see if there were any opportunities…	15–20 minutes
Summary and closure	Review objectives and key learning points Have each participant state one take-away lesson learned Repeat simulation if time permitting Document "parking lot issues," and assure follow-up Thank everyone for participating, and invite them to future simulations	Let's go back to our objectives, and see if we covered all of them… Please state one take-home point from today's simulation Let's use the lessons learned and repeat the simulation. Are there any other issues you would like us to address with leadership? Thanks for playing, hope to see you next time	5–10 minutes

Table 4.2 Simulation debriefing best practices

Always do a debrief after a simulation, and try to do it as soon as possible
Plan the debrief to be two to three times the amount of time as the actual simulation
Address the learning environment both physically and emotionally
State or display the ground rules of simulation during the debrief; basic assumptions that everyone is well-trained and wants to do their best for patient care, psychological safety, and "Vegas rules"
Use a structured format for debriefing
Provide objectives stated in the simulation brief
Make sure to diffuse emotions prior to debriefing to move participants into learning mode
Make sure each participant has a chance to reflect and talk
Let participants do most of the talking, and avoid giving a lecture
Address any clinical skills or protocol checklist items early in debrief
Use a checklist or protocol for performance assessment
Focus most of debrief on teamwork and communication because this is where most patient safety events occur
Use expertise to provide specific feedback and not just "good job everyone"
Participants must be encouraged to reflect during the debrief for learning to occur
The use of video is powerful but must ensure psychological safety (video will be destroyed, etc.)
Focus on 5–8 objectives in the debrief; not everything can be debriefed
"Parking lot issues" on a clipboard or tripod help to defer issues that cannot be resolved in the debrief but will be addressed and followed up at a later time
Relate events in the simulation to real life at every opportunity
Encourage learners not to leave a simulation having incomplete knowledge or skills; repeat, do rapid cycle deliberate practice, or set up a time for repeated simulation
If time permits, let the participants repeat the simulation, so they leave with doing it "the right way"
Always thank learners for participating and welcome them back to simulations in the future
Provide value to time spent in simulation by following up with articles, checklists, or protocols provided to learners based on identified performance gaps
Facilitators must acquire and practice skills in debriefing

cific clinical issues on paper or tag video during the simulation and refer to these. Review any issues related to medical equipment use or availability. Ask the learners if they have any clinical questions, and address them at this time. This is also a good opportunity for coaching through rapid cycle deliberate practice for clinical skills and coordinated teamwork required during emergency events.

Teamwork Debrief

Facilitators will debrief with the method that they are most comfortable. Advocacy-inquiry, plus-delta, and facilitated reflection are a few examples described earlier in this chapter. An important aspect of the team debrief is to use the term "we" such as "how well did we work as a team?" This reinforces team actions and communication. When addressing specific teamwork skills, it is

helpful to focus on TeamSTEPPS® concepts. Posters or cards describing the acronyms and concepts of TeamSTEPPS® such as in Table 4.3 are useful visual aids during this phase of the debrief. Allow each person to speak about how they felt in their role during the simulation and if there was any information that they were missing or needed clarified. Suggest or have team members suggest TeamSTEPPS® concepts or tools that would have made the teamwork and communication more effective.

Summary and Closure

As the time approaches for the conclusion of the debrief, summarize concepts that were learned. This is a good time to review the objectives of the simulation and how they were met. The facilitator may want to list the key principles learned during the debrief or have each participant state

Table 4.3 TeamSTEPPS® concept card (Agency for Healthcare Research and Quality (AHRQ) http://team-stepps.ahrq.gov/)

Concept	Definition
SBAR	*Situation, Background, Assessment, Recommendation*
Call-Out	Communicate critical information
Check-back	Closed-loop communication between sender and receiver
IPASS	*Introduction, Patient, Assessment, Situation, Safety Concerns*
Brief	Short planning session prior to start
Huddle	Team regroup to establish awareness and plan
Debrief	Informal meeting to review team performance
Two-challenge rule	Assertively voicing a concern at least two times to ensure it has been heard
CUS	I'm *Concerned*; I'm *Uncomfortable*; This is a *Safety* Issue!

their take-home points. Ensure that any "parking lot issues" are documented, and provide the group with assurance that items will be provided to the appropriate leaders as well as a follow-up communication. At the closure of the debrief, it is always a nice gesture to thank everyone for their participation and invite them to return for future simulation programs. If time permits, many facilitators prefer to repeat the simulation in order for learning concepts to be reinforced and for participants to leave the simulation feeling they performed "the ideal way."

Examples of Debriefing Assessment Tools

There are a number of debriefing tools and checklists available to facilitators. Several are highlighted here. These include performance assessments of debriefing by raters and students and self-evaluation.

The Debriefing Assessment for Simulation in Healthcare (DASH©) tools were designed by the Center for Medical Simulation [15]. It is a six-element behaviorally anchored rating scale that provides feedback on evidence-based debriefing

behaviors of the simulation facilitator. There are three versions of the tools: rater, instructor, and student (Figs. 4.1, 4.2, and 4.3). The DASH© tools are useful for faculty development in the skills of debriefing which take years of practice to become competent.

Six Elements of the Debriefing Assessment

Element 1 – Establishes an engaging learning environment
Element 2 – Maintains an engaging learning environment
Element 3 – Structures the debriefing in an organized way
Element 4 – Provokes an engaging discussion
Element 5 – Identifies and explores performance gaps
Element 6 – Helps a trainee achieve/sustain good future performance

Special Circumstances

There are several special circumstances that should be addressed in debriefing. Facilitators often become passionate about a particular topic and can hijack the debrief, which rapidly becomes a lecture. Facilitators much be cognizant of this pitfall and avoid it by using a structured format for the debrief.

When a facilitator notices a critical error that would impact patient safety, it is important to make this known during the debrief and immediately remediate. The ultimate goal of simulation is to improve patient safety, and despite the need for psychological safety, learners need to be corrected if there are performance gaps that may lead to patient harm. The facilitator may wish to spare the learner embarrassment in front of others by remediating in private; however it is more likely that other participants would benefit from the correction. Focusing specifically on the task and not the individual is a good way to address a critical error during a group debrief.

Occasionally there are difficult participants such as those who hijack the conversation, blame

a

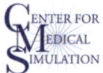

Debriefing Assessment for Simulation in Healthcare (DASH)© Score Sheet

Directions: Rate the quality of the debriefing using the following effectiveness scale on six Elements. Element 1 allows you to rate the introduction to the simulation course and will not be rated if you do not observe the introduction. The Elements encompass Dimensions and Behaviors pertinent to the debriefing as defined in the DASH Rater's Handbook. Within each Element, the debriefing may range from outstanding to detrimental. Please note that the overall Element score is *not* derived by averaging scores for individual Dimensions or Behaviors. Think holistically and not arithmetically as you consider the cumulative impact of the Dimensions, which may not bear equal weight. You, the rater, weight dimensions as you see fit based on **your holistic view of the Element**. If a Dimension is impossible to assess (e.g., how well an upset participant is handled during a debriefing if no one got upset), skip it and don't let that influence your evaluation.

Rating Scale

Rating	1	2	3	4	5	6	7
Descriptor	**Extremely Ineffective / Detrimental**	Consistently Ineffective / Very Poor	Mostly Ineffective / Poor	Somewhat Effective / Average	Mostly Effective / Good	Consistently Effective / Very Good	**Extremely Effective / Outstanding**

Element 1 assesses the introduction at the beginning of a simulation-based exercise.

(This element should be skipped if the rater did not observe the introduction to the course.)

Element 1 **Establishes an engaging learning environment.**	**Element 1 Rating:**

• Clarifies course objectives, environment, confidentiality, roles, and expectations.
• Establishes a "fiction contract" with participants.
• Attends to logistical details.
• Conveys a commitment to respecting learners and understanding their perspective.

Elements 2 through 6 assess a debriefing.

Element 2 **Maintains an engaging learning environment.**	**Element 2 Rating:**

• Clarifies debriefing objectives, roles, and expectations.
• Helps participants engage in a limited-realism context.
• Conveys respect for learners and concern for their psychological safety.

Fig. 4.1 (**a, b**) DASH© tool for rater [16]. (Copyright 2018 Center for Medical Simulation, Inc., Boston, MA, USA, https://harvardmedsim.org/. All rights Reserved, used with permission)

b

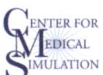

Element 3	
Structures the debriefing in an organized way.	**Element 3 Rating:**

- Encourages trainees to express their reactions and, if needed, orients them to what happened in the simulation, near the beginning.
- Guides analysis of the trainees' performance during the middle of the session.
- Collaborates with participants to summarize learning from the session near the end.

Element 4	
Provokes engaging discussion.	**Element 4 Rating:**

- Uses concrete examples and outcomes as the basis for inquiry and discussion.
- Reveals own reasoning and judgments.
- Facilitates discussion through verbal and non-verbal techniques.
- Uses video, replay, and review devices (if available).
- Recognizes and manages the upset participant.

Element 5	
Identifies and explores performance gaps.	**Element 5 Rating:**

- Provides feedback on performance.
- Explores the source of the performance gap.

Element 6	
Helps trainees achieve or sustain good future performance.	**Element 6 Rating:**

- Helps close the performance gap through discussion and teaching.
- Demonstrates firm grasp of the subject.
- Meets the important objectives of the session.

Fig. 4.1 (continued)

a

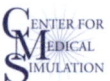

CENTER FOR
MEDICAL
SIMULATION

Debriefing Assessment for Simulation in Healthcare (DASH) Instructor Version©

Directions: Please provide a self-assessment of your performance for the introduction and debriefing in this simulation-based exercise. Use the following rating scale to give a score to each of the six "Elements." For each Element, component Behaviors are given that would indicate positive performance in that Element. Do your best to rate your *overall effectiveness for the whole Element* guided by the Behaviors that define it. If a listed Behavior is not applicable (e.g. how you handled upset people if no one got upset), just ignore it and don't let that influence your evaluation. You may have done some things well and some things not so well within each Element. The Element rating is your *overall* impression of how well you executed that particular Element.
Element 1 assesses the introduction at the beginning of the simulation-based exercise. Elements 2 through 6 assess the debriefing.

Rating Scale

Rating	1	2	3	4	5	6	7
Descriptor	Extremely Ineffective / Detrimental	Consistently Ineffective / Very Poor	Mostly Ineffective / Poor	Somewhat Effective / Average	Mostly Effective / Good	Consistently Effective / Very Good	Extremely Effective / Outstanding

Skip this element if you did not conduct an introduction.

Element 1	Rating Element 1
I set the stage for an engaging learning experience	_____

- I introduced myself, described the simulation environment, what would be expected during the activity, and introduced the learning objectives, and clarified issues of confidentiality
- I explained the strengths and weaknesses of the simulation and what the participants could do to get the most out of simulated clinical experiences
- I attended to logistical details as necessary such as toilet location, food availability and schedule
- I stimulated the participants to share their thoughts and questions about the upcoming simulation and debriefing and reassured them that they wouldn't be shamed or humiliated in the process

Element 2	Rating Element 2
I maintained an engaging context for learning	_____

- I clarified the purpose of the debriefing, what was expected of the participants, and my role (as the instructor) in the debriefing
- I acknowledged concerns about realism and helped the participants learn even though the case(s) were simulated
- I showed respect towards the participants
- I ensured the focus was on learning and not on making people feel bad about making mistakes
- I empowered participants to share thoughts and emotions without fear of being shamed or humiliated

Fig. 4.2 (**a**, **b**) DASH© tool for instructor [17]. (Copyright 2018 Center for Medical Simulation, Inc., Boston, MA, USA, https://harvardmedsim.org/. All rights Reserved, used with permission)

b

Element 3	Rating Element 3
I structured the debriefing in an organized way	_____

- I guided the conversation such that it progressed logically rather than jumping around from point to point
- Near the beginning of the debriefing, I encouraged participants to share their genuine reactions to the case(s) and I took their remarks seriously
- In the middle, I helped the participants analyze actions and thought processes as we reviewed the case(s)
- At the end of the debriefing, there was a summary phase where I helped tie observations together and relate the case(s) to ways the participants could improve their future clinical practice

Element 4	Rating Element 4
I provoked in-depth discussions that led them to reflect on their performance	_____

- I used concrete examples—not just abstract or generalized comments—to get participants to think about their performance
- My point of view was clear; I didn't force participants to guess what I was thinking
- I listened and made people feel heard by trying to include everyone, paraphrasing, and using non-verbal actions like eye contact and nodding etc
- I used video or recorded data to support analysis and learning
- If someone got upset during the debriefing, I was respectful and constructive in trying to help them deal with it

Element 5	Rating Element 5
I identified what they did well or poorly – and why	_____

- I provided concrete feedback to participants on their performance or that of the team based on accurate statements of fact and my honest point of view
- I helped explore what participants were thinking or trying to accomplish at key moments

Element 6	Rating Element 6
I helped them see how to improve or how to sustain good performance	_____

- I helped participants learn how to improve weak areas or how to repeat good performance
- I was knowledgeable and used that knowledge to help participants see how to perform well in the future
- I made sure we covered the most important topics

Fig. 4.2 (continued)

a

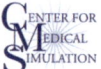

Debriefing Assessment for Simulation in Healthcare (DASH) Student Version©

Directions: Please summarize your impression of the introduction and debriefing in this simulation-based exercise. Use the following scale to rate each of six "Elements." Each Element comprises specific instructor behaviors, described below. If a listed behavior is impossible to assess (e.g., how the instructor(s) handled upset people if no one got upset), don't let that influence your evaluation. The instructor(s) may do some things well and some things not so well within each Element. Do your best to rate the *overall effectiveness* **for the whole Element** guided by your observation of the individual behaviors that define it.

Rating Scale

Rating	1	2	3	4	5	6	7
Descriptor	**Extremely Ineffective / Detrimental**	Consistently Ineffective / Very Poor	Mostly Ineffective / Poor	Somewhat Effective / Average	Mostly Effective / Good	Consistently Effective / Very Good	**Extremely Effective / Outstanding**

Element 1 assesses the introduction at the beginning of a simulation-based exercise.

Skip this element if you did not participate in the introduction.
If there was no introduction and you felt one was needed to orient you, your rating should reflect this.

Element 1	Overall Rating Element **1**
The instructor set the stage for an engaging learning experience.	_____

- The instructor introduced him/herself, described the simulation environment, what would be expected during the activity, and introduced the learning objectives.
- The instructor explained the strengths and weaknesses of the simulation and what I could do to get the most out of simulated clinical experiences.
- The instructor attended to logistical details as necessary such as toilet location, food availability, schedule.
- The instructor made me feel stimulated to share my thoughts and questions about the upcoming simulation and debriefing and reassured me that I wouldn't be shamed or humiliated in the process.

Elements 2 through 6 assess a debriefing.

Element 2	Overall Rating Element **2**
The instructor maintained an engaging context for learning.	_____

- The instructor clarified the purpose of the debriefing, what was expected of me, and the instructor's role in the debriefing.
- The instructor acknowledged concerns about realism and helped me learn even though the case(s) were simulated.
- I felt that the instructor respected participants.
- The focus was on learning and not on making people feel bad about making mistakes.
- Participants could share thoughts and emotions without fear of being shamed or humiliated.

Fig. 4.3 (**a**, **b**) DASH© tool for student [18]. (Copyright 2018 Center for Medical Simulation, Inc., Boston, MA, USA, https://harvardmedsim.org/. All rights Reserved, used with permission)

b

Element 3	Overall Rating Element **3**
The instructor structured the debriefing in an organized way.	_____

- The conversation progressed logically rather than jumping around from point to point.
- Near the beginning of the debriefing, I was encouraged to share my genuine reactions to the case(s) and the instructor seemed to take my remarks seriously.
- In the middle, the instructor helped me analyze actions and thought processes as we reviewed the case(s).
- At the end of the debriefing, there was a summary phase where the instructor helped tie observations together and relate the case(s) to ways I can improve my future clinical practice.

Element 4	Overall Rating Element **4**
The instructor provoked in-depth discussions that led me to reflect on my performance.	_____

- The instructor used concrete examples—not just abstract or generalized comments—to get me to think about my performance.
- The instructor's point of view was clear; I didn't have to guess what the instructor was thinking.
- The instructor listened and made people feel heard by trying to include everyone, paraphrasing, and using non verbal actions like eye contact and nodding, etc.
- The instructor used video or recorded data to support analysis and learning.
- If someone got upset during the debriefing, the instructor was respectful and constructive in trying to help them deal with it.

Element 5	Overall Rating Element **5**
The instructor identified what I did well or poorly – and why.	_____

- I received concrete feedback on my performance or that of my team based on the instructor's honest and accurate view.
- The instructor helped explore what I was thinking or trying to accomplish at key moments.

Element 6	Overall Rating Element **6**
The instructor helped me see how to improve or how to sustain good performance	_____

- The instructor helped me learn how to improve weak areas or how to repeat good performance.
- The instructor was knowledgeable and used that knowledge to help me see how to perform well in the future.
- The instructor made sure we covered important topics.

Fig. 4.3 (continued)

others, or refuse to participate. The skilled facilitator learns to read these signs and adjust the debrief accordingly. Steering the conversation away from hijackers, using "parking lot issues" boards, asking each participant to speak, and depersonalizing the discussion points are strategies that facilitators often use to help diffuse difficult situations.

Co-debriefing has its benefits and challenges. For interprofessional educational programs it is beneficial to have co-debriefers that can provide expertise to the learner groups. For example, physicians and nurses may be able to provide tips in practical skills and model professionalism in team behavior while co-debriefing. Best practices in co-debriefing include planning ahead, clarifying roles and methodology, common objectives, comparing notes on simulation observation, maintaining eye contact and strategic positioning during the debrief, asking questions through open negotiation, and conducting a co-facilitator debrief.

Summary

Debriefing in healthcare simulation is essential to learning but one of the most difficult components of a simulation. Learning achieved through simulation has improved retention due to the debriefing. Becoming a skilled facilitator takes significant expertise, patience, and practice. Debriefing is well grounded in educational theory including experiential learning and reflective practice. Active listening and a structured approach are best practices in debriefing. Though methodologies in debriefing may vary, the common themes include psychological safety of the learners, diffusion of emotion, standards of expertise, reflection and reframing, repeated practice, and optimizing teamwork dynamics. The purpose of simulation in healthcare is the guiding principle of improved patient safety. Debriefing solidifies this concept by identifying the gaps, finding the causes, and improving the healthcare team's knowledge, skills, and attitudes.

References

1. Kolb DA. Experiential learning: Experience as the source of learning and development. Upper Saddle River: FT Press; 2014.
2. Schön DA. Educating the reflective practitioner: Toward a new design for teaching and learning in the professions. San Francisco: Jossey-Bass; 1987.
3. Ericsson KA. Deliberate practice and the acquisition and maintenance of expert performance in medicine and related domains. Acad Med. 2004;79(10):S70–81.
4. King HB, Battles J, Baker DP, Alonso A, Salas E, Webster J, Toomey L, Salisbury M. In: Henriksen K, Battles JB, Keyes MA, Grady ML, editors. Advances in patient safety: new directions and alternative approaches (Vol. 3: Performance and Tools). Rockville: Agency for Healthcare Research and Quality (US); 2008.
5. Rudolph JW, et al. Debriefing with good judgment: combining rigorous feedback with genuine inquiry. Anesthesiol Clin. 2007;25(2):361–76.
6. Eppich W, Cheng A. Promoting excellence and reflective learning in simulation (PEARLS): development and rationale for a blended approach to health care simulation debriefing. Simulation in Healthcare. 2015;10(2):106–15.
7. O'Donnell J, et al. Structured and supported debriefing. Dallas: American Heart Association; 2009.
8. Dreifuerst KT. Debriefing for meaningful learning: Fostering development of clinical reasoning through simulation. Bloomington: Indiana University; 2010.
9. Kolbe M, et al. TeamGAINS: a tool for structured debriefings for simulation-based team trainings. BMJ Qual Saf. 2013;22(7):541–53. https://doi.org/10.1136/bmjqs-2012-000917.
10. Flin R, et al. Anaesthetists' non-technical skills. Br J Anaesth. 2010;105(1):38–44.
11. Hunt EA, et al. Pediatric resident resuscitation skills improve after "rapid cycle deliberate practice" training. Resuscitation. 2014;85(7):945–51.
12. https://www.acog.org/-/media/Patient-Safety-Checklists/psc006.pdf?dmc=1.
13. https://www.cmqcc.org/resources-tool-kits/toolkits/ob-hemorrhage-toolkit.
14. https://www.mededportal.org/.
15. Brett-Fleegler M, et al. Debriefing assessment for simulation in healthcare: development and psychometric properties. Simul Healthc. 2012;7(5):288–94.
16. http://harvardmedsim.org/wp-content/uploads/2017/01/DASH.handbook.2010.Final.Rev.2.pdf.
17. http://harvardmedsim.org/wp-content/uploads/2017/01/DASH.IV.ShortForm.2012.05.pdf.
18. http://harvardmedsim.org/wp-content/uploads/2017/01/DASH.SV.Short.2010.Final.pdf.

Communication and Teamwork Training in Obstetrics and Gynecology

5

Christopher G. Goodier
and Bethany Crandell Goodier

Introduction

Teamwork in healthcare is inherently interdisciplinary. Labor and delivery units are staffed with nurses, patient care technicians, delivering providers, and anesthesiologists. Often other specialists such as pediatric providers (physicians and nurses) as well as respiratory therapists are needed. In the late 1990s, the Pew Health Professions Commission released an analysis recommending interdisciplinary competence in all medical professionals. The report noted that with interdisciplinary team training, resources are used efficiently, mistakes are minimized, and valuable expertise is maximized [1].

Outside of healthcare, especially in aviation and the military, there has been research that suggests teams working in high-risk and highly intense arenas make fewer mistakes than individuals in the same setting. Highly effective teams improve overall task-specific performance by exhibiting qualities such as flexibility and adaptability, as well as resistance to stress [2, 3].

C. G. Goodier (✉)
Department of Maternal Fetal Medicine, Medical University of South Carolina, Charleston, SC, USA
e-mail: goodier@musc.edu

B. C. Goodier
Department of Communication, College of Charleston, Charleston, SC, USA

Key Learning Points

This chapter focuses on teamwork and communication in healthcare by:

- Defining teams and teamwork
- Introducing team training in healthcare
- Utilizing simulation in teamwork training
- Building a team-based culture

Background

Patient safety and medical errors have come to the forefront of healthcare since the Institute of Medicine released *To Err Is Human: Building a Safer Health System* in 1999 [4]. The Institute of Medicine recognized that healthcare was not as safe as it should be due to a complex and often fragmented delivery model leading to challenges in making change, often leading to stagnation. The goal was to force change by publicly recognizing the magnitude of the problem, develop resources, and set aggressive goals and monitoring systems to improve safety.

The Joint Commission on Accreditation in Healthcare Organizations (JCAHO) is an independent, not for profit organization founded in 1951. The mission of the JCAHO is to improve healthcare by evaluating healthcare organizations' ability to provide safe and effective high-quality healthcare. Toward this end, JCAHO has set standards and survey processes designed to help organizations reduce variation in healthcare delivery as well as risk reduction to deliver the safest care possible. They identified communication as the root cause of the majority of sentinel events (defined as an unexpected occurrence involving death or serious physical or psychological injury) in hospitals [5, 8]. Specifically in obstetrics, there was a sentinel alert published that suggested failures of communication and organizational culture were associated with increased perinatal morbidity [6].

In 2011, the American College of Obstetrics and Gynecology (ACOG) put out a call to action for quality patient care in labor and delivery. The statement acknowledged that childbirth is a dynamic process and effective care requires shared decision-making and highly reliable teams in order to reduce errors, increase satisfaction, and improve outcomes. ACOG recognized that highly skilled clinical expertise does not equal expert teamwork [7]. Because labor and delivery teams are often assembled ad hoc due to the nature of the work, it is essential that each team member understands his/her role and responsibility to affect the best outcome for the patient and her baby.

Despite these reviews, there remain many opportunities in medical education to emphasize or strengthen this kind of training. In many instances clinicians, especially clinicians in training, do not typically receive team-based skills training during the course of their education. Communication and teamwork are nontechnical skills which supplement the technical skills required to deliver care safely and effectively. In medicine we reward individual accomplishment and clinical excellence but rarely reward group skills or collaboration. While communication skills are taught, they often focus on patient interviewing to develop a differential diagnosis rather than communication among team members. In addition, nurses and physicians are trained separately, and the communication skills emphasized in these trainings are different. McConaughey acknowledges that "physicians learn a concise, headline, problem-focused approach whereas nurses use narrative, descriptive language often

careful not to diagnose" [8]. She argues for a standardized communication process that leads to shared goals, mutual understanding, and common frame of reference to minimize opportunities for miscommunication. We contend that not only should the process be standardized but also integrated with formal communication and team training across the education continuum.

Teams and Team Development

While the definition of teams varies across contexts and disciplines, it is generally assumed that a team is two or more individuals working together toward a shared goal. Manser defines teams as "two or more individuals who work together to achieve specified and shared goals, have task specific competencies, and specialized work roles, use shared resources, and communicate to coordinate and adapt to change" [9]. Ilgen further distinguishes the difference between a team and a group, arguing that while groups "may be comprised of autonomous individuals working concurrently on some task or goal, teams represent a system of interconnected individuals with unique roles, working collaboratively to attain a common goal" [10]. In healthcare, teams are often physician-directed and hierarchical but require the deliberative participation and interaction of multiple members including a wide variety of healthcare professionals, patients, and caregivers. Compared to other industries, healthcare teams often work under conditions that change frequently. In many, but not all clinical scenarios, teams may be assembled in an ad hoc fashion. The situation may require a dynamically changing membership that must work together for a short period of time consisting of different specialty areas. In the team literature, such teams are known as "action teams." Action teams consist of members with specialized skills who must improvise and coordinate their actions in intense, unpredictable situations [11]. As teams form, communication among members creates and sustains team structures and processes. It is especially critical to attend to the ways these teams form and the patterns of interaction that emerge [12].

While not all scholars endorse the stage model of group development, most agree that high-performing teams tend to cycle through some variation of Tuckman's model of group development. In stage one (forming), team members are brought together to form a structural group, but they may lack confidence in one another, the goals of the team, or a sense of shared vision [13]. In stage one, members seek information about roles, expectations, and intended outcomes. In stage two (storming), the group becomes more familiar with one another, clarifies roles, and may address past conflicts which might limit future effectiveness. In stage three (norming), members gain experience working together as a team, form opinions about the strengths and weaknesses of each member, and clarify roles. The final stage (performing) is characterized by peak performance; group members trust one another explicitly, demonstrate shared decision-making, open communication, and have relational and professional knowledge of one another based on previous experiences working together as a team. While all teams move in and out of these stages based on contextual factors, static teams tend to remain in "performing mode" longer than ad hoc teams because they have established trust, confidence in one another, and a sense of shared goals and processes [13]. Put simply, static teams know what to expect of the situation and one another. Action teams, whose memberships change often, have to cycle through these stages (in some variation) each time the members change making it more challenging to reach peak performance levels. These teams benefit from increased opportunities to build interpersonal competence, strengthen relationships, and build trust. Communication skills training and simulations provide opportunities for ad hoc or action teams to work through these early stages in low-risk circumstances.

Teamwork and Communication in Healthcare

The Institute of Medicine recommended that the healthcare industry adopt an approach, already in place in the aviation industry, known as crew resource management (CRM). The concept utilizes a didactic approach to improve outcomes by focusing on safety and effectiveness by enhancing communication and collaboration. CRM relies on strong leadership breaking down barriers to communication and empowering each team member to enhance cohesion. While the concept of CRM is beyond the scope of this chapter, it can be an integral step to improve communication and collaboration among healthcare team members working together to improve patient safety [14].

In November 2006, the Agency for Healthcare Research and Quality (AHRQ), in collaboration with the Department of Defense, released an evidence-based teamwork system called Team Strategies and Tools to Enhance Performance and Patient Safety (TeamSTEPPS™) as the national standard for team training in healthcare. Information can be found at the following website https://www.ahrq.gov/teamstepps/index.html. ACOG, in Committee Opinion #447 on patient safety in obstetrics and gynecology, recognized the importance of teamwork training and identified TeamSTEPPS™ as a way to increase awareness and enhance communication to improve patient safety [15].

Based on over 30 years of research, the TeamSTEPPS™ training program focuses on:

- *Team Structure:* the components of the team or teams that must be assembled to ensure patient safety
- *Communication:* the exchange of information among team members
- *Team Leadership:* the ability to coordinate among team members, secure resources, help others understand actions needed
- *Situation Monitoring*: the process for scanning and assessing situational elements to gain information understanding or to maintain awareness to support functioning of the team
- *Mutual Support*: anticipating and supporting other team members' needs through accurate knowledge about their responsibilities and workload

In a study published in the *Journal of Perinatology*, Thomas et al. performed a randomized trial looking at teamwork training and impacts on neonatal resuscitation. They identified that approximately 30% of standard neonatal resuscitation steps are either missed or not performed correctly and that team training resulted in improved team behaviors [16].

While team training has been shown to improve team behaviors, it is often taught via traditional didactic lectures which leave it up to the individual learner to apply the concepts in their day-to-day activities. Simulation has been used for decades in other industries and has been increasingly adopted in healthcare as a bridge to apply these tools in clinical scenarios.

The Joint Commission Journal on Quality and Patient Safety published a report on teamwork and communication on obstetric birth trauma and found a statistically significant and persistent improvement in perinatal outcomes utilizing simulation in addition to didactic training [17]. They recognized that while team training can improve teamwork, simulation guides decision-making through interactive multidisciplinary collaboration. This prospective study compared three scenarios, a control with no intervention, didactic training only, and didactic training augmented with simulation exercises. The primary outcome chosen was perinatal morbidity and mortality using a Weighted Adverse Outcome Score (WAOS). In addition they looked at a perceived culture of safety as measured subjectively by a Safety Attitudes Questionnaire (SAQ). There was a 37% improvement in weighted perinatal outcome (WAOS) in the group that utilized both didactic training and simulation exercises from pre-intervention to post-intervention measurements. The perception of safety did not show significant improvement, however [17]. This study argues for dual modality, including experiential exposure with simulation training to improve outcomes.

Teamwork and Simulation

In April of 2011, ACOG published a committee opinion entitled "Preparing for Clinical Emergencies in Obstetrics and Gynecology." The use of drills and simulation was identified to address "the principle that standardized care can

result in safer care" [18]. Team drills, high fidelity simulation, and in situ simulation can identify common errors and deficiencies in communication and aid in the identification and assigning of roles and personnel. Practicing for both common and uncommon events allows experiential learning in a fluid environment and the practice of communication among providers. Protocols, workflows, and emergency supply needs can be identified, and the most efficient processes can be developed to aid in accurate and effective care delivery in a low-stakes environment.

Notably, research suggests that teams whose work is fairly standardized experience less role confusion requiring less directive leadership styles with implicit direction. Simply put, everyone understands their role and how their work contributes to progress toward the goal. In urgent, emergent, or rare scenarios, the team requires a strong sense of structure, explicit directions, and more directive leadership behavior [19–22].

Simulation can bring together multiple stakeholders and foster building trust, clarify roles, and enhance shared decision-making. These team development opportunities create a shared frame of reference for those who participate in them regardless of team membership which creates certainty and reduces communication errors when they are assembled ad hoc in high-stakes situations. The process described below offers one such model for directive leadership with explicit role identification and process mapping. When practiced repeatedly in simulations, it creates a shared mental model and a common frame of reference for managing these scenarios in real-life situations [19, 22].

Problem Identification The initial provider (regardless of his/her role) should acknowledge the problem, assess the situation, determine what, if any, additional resources are necessary (e.g., staff, medications, equipment, etc.), and call those items/individuals to the room.

Attend to the Patient While awaiting additional resources or actions, explain to the patient the current situation and what steps are being taken to resolve the problem. Ensure that the care space is clear of additional distractors (e.g., visitors, nonessential personnel).

Organize the Team Once the physician is present, the problem should be clearly stated. The Institute for Healthcare Improvement and the Joint Commission both support the use of SBAR (situation, background, assessment, and recommendation) as a form of structured communication. The initial provider should clearly and *briefly* define the situation; then provide clear, relevant background information that relates to the situation; and then provide an assessment and what he/she needs from the individuals on the team. SBAR is especially important in urgent or high-acuity situations where clear and effective interpersonal communication is critical to patient outcomes. This provides a consistent language and framework to ensure effective communication and transfer of information.

Assign Roles The leader should restate the problem and clearly identify roles while determining if additional resources are required.

Close the Loop Once specific orders are placed (testing, labs, imaging, etc.), closed-loop communication should be utilized by restating the orders to minimize errors. Ask for questions and encourage continued cross talk. The briefing leader should ask for any questions regarding the patient and procedure just discussed and encourage team members to continue to speak up if they have any questions or concerns during the procedure or to report on progress.

Reassess The team leader should reassess the situation once orders have been completed and results are reviewed to determine if resolution or improvement has occurred. Team members should feel empowered to ask questions and add information as needed.

Communicate with the Patient The patient (and/or patient's family) should be informed of the findings and treatment, as well as if the problem is resolved or ongoing and what the next steps are.

Debrief An essential component of effective teams and patient safety is debriefing in which performance feedback can be provided. This includes what went well and what could be improved upon.

Be sure to acknowledge that the debrief process allows us to understand one another's perspective and frame of reference. Doing so regularly helps to build teamwork and communication skills. Were roles clear? Was communication effective throughout? What went well? What should improve? In simulated environments, the use of checklists or frequency charts can be utilized to determine if appropriate actions were taken and reinforce the use of common language, behavior, or action that was performed. Multiple authors have addressed both the importance of debriefing and specific strategies to promote its effectiveness [23–25].

It is important to note that while team members should attend to the verbal elements of process described above, they should also attend to the nonverbal aspects of their message. Communication research suggests that a significant portion of what is remembered or conveyed in all interactions is nonverbal, conveyed through eye contact, body language, tone of voice, as well as pace and volume of speech [26]. Throughout the interactions described above, all participants should speak clearly and calmly, establish and maintain eye contact when speaking, and make sure there are no physical barriers limiting communication.

As an example of the framework described above, a simulation of a vaginal delivery that results in a shoulder dystocia may proceed as shown in Box 5.1:

Where Should Simulation Training for Teamwork Training Be Performed?

Simulation training can occur at the location of the learner (in situ) or in a dedicated training center. Deering et al. note that each has unique advantages and disadvantages [27]. Dedicated simulation centers offer a controlled, standard-

Box 5.1 Example Simulation

Delivering provider – We have a shoulder dystocia. Nurse A we need to call additional help to the room. Please call additional resources (nurse(s), patient care tech, additional physician, etc.) as well as notify pediatrics. Please mark the time and ensure there is a stool available.	*Problem Identification*
Ms. X, your baby has not been delivered due to one of the shoulders being positioned behind a bone in your pelvis. I would like you to stop pushing, remain calm, and carefully listen to the instructions we provide so that we can deliver your baby. Additional resources will be arriving to help. (Visitors may need to leave the room to allow for space.)	*Attend to the patient*
We have a shoulder dystocia. The head was delivered "x" seconds ago. This is Ms. X and it is her first baby. She has diabetes and the estimated fetal weight was 7 pounds. I would like to place the patient in McRobert's position and utilize suprapubic pressure to try and resolve the problem.	*Organize the team*
Nurse A and B will you please place the patient in McRobert's position. Nurse B please apply suprapubic pressure in "x" direction. Patient care tech please call out the time in __ increments. Please ensure that the pediatric resuscitation equipment is available, and if not, please ask "x" to gather it, while we await the pediatricians.	*Assign roles*
Nurse B confirms the position for suprapubic pressure with the delivering physician. The patient care tech acknowledges the time from onset of shoulder dystocia and confirms the equipment request. Time is called out every __ seconds.	*Close the loop*
The physician notes that the anterior shoulder has/has not resolved after the initial maneuvers and states this to the team. Additional instructions are provided as a next step. Team members should feel empowered to speak up with any concerns.	*Reassess*
Ms. X, the problem has been resolved, and I need you to push again, and you will deliver your baby. Once delivered we will assess your baby to ensure he/she is healthy and vigorous, and the pediatric team will be here to assist us.	*Communicate with the patient*
The physician leads the debriefing episode. How do you all think the simulation went? Did we recognize the problem? What steps did we take to resolve the problem? Were there any stumbling blocks to success? What ideas do you have to improve for the next event? Remember, our goal is to review all aspects of the event to find opportunities for improvement.	*Debrief*

ized environment with skilled trainers and technicians to offer the most seamless experience with minimal complications. They often have dedicated AV equipment allowing for detailed feedback. Disadvantages include an artificial environment that may not explicitly highlight or identify process or communication barriers which is where in situ drills have a distinct role. In addition it is often challenging to get staff to go off-site given busy patient care environments. Attention should be given to the optimal way to ensure staff from all shifts and representatives from each discipline have the opportunity to participate and learn.

Building a Culture of Teamwork

Healthcare organizations emphasize patient safety through teamwork. Effective teamwork does not occur as a result of placing people together when a problem arises. Teams require competent members who utilize a common set of tools and training to improve performance [28]. In order to adopt a collaborative, interdisciplinary model of teamwork, there needs to be significant buy-in from the institutional leadership, including the identification of a champion. Resources, training, and time need to be allocated to optimize successful implementation.

The champion should be empowered to seek opportunities to constantly query departmental management and staff regarding opportunities to reeducate staff and practice the model in all activities. To further this, organizations should consider adding simulation opportunities to reinforce concepts and language from team training in an organized or ad hoc fashion, in a simulation lab or in situ. The language and techniques should be utilized in every aspect of care, and drills should be repeated regularly to reinforce the process and shared framework. Organizational processes should be aligned to support and reward effective communication and teamwork.

Summary

Interdisciplinary teamwork and communication skills training are essential to improve patient safety. Healthcare teams are dynamic and often formed ad hoc increasing the risk for unintentional adverse outcomes. Well-researched team training methodologies are available and require a strong commitment from all levels of the organization to build and foster a culture by providing the resources and time to succeed. Simulation training provides an outstanding opportunity for team training by creating a space to practice effective communication skills and providing a shared frame of reference for all caregivers during low-stakes scenarios that create a structure to maximize outcomes when the stakes are high.

References

1. O'Neil EH and The PEW Health Professions Commission. Recreating health professional practice for a new century. San Francisco: PEW Health Professionals Commission; 1998.
2. Baker D, Gustafson S, Beaubien J, Salas E, Barach P. Medical teamwork and patient safety: the evidence-based relation. Rockville: Agency for Healthcare Research and Quality, Center for Quality Improvement and Patient Safety; 2005.
3. Gully SM, Incalcaterra KA, Joshi A, Beaubien JM. A meta-analysis of team efficacy, potency, and performance: interdependence and level of analysis as moderators of observed relationships. J Appl Psychol. 2002;87(5):819–32.
4. Kohn L, Corrigan J, Donaldson MS. To err is human: building a safer health care system. Washington, DC: National Academy Press; 1999.
5. Salas E, DiazGranados D, Weaver SJ, King H. Does team training work? principles for health care. Acad Emerg Med. 2008;15:1002–9.
6. Joint Commission on Accreditation of Healthcare Organizations: Preventing Maternal Death. The Joint Commission, Sentinel Event Alert 30. http://www.jointcommission.org/.
7. American College of Obstetrics and Gynecology. Quality patient care in labor and delivery: a call to action. Available from https://www.acog.org/-/media/Departments/Patient-Safety-and-Quality-Improvement/Call-to-Action-Paper.pdf. 2011. Accessed 20 Feb 2017.
8. McConaughey E. Crew resource management in healthcare. The evolution of teamwork training and MedTeams®. J Perinat Neonat Nurs. 2008;22(2):96–104.
9. Masner T. Teamwork and patient safety in dynamic domains of healthcare: a review of the literature. Acta Anaesthesiol. 2009;53(2):143–51.
10. Ilgen DR. Teams embedded in organizations: some implications. Am Psychol. 1999;54:129–39.
11. Sundstrom E, de Meuse KP, Futrell D. Work teams: application and effectiveness. Am Psychol. 1990;45(2):120–33.
12. Kilgore RV, Langford RW. Reducing the failure risk of interdisciplinary healthcare teams. Crit Care Nurs Q. 2009;32(2):81–8.
13. Tuckman BW. Developmental sequence in small groups. Psychol Bull. 1965;63:384–99.
14. Miller KK, Riley W, Davis S, et al. In situ simulation: A method of experiential learning to promote safety and team behavior. J Perinat Neonat Nur. 2008;22:105–13.
15. American College of OB/GYN: Committee Opinion #447. Patient safety in obstetrics and gynecology. Obstet Gynecol. 2009;114:1424–7.
16. Thomas EJ, Taggart B, Crandell S, Lasky RE, Williams AL, Love LJ, Sexton JB, Tyson JE, Helmreich RL. Teaching teamwork during the Neonatal Resuscitation Program: a randomized trial. J Perinatol. 2007;27(7):409–14.
17. Riley W, Davis S, Miller K, Hansen H, Sainfort F, Sweet R. Didactic and simulation nontechnical skills team training to improve perinatal patient outcomes in a community hospital. Jt Comm J Qual Patient Saf. 2011;37(8):357–64.
18. American College of OB/GYN: Committee Opinion #487. Preparing for clinical emergencies in obstetrics and gynecology. Obstet Gynecol. 2011;117(4):1032–4.
19. Eisenberg EM, Murphy AG, Sutcliffe K, Wears R, Schenkel S, Perry S, Vanderhoef M. Communication in emergency medicine: implications for patient safety. Commun Monogr. 2005;72:390–413.
20. Grote G, Zala-Mezo E, Grommes P. Effects of standardization on coordination and communication in

high workload situations. Linguistiche Berichte. 2003;12:127–54.

21. Entin EE, Serfaty A. Adaptive team coordination. Hum Factors. 1999;41:312–25.

22. Lingard L, Whyte S, Espin S, Baker GR, Orser B, Doran D. Towards safer interprofessional communication: constructing a model of "utility" from preoperative team briefings. J Interprof Care. 2006;20:471–83.

23. Eppich W, Howard V, Vozenilek J, Curran I. Simulation-based team training in healthcare. Simul Healthc. 2011;6(7):S14–9.

24. Rudolph JW, Simon R, Rivard P, Dufresne RL, Raener DB. Debriefing with good judgment: combining rigorous feedback with genuine inquiry. Anesthesiol Clin. 2007;25:361–76.

25. Hunter LA. Debriefing and feedback in the current healthcare environment. J Perinat Neonatal Nurs. 2016;30(3):174–8.

26. Knapp M, Hall J. Nonverbal communication. Boston: De Gruyter Mouton; 2013.

27. Deering S, Johnston LC, Colacchio K. Multidisciplinary teamwork and communication training. Semin Perinatol. 2011;35:89–96.

28. Lerner S, Magrane D, Friedman E. Teaching teamwork in education. Mt Sinai J Med. 2009;76:318–29.

Competency Assessment in Simulation-Based Training: Educational Framework and Optimal Strategies

6

Etoi A. Garrison and Jessica L. Pippen

Introduction

Simulation-based training can be used to evaluate communication and teamwork competencies among interdisciplinary teams and promote healthcare quality and safety [1–3]. Simulation has been used as an instructional design method to teach medical students, residents, and subspecialty fellows [4, 5]. It is also recognized as a method of evaluating professional competence for practicing physicians [6, 7]. Simulation-based training is most effective when it is designed to successfully capture the knowledge, skills, and clinical reasoning that underlie expected behavior within the framework of the competencies assessed. Accurate and objective evaluation of trainee performance depends on the assessment method and the assessment tools selected. In this chapter, we will review a commonly recommended framework for evaluating the quality of an assessment tool. We end the chapter with examples of checklists and global rating scales, two common assessment tools that can be used during simulation-based training to determine if the expected clinical and procedural performance outcomes for learners have been achieved.

> **Key Learning Points**
> - Simulation-based training is a useful tool for evaluation of communication and teamwork skills.
> - Understanding the concept of validity is important to assessing the usefulness of a simulator and simulation training programs.
> - The assessment tools chosen should be tailored to the simulation objectives with some better suited to checklists and others a more global rating scale.

Reliability

Webster defines reliability as "the extent to which an experiment, test, or measuring procedure yields the same results on repeated trials" [8]. As it relates to assessment, reliability is a property of both the assessment method and the data generated by it [9, 10]. *Test-retest reliability* refers to the ability of one individual learner to be assessed by an assessment method at different times or under different circumstances and produce similar results each time [9]. *Equivalence reliability*

E. A. Garrison (✉)
Department of Obstetrics and Gynecology, Vanderbilt University Medical Center, Nashville, TN, USA
e-mail: Etoi.A.Garrison@VUMC.ORG

J. L. Pippen
Department of Obstetrics and Gynecology, The Ohio State University Wexner Medical Center, Columbus, OH, USA

© Springer International Publishing AG, part of Springer Nature 2019
S. Deering et al. (eds.), *Comprehensive Healthcare Simulation: Obstetrics and Gynecology*, Comprehensive Healthcare Simulation, https://doi.org/10.1007/978-3-319-98995-2_6

refers to the degree to which scores can be reproduced if the assessment is given to different learners with similar skill levels. Equivalence reliability can also be assessed if one learner repeatedly obtains the same score despite the use of different assessment methods that are similar with regard to content, complexity, and structure. This concept can be illustrated by a basketball analogy. For example, let's assume you have two players (each representing two different trainees) whose goal is to sink a basketball into the same basketball hoop. Player A will be assessed by shooting the basketball from the three-point line (method A), and player B will be assessed by shooting the basketball from mid-court (method B). Each player makes the same number of attempts to shoot the basketball through the hoop. One player successfully sinks the basketball through the hoop with every attempt and the other player hits the rim with every attempt but does not score a point. Both players are similarly reliable over time with regard to their ability to make the basketball hit the same target. However, one player will have a higher score than the other. It is also important to note that in this example making a basket from mid-court may require more skill compared to making a basket from the three-point line. This difference suggests that data generated by the assessment must be interpreted cautiously because it will depend in part upon the trainee and the rigor inherent within the assessment method. Scalese and Hatala published a similar analogy using archery as an example [9].

Equivalence is a term used to describe the similarity of test scores if one assessment method is given to several individuals with similar skill and training, and each individual generates similar results. If for example, ten players with similar training and skill failed to make a basket from mid-court, we would surmise that the assessment method (shooting a basket from mid-court) produces equivalent scores that may be independent of the individual player. Equivalence can also be determined if the same individual takes two different forms of an assessment that are matched for difficulty and structure.

Inter-rater reliability can be assessed when one learner is evaluated separately by two trained evaluators who utilize the same assessment tool. *Intra-rater reliability* can be determined when one evaluator performs the same assessment on multiple examinees with similar skill and training and generates equivalent assessment results. Intra-rater reliability can also be used to refer to the ability of one examiner to perform an assessment repeatedly at different time points on the same individual and generate similar results.

The reliability of an assessment method may be influenced by the circumstances in which the assessment tool is used. McEvoy et al. published a study to determine the reliability of an assessment tool used to evaluate residents during the management of simulated perioperative anesthetic emergencies. Trained expert and trained non-expert faculty members were asked to view videotaped simulations twice allowing the rater to stop the video ("with pauses") and twice without the ability to pause during grading ("continuous") [11]. In this study, they found that the assessment scores were reliably reproduced by trained faculty regardless of their innate expertise. They also found that assessment scores were reliably reproduced despite variability in the method of videotape review. It is unknown, however, if assessment scores for examinees with similar training can be reproduced if the assessment is given to trainees at another academic center. Further, it is unknown if the assessment tool can produce reliable results if the assessment method is applied during an in situ simulation or an actual patient care encounter.

The variables that influence the reliability of a simulation-based training assessment tool are depicted in Fig. 6.1.

Validity

Validity is defined by Merriam-Webster as "the quality of being logically or factually sound; soundness or cogency" [12]. An assessment tool is valid when there is an evidence basis to support the conclusions drawn about the data generated. With regard to simulation-based evaluations in medicine, competency-specific performance data must be interpreted within the context of both the

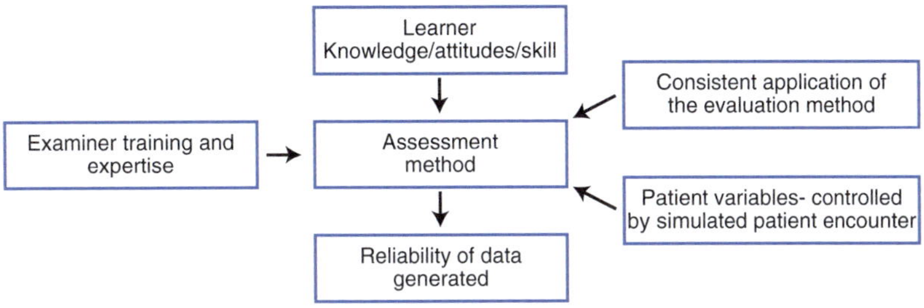

Fig. 6.1 Assessment reliability can be influenced by (1) examinee factors, (2) examiner factors, (3) the assessment method, (4) consistent application of the assessment method, and (5) patient variability + environmental factors

competency and the learner being evaluated. Andreatta, Downing, Cook, and Messick are just a few of the authors who can be credited with articulating current concepts regarding validity as it relates to assessment and simulation-based training in healthcare [13–17]. They argue that validity is not a property that is unique to the assessment tool, and it cannot be directly attributed to the scores generated by the assessment. It is directly related, however, to the decisions made about the assessment data and how the data is interpreted within the construct evaluated. According to Andreatta, validity is a function of the following: (1) what is being measured ("the construct"), (2) how the "construct" or competency is measured via the assessment tool, (3) the clinical context in which the assessment tool is applied, and (4) the evidence used to support conclusions made about the resulting data [14]. In a clinical opinion by Andreatta et al. published in 2011, the word "construct" is used as a term referring to what is being assessed [14]. Within the field of medical education, the construct can be either a broad or a more specific component of the competency assessed. The construct can refer to broad topics such as family planning or normal labor. The construct can also refer to more specific topics such as IUD placement or fourth-degree laceration repair. Within the ACGME patient care and procedural skill competencies for example, the identification and management of normal labor is a broad construct, while performance of a spontaneous vaginal delivery would be more specific. The knowledge, attitudes, skills, and behaviors that define each construct also determine the key components of the assessment tool. For simulation-based training, the challenges lie however, in the identification of the construct components and determining if key elements of the construct can be observed and measured by the assessment tool. Constructs that include observable behaviors can be measured easily. Within the construct of normal vaginal delivery, for example, correct knowledge of fetal OA vs OP position and appropriate hand placement on the perineum are measureable behaviors readily assessed. The clinical reasoning underlying the decision to abandon a vaginal delivery attempt and proceed with delivery by cesarean is an important component of the construct but may be more difficult to infer from the behaviors observed unless it is explicitly stated by the learner (see Fig. 6.2).

The term *construct validity* refers to how well the assessment tool captures the key components of the construct and how the data is interpreted within the context of the construct. In Fig. 6.2, several of the key components involved in the performance of a normal vaginal delivery are listed. The construct elements must be defined with sufficient detail such that desired knowledge, behaviors, and skills observed during the simulation provide evidence of clinical and procedural competence. The ideal assessment tool is mapped to the construct components in order to accurately capture performance measures and provide a general impression regarding the learner's ability to integrate information from various sources during patient care. If the assessment tool accurately reflects the construct, logical assumptions can be made about the data generated by the tool. If, for example, the simulation assessment tool accu-

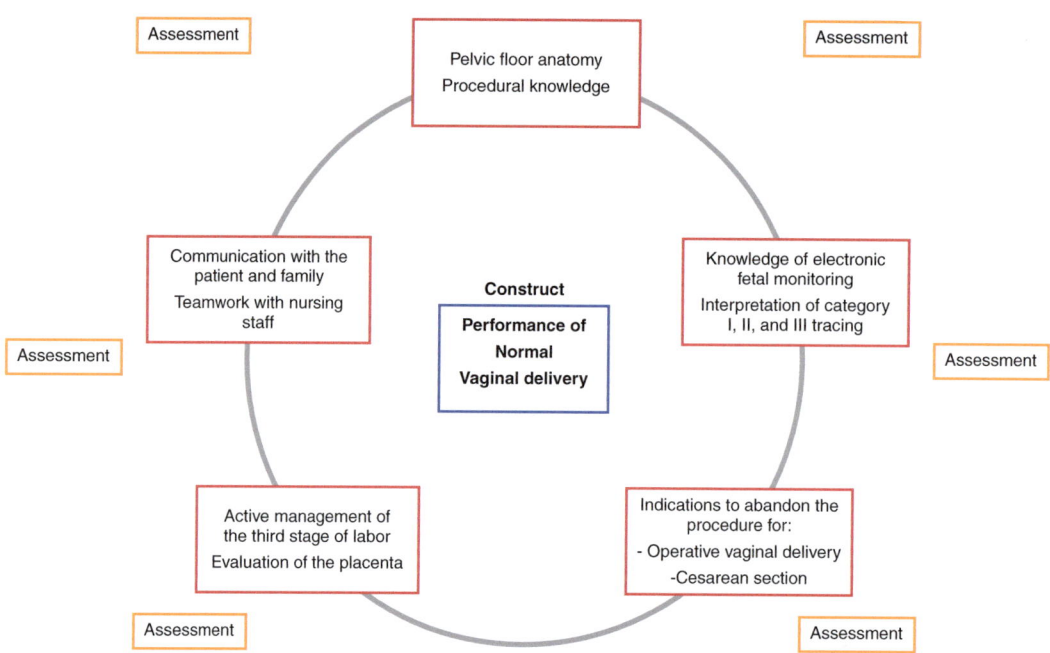

Fig. 6.2 Construct components and assessment. The ideal assessment accurately represents the construct and its individual components. Modified from Andreatta et al. Validity and assessment. Am J Obstet Gynecol 2011 [14]

rately captures all of the knowledge/behavior/skill components associated with the performance of an actual vaginal delivery, a low assessment score during the simulation may correlate with poor clinical performance during an actual vaginal delivery. A trainee who does not properly position the patient and communicate with her during maternal pushing would score poorly on the assessment tool compared to the trainee who appropriately performs these tasks. If the assessment tool does not capture information about trainee communication with the patient and nursing staff, the learner may score well during the simulation; however the assessment underrepresents the breadth of the construct and could lead to a misrepresentation of clinical competence as it relates to appropriate performance of the actual procedure. Similarly, if a simulated vaginal delivery construct fails to include information about electronic fetal monitoring and the management of a category I, II, or III tracing, the assessment data generated will match the construct but may have limited applicability to the management of an actual patient. Validity evidence would be necessary to justify any decisions made regarding the

learner's ability to perform the construct during a patient encounter. The reader is referred to texts by Andreatta, Shields, Downing, and Messick for a more in-depth review of the relationship between construct and assessment tool [14–16].

According to Scalese and Hatala, validity is the degree to which a test measures what it is intended to measure [9]. Using the basketball analogy, let's assume that the goal is to score a point by sinking a basketball through the basketball hoop. Player A shoots the ball and always hits the rim. Player B shoots the ball and consistently passes the ball through the net. Only the method utilized by player B resulted in the accumulation of points, and as such it would be considered a more valid approach compared to the method utilized by player A. Validity refers to accurate interpretation of the data within the constraints of the subject matter assessed. It is not considered to be a dichotomous yes-or-no variable that can be attributed to the instrument (player) or assessment method that in this example would be standing at the three-point line. Validity is a process by which a structured argument can be developed that supports the inferences and decisions made about the data collected. Conversely, if the goal of basketball is to touch the rim of the basketball hoop one would argue that player A has a more valid approach.

It has been argued that validity determination is a process by which evidence can be gathered to either support or refute the interpretation of the assessment data and the decisions made as a result [10, 14]. Evidence to support validity arguments may be broadly divided into five categories: content validity, response process validity, measurement or internal structure validity, relational validity, and consequential validity. A five-component framework to define validity evidence was initially proposed by Messick in 1989 [16, 18]. It was adopted as standard by the American Psychological Association in 1999 and again in 2014 [18, 19]. Table 6.1 lists the sources of evidence and provides representative examples of each.

Content validity evidence refers to the degree to which the construct components realistically reflect the construct and the degree to which key construct elements are represented in the assessment tool.

Content validity evidence for the simulation assessment methodology can be determined by a panel of expert reviewers. A description of the procedures used to determine if the simulated case and the assessment tool realistically capture the construct, curriculum content, and the clinical/procedural learning objectives can be used to provide

Table 6.1 Definitions and representative examples of validity evidence

Type of validity evidence	Definition	Examples of evidence (Cook, what counts as validity evidence)
Content validity	The relationship between the assessment tool and the construct is designed to measure APA (Cook/Hatala validation)	Group consensus or expert review of construct elements and assessment tools Modification or adaptation of an assessment tool that was previously validated and will be used in a similar context with the current study Description of pilot testing and revision of assessment tool Use of clinical guidelines or other high-quality evidence to support construct development and the assessment tool
Response process validity	The correlation between simulated performance of the construct and actual performance of the construct	Analysis of expert opinion and trainee feedback during the assessment process Quality control – video capture of trainee performance Standardized training on use of the assessment tool for examiners
Measurement validity or internal structure reliability	Relationship among data items within the assessment and how these relate to the construct	Interrater reliability – reproducibility of scores across different raters Test-retest reliability – reproducibility of scores across different versions of the test Item analysis – evaluation of scoring, inter-item correlation, and item discrimination
Relational validity	Relationship between the assessment score and other variables or factors that are predictive of construct performance	Association (positive or negative) between simulation-based assessment score and the score obtained on an independent measure of performance Association between the simulation assessment score and the observed level of performance in clinical practice Association between the simulation assessment score and the level of performance by computer, written, or oral exam Association between assessment score and training level (novice/expert) or status (trained/untrained)
Consequences	Impact beneficial or harmful of the assessment itself	Pass/fail threshold using established procedures (ROC curve) Comparison of actual vs expected pass/fail rate Description of anticipated impact (positive, negative, or neutral) on students or patients

See the following references for additional information regarding examples of evidence that can be used to support the validity elements above [10, 15, 17, 20]

evidence to support content validity. The process by which the assessment tool is piloted and revised based upon content expert review and learner feedback can also be used as content validity evidence [15]. An additional source of content validity evidence includes the appropriate use of a previously described instrument [20]. It is important to note that construct validity arguments based upon a previously validated assessment tool can only apply to cases in which the tool is utilized under the same testing conditions for which it was originally developed and previously validated.

Process validity is a term that refers to whether or not the cognitive and physical processes required during the simulation realistically approximate the cognitive and physical tasks that are actually required by the construct. Simulation has gained broad appeal as a platform for clinical assessment because it provides more realistic opportunities to assess the cognitive and physical processes required for patient care compared to the standard oral or written examination [14]. Process validity evidence can be provided by opinions culled from content experts and examinee feedback [13, 20]. Process validity can also be used to refer to methods that maintain data integrity. Evidence used to support process validity includes description of how sources of error were minimized during test administration and a description of quality control measures. An example of data-driven quality control for simulation-based exercises includes analysis of examiner rating disagreements in order to better facilitate consensus.

Measurement validity can be provided by demonstrating strict adherence to established scoring algorithms and criteria [14]. There should be clear evidence of the association between the data generated by the algorithm and applicable construct. The reproducibility of scores given variability in trainee or examiner can be used to support the strength of the association between the score, the assessment tool, and the construct. The data elements that can be used to provide internal structure validity arguments include: reproducibility of scores across different raters (inter-rater reliability), reproducibility of scores across different stations or tasks (interstation reliability), and reproducibility across different items on the test (internal consistency).

Relational validity refers to the evidence supporting a positive or negative relationship between the assessment data and independent variables that can be used to predict performance within the construct [14, 17]. Assessment scores that can be replicated across multiple trainees of varying skill is an example of reliability but can also be used to provide evidence regarding the relational validity of the assessment tool. For example, one would expect a positive relationship between the simulation assessment score and trainee experience. A positive correlation between the simulation-based assessment of a vaginal delivery and novel, intermediate, and advanced resident trainees would support validity arguments regarding the accuracy of the assessment.

Consequential validity evidence refers to the intended or untended results that occur after decisions are made on the basis of assessment results [13, 14]. For example, resident scores on a vaginal delivery curriculum can be used along with additional clinical data to determine a threshold by which the resident is given independent responsibility for performing vaginal deliveries and teaching junior residents. Downstream measures of patient care can then be used to determine if the decision to provide residents with independent practice opportunities based upon the simulation-based assessment method and scoring process was appropriate and resulted in intended or unintended consequences.

Arguments made about the extrapolation of assessment data to determine trainee competence should be made with care as they are dependent upon trainee expertise, clinical context, and the formative vs summative nature of the assessment [13].

Assessment Tools in Obstetrics: Checklists and Global Ratings Scales

Simulation performance checklists and global ratings scares are frequently used in a summative or formative manner to identify performance deficits and direct trainee learning. Checklist instruments and global rating scale results may be used by course faculty to identify the curricular elements that require dedicated teaching and/or practice-based improvement.

Table 6.2 shows an example of the checklist used in The Department of Obstetrics and Gynecology at MedStar Washington Hospital Center and MedStar SiTEL to assess trainee knowledge, skills, and attitudes regarding the management of eclampsia.

This checklist clearly outlines the learning objectives for the trainee, preceptor, and observer. Trainees will be assessed on their ability to make an accurate diagnosis, communicate an appropriate treatment plan to the patient and nursing staff, and escalate the level of care if the patient does not clinically improve. Dichotomous "yes" or "no" options were used to document trainee per-

formance of key tasks. If the simulation is used for formative assessment, it may be appropriate to modify the checklist by stratifying the yes/no columns into unsatisfactory/satisfactory/superior framework (Table 6.3). A trainee, for example, may be able to identify the name, dose, and route of the antihypertensive but may not understand the criteria for initiation or cessation of therapy. This distinction would help to differentiate satisfactory from superior performance.

Global rating scales can be used to assess trainee performance. Trainee assessment when utilizing a global rating scale demands a greater level of skill and expertise by the examiner [21]. An example of a global rating scale is detailed below (Box 6.1).

Table 6.2 MedStar Health Simulation Training and Education Lab. Eclampsia Checklist

Eclampsia Obstetrics Emergency-Assessment Tool

Participant Name:				Affiliation:	
☐ PGY1	☐ PGY2	☐ PGY3	☐ PGY4	☐ Fellow	☐ Staff
Learning Outcomes: At the end of this session the participant will be able to:					
Identify risk factors associated with eclampsia.					
Discuss potential complications related to eclampsia.					
Recognize an eclamptic seizure.					
Demonstrate the management of an eclamptic seizure.					
Demonstrate the proper counseling of a patient experiencing eclampsia.					
Demonstrate the proper documentation of an eclamptic patient.					

Checklist Items(from ACOG Simulation Consortium)	ACGME Core Competency	Rating		Comments
		Yes	No	
1. Recognize situation as eclampsia	MK	☐	☐	
2. Calls for additional OB help	IC	☐	☐	
3. Calls for anesthesia	IC	☐	☐	
4. Orders magnesium sulfate with correct dose.	PC	☐	☐	
5. Orders Ativan or Valium with correct dose	PC	☐	☐	
6. Orders antihypertensive medication with correct dose	PC	☐	☐	
7. Assure patient airway is patent	PC	☐	☐	
8. Monitors vital signs closely	PC	☐	☐	
9. Assess patient properly after seizure	PC	☐	☐	
10. Demonstrate appropriate counseling to the patient/family	IC	☐	☐	
11. If needed calls a "Rapid Response"	PC	☐	☐	

Comments:

Table 6.3 Revised Eclampsia Checklist with the addition of a three-tier system

Task	ACGME Competency	Rating (select one category)	Comment
Recognize eclampsia	MK	*Unsatisfactory:* Does not state diagnosis *Satisfactory:* States correct diagnosis *Superior:* States correct diagnosis. Utilizes patient history to consider other diagnoses on differential	
Calls for additional OB help	IC	*Unsatisfactory:* Does not call for help *Satisfactory:* Calls for help *Superior:* Calls for help. Delegates responsibility as team members arrive. Communicates effectively with staff	
Calls for anesthesia	IC	*Unsatisfactory:* Does not call for anesthesia *Satisfactory:* Calls for anesthesia *Superior:* Calls for anesthesia. Provides respiratory support until anesthesia arrives. Gives appropriate SBAR. Demonstrates effective communication regarding plan of care	

Descriptive terms can be used to anchor performance expectations for the trainee and faculty examiner

---

Box 6.1 Areas to consider (there may be others in addition)

1. History taking: Completeness, logic, focus
2. Physical examination skills: Approach to patient, technical skill, interpretation of findings
3. Counseling skills: Patient-friendly, questioning style, empathy, clear explanation
4. Clinical judgment: Use of clinical knowledge, correct interpretation, logical approach, recognizing limits, and appropriate advice sought
5. Professionalism: Respectful, courteous, confident
6. Organization/efficiency: Efficient, logical, and ordered approach
7. Overall clinical competence: Demonstrates judgment, synthesis, caring, effectiveness, efficiency

History Taking

1	2	3	4	5	6	7	8	9	NA
Unsatisfactory			Satisfactory			Superior			

Physical Examination

1	2	3	4	5	6	7	8	9	NA
Unsatisfactory			Satisfactory			Superior			

Clinical Judgment

1	2	3	4	5	6	7	8	9	NA
Unsatisfactory			Satisfactory			Superior			

Professionalism

1	2	3	4	5	6	7	8	9	NA
Unsatisfactory			Satisfactory			Superior			

Organizations/Efficiency

1	2	3	4	5	6	7	8	9	NA
Unsatisfactory			Satisfactory			Superior			

Overall Clinical Competency

1	2	3	4	5	6	7	8	9	NA
Unsatisfactory			Satisfactory			Superior			

Like checklists, global rating scales can be used as either a primary or secondary assessment method for simulation-based training. Global rating scales are often more generalizable compared to checklists as they can be used to assess a variety of clinical performance tasks. It has been argued that global rating scales require greater expertise by the examiner because they are designed to capture more subtle nuances of performance [10]. Checklists, by their very structure, can be designed for use by examiners who are not content experts. The step-by-step format of the checklist permits a very regimented approach to assessment and facilitates ease of use; however it may not permit the observer to capture and reward subtle differences in clinical performance that are significant indicators of clinical competence [21]. It has been argued that checklists reward thoroughness but may not sufficiently recognize alternate approaches to patient care that can distinguish novice from more expert trainees [10, 20–22]. The reader is referred to Ilgen et al. for an excellent review on the benefits and limitations of checklist vs global rating scale. Both tools can be used to assess clinical performance during simulation-based training [21].

Interpretation of simulation-based training results requires basic information about the reproducibility of the assessment method, ability of the simulation tool to accurately evaluate the construct in question, and validity arguments that will better enable the translation of simulation-based testing scores to clinical practice.

References

1. Rosen MA, Salas E, Wilson KA, et al. Measuring team performance in simulation-based training; adopting best practices for healthcare. Sim Health Care. 2008;3:33–41.
2. Guise J, Deering SH, Kanki BG, et al. Validation of a tool to measure and promote clinical teamwork. Sim Healthcare. 2008;3:217–23.
3. Goffman D, Lee C, Bernstein PS. Simulation in maternal–fetal medicine: making a case for the need. Semin perinatol. 2013;37:140–2.
4. Medical simulation in medical education: results of an AAMC survey. https://www.aamc.org/download/259760/data/medical simulation in medical education an aamc survey.pdfS.
5. Deering S, Auguste T, Lockrow E. Obstetric simulation for medical student, resident, and fellow education. Semin Perinatol. 2013;37:143–14.
6. Sidi A, Gravenstein N, Lampotang S. Construct validity and generalizability of simulation-based objective structured clinical examination scenarios. J Grad Med Educ. 2014;6(3):489–94.
7. Chiu M, Tarshis J, Antoniou A. Simulation-based assessment of anesthesiology residents' competence: development and implementation of the Canadian National Anesthesiology Simulation Curriculum (CanNASC). Can J Anesth. 2016;63:1357–63.
8. Webster- Reliability. https://www.google.com/search?q=reliability&oq=reliability&aqs=chrome..69i57j0l5.2916j0j8&sourceid=chrome&ie=UTF-8.
9. Scalese, RJ, Hatala R. Competency assessment. The comprehensive textbook of healthcare simulation. Chapter 11. Springer Science Media: New York 2013. 135–160.
10. Cook DA, Hatala R. Validation of educational assessments: a primer for simulation and beyond. Adv Simul. 2016;1:31.
11. McEvoy MD, Hand WR, Furse CM, et al. Validity and reliability assessment of detailed scoring checklists for use during perioperative emergency simulation training. Simul Healthc : J Soc Simul Healthc. 2014;9(5):295–303.
12. Webster- Validity. https://www.google.com/#q=definition+of+validity+as+a+noun.
13. Andreatta PB, Gruppen LD. Conceptualising and classifying validity evidence for simulation. Med Educ. 2009;43:128–03.
14. Andreatta PB, Marzano DA, Curran DS. Validity: what does it mean for competency based assessment in obstetrics and gynecology? Am J Obstet Gynecol. 2011;204:384 e1–6.
15. Downing S. Validity: on the meaningful interpretation of assessment data. Med Educ. 2003;37:830–7.
16. Messick S. Validity of psychological assessment: validation of inferences from persons' responses and performances as scientific inquiry into score meaning. Am Psychologist. 1995;50:741–9.
17. Cook DA, Zendeja B, Hamstra SJ, Hatala R, Brydges R. What counts as validity evidence? Examples and prevalence in a systemic review of simulation based assessment. Adv Health Sci Educ. 2014;19:233–50.
18. Messick S. Standards of validity and the validity of standards in performance assessment. Educ Measure Issues Prac. 1995;14:50–8.
19. American Educational Research Association, American Psychological Association, National Council on Measurement in Education. Validity. Standards for educational and psychological testing.

Washington, DC: American Educational Research Association. 2014. pp. 11–31.

20. Cook DA, Brydges R, Zendejas B, et al. Technology-enhanced simulation to assess health professionals: A systematic review of validity evidence, research methods, and reporting quality. Acad Med:872–83. https://doi.org/10.1097/ACM.0b013e31828ffdcf.

21. Ilgen JS, Ma IWY, Hatala R, Cook DA. A systematic review of validity evidence for checklists versus global rating scales in simulation-based assessment. Med Educ. 2015;49:161–73.

22. Norman GR, Van der Vleuten CP, De Graaff E. Pitfalls in the pursuit of objectivity: issues of validity, efficiency and acceptability. Med Educ. 1991;25:119–26.

Licensure, Certification, and Credentialing

7

E. Britton Chahine

Introduction

This chapter will explore the basis for use of simulation in licensure, certification, and credentialing, discuss where the specialty of Obstetrics and Gynecology is currently with regard to these, and discuss challenges regarding its implementation and future directions.

> **Key Learning Points**
> - Current licensure, certification, and credentialing are still primarily based on didactic test scores and subjective clinical evaluations.
> - Simulation can provide a more objective assessment than current methods, although additional work is needed and underway to develop and validate simulation assessments.
> - Simulation assessment of skills is increasingly being used in high-stakes exams to establish standardized level of skills and knowledge.

Background

Before discussing simulation as it applies to licensure, certification, and credentialing, it is important to begin with some definitions. Licensure is a time-limited permit granted by a governmental agency ensuring that preexisting requirements have been met in order to use the professional degree obtained. Certification is a voluntary time-limited verification that an individual has obtained training beyond or in addition to their primary degree [1, 2]. Credentialing is a local action by an organization that a professional has fulfilled the requirements and has the necessary expertise to practice in their specialty at the institution. The purpose of all of these qualifications is to ensure that physicians and other health professionals are competent to perform within their scope of practice. Competence requires didactic knowledge, hands-on skills, and communication and lies within the intersection of these specific components (Fig. 7.1). Within this as a foundation, clinical decision-making, correct implementation and execution, and clear communication with the health team and the patient are imperative to ensure the desired outcome. When one considers these different components, it becomes obvious that the measures used most commonly at this time, standardized multiple-choice examinations, completed degrees, and documented case logs, are more suited to only

E. Britton Chahine (✉)
Department of Gynecology and Obstetrics, Emory University School of Medicine, Atlanta, GA, USA
e-mail: e.britton.chahine@emory.edu

© Springer International Publishing AG, part of Springer Nature 2019
S. Deering et al. (eds.), *Comprehensive Healthcare Simulation: Obstetrics and Gynecology*,
Comprehensive Healthcare Simulation, https://doi.org/10.1007/978-3-319-98995-2_7

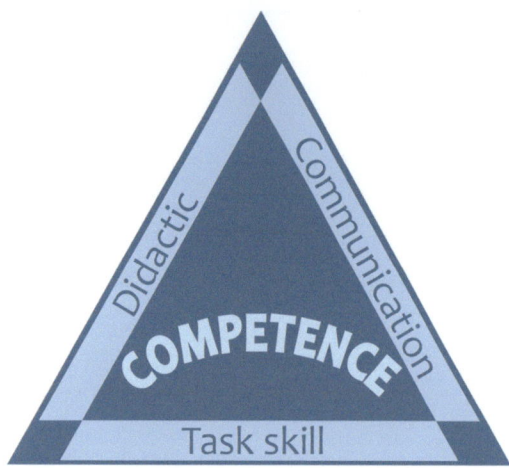

Fig. 7.1 Competence requires didactic knowledge, hands-on skills, and communication and lies within the intersection of these specific components

the didactic knowledge part and do little to assess technical and communication skills.

Currently the most accepted determinant of competency is time served in training. This may include undergraduate and graduate work, medical or nursing school, residency, and/or fellowship in conjunction with the successful completion of a standard didactic knowledge-based assessment. As an example, the United States Medical Licensing Exam (USMLE), initially implemented in 1992, is required before physicians can obtain a license to practice medicine in the United States [3]. In Obstetrics and Gynecology, the CREOG (Council on Resident Education in Obstetrics and Gynecology) exam during residency and the American Board of Obstetrics and Gynecology (ABOG) written exam with completion of residency are paramount for board certification. These written assessments establish the didactic basis of competency and are standardized within Obstetrics and Gynecology as well as the subspecialties within our discipline.

For nursing, an example of additional certification is inpatient obstetric nursing (RNC-OB), and this can be accomplished by taking the National Certification Corporation (NCC) certification exam. Similar to the CREOG and ABOG written examinations, this is a multiple-choice test that can be taken after the candidate has obtained their RN license and has additional experience and contact hours in obstetrics.

Skills assessment during residency training in Obstetrics and Gynecology is determined by reaching a certain case threshold for surgical and obstetric procedures with faculty feedback regarding residents' technical abilities. There is currently no standardized assessment other than this apprentice-based model although ACGME (Accreditation Council for Graduate Medical Education) milestones, which will be discussed more later in the chapter, have been put into place in an attempt to standardize some of the core experiences. Skills acquisition is still dependent on the innate abilities of the learner since every individual masters skills at different rates. Given that some individuals may not achieve competency when the current set number of cases is reached and others achieve competency much faster, it is difficult to set minimum case volumes and to know when a skill has been mastered. To address this, some global and checklist scoring have been validated in different contexts in an attempt to better define this, though they have some limitations [4]. In general, technical checklists reflect that the operator has knowledge of the key steps to a procedure but may not completely assess the actual technical skill. Global assessments are much better at assessing technical skills but may be affected by recall and subjectivity bias. In general, faculty have often not been taught how to assess, i.e., what specific skills constitute a better score and what the scoring anchors should reflect, which can increase the scoring error and decrease the inter-rater reliability between assessors.

Additionally, assessment of performance in our specialty usually occurs after case completion, increasing the risk of recall bias unless a procedure or surgery is videotaped and reviewed. More importantly, as the number of clinical cases has decreased with ACGME work hour restrictions, the number of operative exposures and learning opportunities has also decreased. With less experienced providers, there is understandably less autonomy to exercise clinical intraoperative decision-making which only exacerbates the challenge of real-time assessment. Thus current technical assessments tend to be based on the general impression of the evaluator often without clear reproducible or reliable data.

The assessment of communication skills, including interactions with patients, other providers, and the healthcare team, is probably the least developed area of assessment of competence, yet miscommunication between healthcare providers is one of the leading causes of preventable medical error [5]. Currently, most communication assessments are based on recall by attending faculty involving their own interactions or those observed with patients. The American College of Obstetrics and Gynecology (ACOG) has endorsed teamwork training, which may include the TeamSTEPPS program, to facilitate a standardized communication system to decrease errors when relaying patient information between healthcare providers [6]. While the emphasis on teamwork and communication training is an important step in improving patient safety, implementation requires practice and a commitment from leadership in order for it to become an integral part of transitions of care. And, with regard to measurement, this area is even more challenging to assess and not something that lends itself to a multiple-choice test.

The benefit of simulation as a teaching and evaluation tool is that it allows for integration and assessment of the three components of competence: knowledge, technical skills and communication, and provides a more comprehensive insight into what actual clinical practice looks like. The incorporation of simulation in the process of licensure, certification, and credentialing has evolved slowly as this understanding has evolved. The use of Resusci Anne is one of the earliest simulation-based certifications, i.e., Basic Life Support (BLS) certification. The development of Resusci Anne in the 1960s as a task trainer was to initially teach and then assess basic life support skills. Subsequent creation of Harvey the cardiology mannequin and the Gainesville Anesthesia Simulator continued the trend to use simulators to both teach and evaluate

specific skills [7]. In 1979, Advanced Cardiac Life Support (ACLS) was introduced as a certification course that incorporated didactics, technical skills, and team training utilizing a mannequin-based curriculum to teach and assess participants [7]. Then, in 1999, the American Institute of Medicine released the *To Err is Human* report that outlined the large number of patients who die each year from medical errors. This report significantly increased interest and incorporation of simulation into training programs and institutions because of the realization that the current standard of assessment and education was lacking [8].

Following the *To Err is Human* report, the ACGME (Accreditation Council for Graduate Medical Education) endorsed six core competencies that every physician should possess (see Box 7.1). These competencies focused on global skills that were eventually incorporated into the Obstetrics and Gynecology Milestones Project. The milestones provide a more explicit definition of expected resident knowledge, skills, attributes, and performance to better assess competency [9]. With this change in focus, the importance of simulation-based assessment to help set basic standards has expanded with integration of simulation into licensure, certification, and credentialing in most disciplines.

In general, there are several points at which simulation can be introduced into the licensure/certification/credentialing process. The first is as a prerequisite for a provider to be eligible to sit for an examination. The second is as part of the examination itself, and a third is for maintenance of certification. The final place it can be used is as

Box 7.1 ACGME Core Competencies
- Patient care
- Medical knowledge
- Practice-based learning and improvement
- Systems-based practice
- Professionalism
- Interpersonal skills and communication

part of credentialing or the granting of privileges at the local institution.

With respect to simulation training as a prerequisite for certification, this process is now beginning in medical school. Many schools have been incorporating Objective Structured Clinical Examinations (OSCEs) that utilize standardized patients (SPs) to simulate clinical encounters on an increasing basis. Since 2004, the USMLE has incorporated simulation into the Clinical Skills portion of their exam by utilizing SPs to assess professionalism and communication skills. For residents, the American Board of Surgery requires Fundamentals of Laparoscopic Surgery (FLS), a simulation-based training and assessment certification, before being eligible to sit for board certification in general surgery. Additionally, the Society of American Gastrointestinal and Endoscopic Surgeons (SAGES) has developed a simulated-based Fundamentals of Endoscopic Surgery (FES) program as a comprehensive educational and assessment tool designed to teach and evaluate the fundamental knowledge, clinical judgment, and technical skills required in the performance of basic gastrointestinal (GI) endoscopic surgery for gastroenterologists, general surgeons, and other physicians [10]. This program is now also a prerequisite for eligibility for board certification in general surgery. While the specialty of OB/GYN has not yet created simulation courses that are a requirement for providers prior to certification boards, with the obvious overlap in surgical skills, this may occur in the near future. In terms of use for board examination, the American Board of Anesthesiology has already incorporated simulation into their testing process, including simulation-based OSCEs with standardized patients and high-fidelity simulation scenarios to demonstrate technical skills. In our specialty, the American Board of Obstetrics and Gynecology (ABOG) has started to offer simulation courses as an option for ACOG diplomats to fulfill requirements for Part IV of the Maintenance of Certification (MOC) process and has also created a simulation committee to evaluate the potential to expand the use of simulation in other aspects of the certification process [11].

Recently, ABOG has even entered into an agreement with a simulation company to work on sonogram simulation for potential incorporation into their board examination process [12].

In terms of credentialing, which is a local institutional action, robotic surgery is an example where simulation training may be required to have operative privileges. At this time a high-fidelity simulation robotic surgery skills program with vendor-sponsored training on a simulator is part of the process at many hospitals. Another example of simulation training requirements for credentialing can be found in the Military Healthcare System (MHS) in the United States, which includes 50 hospitals that provide maternity care services. As of 2017, all nurses, midwives, and physicians that work on labor and delivery are required to attend a simulation-based obstetric emergencies simulation course every 2 years. Options for this training include either the Emergencies in Clinical Obstetrics (ECO) Course from ACOG or Advanced Life Support in Obstetrics (ALSO) from the American Academy of Family Practice.

Although simulation is starting to be utilized in both high-stakes assessments and credentialing, standardization of simulation at all levels of training is still a work in progress, although there has been more progress at the resident/fellow training level. The Obstetrics and Gynecology Milestones Project, endorsed by ACGME, ABOG, and ACOG, has helped to make progress in delineating critical knowledge and skills required by level of training and provides a target for simulation training goals. Similarly, ACGME-accredited fellowships (Maternal-Fetal Medicine, Female Pelvic Medicine and Reconstructive Surgery, Reproductive Endocrinology and Infertility and Gynecologic Oncology) also have milestones associated with the didactic and skills required for each particular subspecialty. In an attempt to provide simulation training options that can be applied to the milestones, the ACOG Simulation Working Group and the CREOG Surgical Skills Task Force have created standardized curricula that provide low-fidelity, affordable simulation models along with didactic content and evaluation tools that can be utilized [11, 13]. How the milestones and related simulations are incorporated into programs is still very much individualized to each particular residency and fellowship, as is the assessment of technical and communication skills. There is still a lack of formal simulation curricula for physicians who are reentering the workforce or who have identified areas of weakness that need addressing, although there are efforts to create these. Looking toward the future, it appears certain that simulation will become more universal in assessments of all levels of providers. However, for this to happen, the barrier of being able to provide standardized and validated evaluation tools must be overcome.

Before using simulation as a high-stakes evaluation, it is necessary to ensure that the evaluation tools are valid measures of performance. Additionally, as compared to a multiple-choice test, faculty need to be specifically trained how to evaluate objectively in order for specific feedback and instruction to benefit the learner and for the assessment to be a reproducible and reliable evaluation tool. By establishing construct validity and incorporating assessments for the milestones, different levels of providers can have a competency target as well as a defined mastery score for each core procedure and skills [14]. This feedback enables an individual to be objectively evaluated, and deficiencies can be more easily identified and addressed, and this is a rational place to begin the process of validation before moving on to certification.

Summary

Simulation provides an opportunity to observe providers' knowledge, technical skills, and communication skills and has the potential to provide a much better assessment of competence compared to current methods. With continued development and validation of assessment tools, the extent to which it is incorporated into licensure, certification, and credentialing will most certainly continue to expand. While there may be some hesitation and resistance to these changes, it is difficult to argue that a multiple-choice test is a better assessment of competency when these simulation methods are available.

References

1. Astho [Internet]. Arlington: Association of State and Territorial Health Officials; c1999–2017 [cited 2016 Dec 19]. Understanding licensing, credentialing, certification, and privileging; [about 1 p.]. Available from: http://www.astho.org/Programs/Preparedness/Public-Health- Emergency-Law/Scope-of-Practice-Toolkit/Understanding-Licensing,-Credentialing,-Certification,-and-Privileging(2)/.
2. Silvis J. Accreditation, certification, licensure, registration. 2011 Nov 22 [cited 2017 Apr 9]. In: Healthcare Design Magazine [Internet]. Ontario: Healthcare Design. c2002–2017 [about 7 screens]. Available from: http://www.healthcaredesignmagazine.com/architecture/accreditation-certification-licensure-registration/.
3. USMLE [Internet]. Philadelphia: United States Medical Licensing Examination; c1996–2017 [cited 2017 Apr 9]. Available from: http://www.usmle.org/.
4. Darzi A, Mackay S. Assessment of surgical competence. Qual Health Care. 2001;10(Suppl 2):ii64–9.
5. Committee on Patient Safety and Quality Improvement. Committee opinion no. 517: communication strategies for patient handoffs. Obstet Gynecol. 2012;119(2 Pt 1):408–11.
6. American College of Obstetricians and Gynecologists, Communication Strategies for Patient Handoffs. Committee Opinion #517, 2012.
7. Cooper J, Taqueti V. A brief history of the mannequin simulators for clinical education and training. Qual Saf Health Care. 2004;13(Suppl 1):i11–8.
8. Ziv A, Berkenstadt H, Eisenberg O. Simulation for licensure and certification. In: Levine, et al., editors. The comprehensive textbook of healthcare simulation. New York: Springer Science+Business Media; 2013. p. 161–2.
9. Bienstock J, Edgar L, McAlister R, Obstetrics and Gynecology Working Group. Obstetrics and gynecology milestones. J Grad Med Educ. 2014;6(Suppl 1):126–8.
10. SAGES-Fundamentals of Endoscopic Surgery [Internet]. Los Angeles: Fundamentals of Endoscopic Surgery; c2017 [cited 2017 May 7]. Available from: http://www.fesprogram.org/.
11. MOC Division. Bulletin for maintenance of certification for basic certification diplomates. Dallas: The American Board of Obstetrics & Gynecologists; 2017. ACOG [Internet]. Simulations working group toolkit. Washington (DC): The American Congress

of Obstetricians and Gynecologists; c1997–2017 [cited 2017 Apr 18]. Available from: http://www. acog.org/About-ACOG/ACOG-Departments/ Simulations-Consortium/Simulations-Consortium-Tool-KitGynecology. 2017. 37p. Available from: https://www.abog.org/bulletins/2017%20MOC%20 Basic%20Bulletin%20Final.pdf.

12. MedaPhor and the American Board of Obstetrics and Gynecology (ABOG) Sign Agreement. Medaphor. com, 1 Mar. 2016, www.medaphor.com/medaphor-and-abog-sign-agreement/. Accessed 8 Sept 2017.

13. American Congress of Obstetricians and Gynecologists [Internet]. Washington, DC: Surgical Curriculum in Obstetrics and Gynecology; c2017 [cited 2017 May 10]. Available from: http://cfweb. acog.org/scog/.

14. Downing S. Validity: on the meaningful interpretation of assessment data. Med Educ. 2003;37:830–7.

Simulation and Patient Safety in Obstetrics and Gynecology

8

Angela Chaudhari

Introduction

The use of simulation in education and subsequent improved patient safety would appear, at first evaluation, to be an apparent assumption. But to discuss the use of simulation and its effect on patient safety, it is first important to discuss briefly the evolution of patient safety in medicine. Physicians and healthcare providers have long held the edict "to do no harm," documented in the Hippocratic oath, and lectured and quoted at medical school graduations across the country. Providers, however, hold different ideas about what constitutes harm to patients making this edict less cut and dry than it initially appears. Charles Vincent, a patient safety expert from the UK, comments in his book on the origins of patient safety and discusses physician and surgeon, Ernest Codman, a pioneer in surgical safety. Dr. Codman created and published on the "assessment of unsuccessful treatment" in the early 1900s, one of the first physicians to publish on surgical errors and their causes, and included on his list were errors of technical knowledge and skill, errors of surgical judgment, errors due to

lack of equipment, errors due to lack of diagnostic skill, patient's unconquerable disease, patient's refusal of treatment, and the calamities of surgery over which we have no control. Codman also challenged fellow surgeons to identify and document errors, demonstrate that their procedures were efficient and efficacious, and "use the methods of science" to evaluate outcomes. It is said that he was initially ridiculed for his ideas, but his proposals were soon adopted by the American Surgical Society, the Minimum Standard for Hospitals, and now have been adapted by the modern Joint Commission on Accreditation of Healthcare Organizations, the largest accrediting body in the USA [1].

Medical errors and patient safety, in the modern era, tend to come into the public eye due to negative press surrounding medical malpractice and litigation cases that are highly publicized due to large payouts or unfortunate outcomes. This focus changed in November 1999 when the Institute of Medicine released the landmark publication entitled *To Err Is Human: Building a Safer Health System*. This report highlighted the findings of two studies, the Utah-Colorado Medical Practice Study and the Harvard Medical Practice Study, and extrapolated from their data estimating that between 44,000 and 98,000 patients die each year as a result of medical error, a staggering number that made both laypeople and those in the healthcare field take notice. This report concluded, however, that most of these

A. Chaudhari (✉)
Division of Minimally Invasive Gynecology,
Fellowship in Minimally Invasive Gynecologic Surgery, Department of Obstetrics and Gynecology, Northwestern University, Feinberg School of Medicine, Chicago, IL, USA
e-mail: achaudha@nm.org

© Springer International Publishing AG, part of Springer Nature 2019
S. Deering et al. (eds.), *Comprehensive Healthcare Simulation: Obstetrics and Gynecology*,
Comprehensive Healthcare Simulation, https://doi.org/10.1007/978-3-319-98995-2_8

errors result from systematic problems in health-care delivery rather than poor performance by individual providers [2]. This report brought patient safety into the forefront of the public eye and called on medical organizations to make system-wide change individually and on larger scales. Since then, patient safety has been redefined by organizations throughout the world. The World Health Organization defines patient safety as "the absence of preventable harm to a patient during the process of health care" [3]. Similarly, the National Patient Safety Foundation defines patient safety as "freedom from accidental or preventable injuries produced by medical care" [4]. The Agency for Healthcare Research and Quality (AHRQ) instead defines patient safety as "a discipline in the health care sector that applies safety science methods toward the goal of achieving a trustworthy system of health care systems; it minimizes the incidence and impact of, and maximizes recovery from, adverse events" [5]. This certainly marks a change from the historical edict: "first do no harm." Patient safety is now considered a discipline in the healthcare sector separate from the treatment of the individual patient that requires documentation and evaluation of causes of medical errors on a regular basis.

Key Learning Points
- Medical errors and adverse events occur with frequency in healthcare; addressing preventable adverse events and near misses is key to improving patient safety.
- Key components of improving patient safety in obstetrics and gynecology are error reporting, team training and crew resource management, and the use of simulation for competency.
- Building an institutional culture of safety is an important piece of improving patient safety that can be facilitated with simulation.

Description and Background

In discussing patient safety, it is, first, important to understand the key definitions of what institutes a medical error versus an adverse event. A medical error is defined by the Institute of Medicine as a "failure of a planned action to be completed as intended or the use of a wrong plan to achieve an aim" [2]. An example of one type of medical error is a patient receiving the wrong blood-typed blood. Alternatively, an adverse event is defined as injury to a patient that occurs due to the management of care, not due to the patient's underlying medical condition. These events may occur with or without a medical error occurring [6]. One example of an adverse event would be deep venous thrombosis (DVT) that occurs due to the lack of appropriate prophylaxis with surgery, an adverse event due to medical error; the patient failed to receive the prophylaxis that was needed. Another example of an adverse event would be a patient who had a postoperative hematoma due to appropriate DVT prophylaxis. Though the patient was managed appropriately to prevent DVT, their anticoagulation caused a postoperative wound hematoma; this is an example of adverse event that was not due to medical error. Alternatively, a near miss is an event that has the potential to cause harm but did not ultimately lead to harm of the patient. One example of a near miss would be a patient receiving the wrong medication, but this medication did not ultimately lead to harm to the patient. Finally, a preventable adverse event is injury that could have been avoided and is due to an error or system flaw, for example, wrong-site surgery that occurs due to inappropriate identification of surgical location or patient that could have been prevented at multiple checkpoints within the surgical check in process. Gluck published a Venn diagram showing the relationships between these terms and describes preventable adverse events as those that fall in the overlap between adverse events and medical error. The "near miss" events are an important area to focus on from a patient safety standpoint as it is these events which can best be learned from and focus strategies to decrease error and improve safety [6].

As described by Gluck, causes of medical errors are due to four factors in healthcare: human fallibility, complexity of care, system deficiencies, and vulnerability of defensive barriers [7].

- Human fallibility: Human fallibility is considered "a part of the human condition" and follows the long proclaimed edict, "To Err is Human" [2]. Certain human conditions, however, have been associated with higher medical error rate such as individual burnout, extended work hours, and lack of rest. Gluck describes the use of forced functions and reminders at points of care to help overcome human fallibility. Forced functions are defined as "physical or process constraints that make errors difficult if not impossible by making the correct action the default mode" [7]. One example of a forced function is the automated order sets embedded within the electronic medical record that default to the correct medications and steps for any given condition. Reminders at points of care can also improve medical errors [8]. A clinical example is the posting of signs reminding providers, patients, and family to wash their hands to reduce the spread of transmissible infections.
- Complexity of healthcare: The complexity of modern healthcare and the technologies that are necessary have also been blamed for medical error [7]. Due to the variety of patients seen, a time-pressured environment, and the many steps needed to take care of any given condition, it is important to standardize care whenever feasible. In obstetrics and gynecology, many departments have begun to standardize their protocols for labor and delivery in hopes of foreseeing and preventing errors before they occur.
- System deficiencies: Another area of medical error is due to deficiencies and a lack of coordination in systems in healthcare. Medical systems are vast and include patients, practitioners, infrastructure, administration, and regulation [7]. An example of a system deficiency that may diminish safety conditions is a nursing shortage or understaffing. With a

lack of nursing staff to cover the workload, errors due to omission or due to too large of a workload may lead to poor patient safety. Errors in this example occur, not due to individuals, but due to systems practices. Patient handoffs are another area of error in this category that have been robustly studied particularly in academic medical centers and across healthcare disciplines [9].
- Vulnerability of defensive barriers: Defensive barriers embedded within healthcare systems are necessary, but deficiencies in these barriers are, unfortunately, inevitable and lead to medical error [7]. One example of the use of defensive barriers in surgery is the use of the consent process, time-out, and sign-in procedure in the operating room. The patient's history is collected by a number of teams: surgery, nursing, and anesthesia. Consents are signed by all groups to ensure the patient is aware of the risks of the procedure. The patient is then marked, and a circulating nurse checks the patient's identity, location of surgery, allergies, and surgical procedure prior to going to the operating room. A sign-in is then done again prior to beginning the surgery to ensure all members of the team are aware and agree on the patient identity, type and location of surgical procedure, and equipment needed. This creates multiple points prior to beginning a surgical procedure to prevent wrong-site surgeries. Unfortunately, despite these regulations being in place, wrong-site surgeries still occur and are reported upon; these errors are due to vulnerability in the defensive barriers in place.

Though quality care and safety are now a key focus in many medical organizations, approaches on how to reduce errors and improve care still are not standardized in the medical community. Many organizations advocate that part of a better system must incorporate a culture of safety, defined by AHRQ in 2009 as "the product of individual and group values, attitudes, perceptions, competencies, and patterns of behavior that determine the commitment to, and the style and proficiency of, an organization's health and safety management." The culture of safety must include acknowledgment of the high-risk nature of the organization's work, commitment from all members of the healthcare team on both an individual and organizational level, and open communication regarding errors without risk of retribution in a blame-free environment [8]. The Joint Commission recently published a statement on the essential role of leadership within the culture of safety citing causes of insufficient support for patient event reporting, lack of feedback or response to staff, allowing intimidation of staff who report, and not addressing staff burnout as potential flaws within leadership in creating a culture of safety [10]. Morello et al. performed a systematic review of over 2000 articles to identify strategies for improving this culture within medical organizations. The strategies that were found were diverse and included leadership walk-rounds, team-based trainings, and simulation-based training programs but, unfortunately, provided no definitive evidence regarding the best types of interventions to improve the culture [11].

The National Patient Safety Foundation recently convened an expert panel to review the literature over the last 15 years since the original Institute of Medicine's report and provide recommendations. The panel identified these eight components in their recommendations:

1. Ensure that leaders establish and sustain a safety culture.
2. Create centralized and coordinated oversight of patient safety.
3. Create a common set of safety metrics that reflect meaningful outcomes.
4. Increase funding for research in patient safety and implementation science.
5. Address safety across the entire care continuum.
6. Support the healthcare workforce.
7. Partner with patients and families for the safest care.
8. Ensure that technology is safe and optimized to improve patient safety [8].
   These are important recommendations for institutional improvements in safety, but

what is the role of the individual obstetrics and gynecology department and provider? And, what role does simulation play in patient safety and the avoidance of medical error and adverse events in the field of obstetrics and gynecology?

The Evidence

With the high rates of maternal and infant morbidity and mortality in many first world countries and the continued increase in medical liability, there has been a resurgence of evidence defining and evaluating obstetrical safety measures. In 2010, Abuhamad and Grobman published on patient safety and medical liability in obstetrics and gynecology and recommended three key components to an obstetrical safety initiative: error reporting, crew resource management (CRM), and simulation training [12].

Error Reporting

Error reporting is one of the key components to improving systems deficiencies in a healthcare organization. Historically and still in many hospitals now, an event that leads to patient harm triggers a system that begins an internal review. These reviews often focus more on identifying the individual cause of an event rather than looking at system deficiencies that could have prevented the original error. It has been shown that most errors occur due to systems complexities and deficiencies rather than the competence of individual providers [13]. Because of this, the reporting of all errors and near misses that don't create harm are just as important to report upon to aid with the creation of system-wide improvements. Other complex, technological industries such as the airlines have used nonpunitive error reporting very successfully to improve and maintain safety standards within their organizations. This industry strives to recognize the limitations of the human condition and, therefore, makes error and near miss reporting more "blame-free" [14]. This aids in development of system-wide changes that help to overcome natural human fallibility and improve aviation safety. If the complexities of both fields are compared, it certainly seems that a similar culture may improve safety in systems in the healthcare industry as well. Penney et al. published a systematic review in 2006 of near miss and adverse event reporting and found that the reporting methods were too diverse to determine the benefits of event reporting [15]. More recently, Fox et al. recently published on an initiative at the Children's Hospital of Pittsburgh educating resident physicians on error reporting. They showed an increase in reporting from 3.6 to 37.8 per month over 4 years and a decrease in serious harm from 15.0 to 8.1 per month over 4 years highlighting the importance of error reporting [16]. Unfortunately, medical systems still need to rely on voluntary reporting by physicians and nurses, so the approach by many institutions is still to perform analysis for the events that lead to harm rather than prevention of error by evaluating near miss events.

Team Training and Crew Resource Management

Errors in obstetrics occur, in part, due to the complexity of the care teams. Care is often provided by obstetrics, anesthesia, and pediatrics as well as their nursing and support teams, and the need to care for both mother and infant makes prioritizing difficult. Often, communication errors between these teams lead to medical errors. Team training and crew resource management are key in prevention of these types of errors. Crew resource management (CRM) is a safety initiative that has been implemented in obstetrics and gynecology and is described as the "organization of individuals into effective teams to perform a common goal with efficient, safe, and reliable interaction" [12]. The common principles of CRM training skills derived from the aviation industry guidelines include know the environment, anticipate and plan, call for help early, exercise leadership and followership, distribute the workload, mobilize all available resources,

communicate effectively, use all available information, prevent and manage fixation errors, cross-check, use cognitive aids, reevaluate repeatedly, apply good teamwork, allocate attention wisely, and set priorities dynamically [17]. Crew resource management, also known as team training, has been used in the aviation industry since the 1970s, and though it has changed over those years, it still remains a vital part of aviation training and maintenance of safety standards.

Hospitals have now incorporated team training on labor and delivery to try to improve practices and decrease errors, and many studies have been published evaluating team training and crew resource management in obstetrics. Haller et al. performed a cross-sectional study to evaluate a crew resource management intervention to improve teamwork and communication skills in the obstetrics setting, therefore improving on the culture of safety. They showed that participants of the study highly valued the team training and showed a positive change in the team and safety climate of the hospital with OR of 2.9 to 4.7, post intervention [18]. Pettker et al. published on the effects of a more comprehensive obstetrics safety program that included crew resource management training as well as the implementation of an obstetrics safety nurse, standardization of protocols, patient safety committee oversight, and anonymous event reporting. With this more comprehensive program, they showed improvements in perception toward teamwork cultures, safety cultures, and job satisfaction, and individual providers reported more congruence between doctors and nursing staff. Their team trainings consisted of a continuing series of seminars from the aviation and defense industries' CRM trainings and then utilized videos, lectures, and role-playing in the different domains of an integrated obstetrics team (physician, resident, nurse, administrators) to try to maximize benefit for all participants [19]. One study evaluated the effect of CRM training on communication during cesarean section. Instead of participant evaluation, they utilized trained observers pre and post intervention and saw improved team communications during cesarean sections in both quality and quantity post training supporting CRM intervention for teamwork communication in obstetrics [20]. Another study by a group from the Netherlands evaluated the impact of obstetric team training on patient perception of quality care. They used a combination of team training, role-playing, and high-fidelity simulation to train their providers and then used a validated questionnaire on term low-risk obstetric patients before and after their intervention. Patient's perception of quality increased significantly after intervention, and, specifically, the domains of communication, clear leadership, involvement of planning, and better provision of information were the largest increases in improvement. These studies would support that CRM interventions aid in improving communication and satisfaction on labor and delivery that functions in teams of providers across disciplines by the necessity of the patient complexity. Based on smaller studies, team training may also aid in improving patient's perception of quality and, therefore, may impact patient satisfaction.

Crew resource management in aviation is not only used because of the impact on team dynamics but instead on the positive impact on safety [14]. Based on available evidence, this seems to hold true for obstetrics teams as well. Nielsen et al. performed a randomized controlled trial in 2007 evaluating more specifically for a decrease in adverse events after didactic team training in the operating room for cesarean sections. They noted no difference in outcomes between groups, but did note that those teams that had undergone training had a shorter time from decision to incision in the cesarean section group [21]. They attributed the lack of difference to their short-term follow-up on their original study so published a follow-up study in 2008. With longer-term evaluation, they showed improvements in the adverse outcomes index, a composite score of clinical outcomes [22]. Phipps et al. also published on a crew resource management-based curriculum implemented on labor and delivery but incorporated both didactic sessions and a high-fidelity simulation. They evaluated the adverse outcomes index for 2 years prior to intervention and 1.5 years after training and showed a significant decrease in the adverse outcomes

index. They concluded that the combination of crew resource management training with simulation techniques for competency improved their outcomes [23].

Many studies have also looked at the use of simulation for more specific obstetric emergencies such as shoulder dystocia. The use of simulation for training is particularly applicable to shoulder dystocia due to its relative infrequency in practice, its risk of both temporary and permanent injury to an infant, and the need for a team-centered approach to improve outcomes [24]. Deering et al. showed that residents who did training on a birth simulator were more likely to utilize maneuvers at the time of a second simulation and have improved performance scores by an external reviewer compared to those residents who did not undergo training [25]. Goffman et al. performed a similar study with both attending and resident physicians and showed resident improvements in both maneuvers and team communications and attending improvement in communication during subsequent simulated dystocia events [26]. Both of these studies were designed to evaluate improvements in performance scores during simulation but did not correlate their findings to clinical outcomes and patient safety. In 2011, Grobman et al. published on a team-based shoulder dystocia protocol that utilized CRM strategies for communication tailored for an obstetrics team and combined this training with the use of low-fidelity simulation. They then evaluated clinical outcomes after implementation of the protocol and simulation and showed the rate of brachial plexus injuries declined at both the time of birth and discharge improving infant safety at the time of dystocia [27]. Kim et al. also reported on the incidence of dystocia outcomes pre and post a simulation protocol and found discrepant outcomes. They found that the rate of dystocia was higher after simulation likely due to increased reporting and recognizing and there was no decrease in birth injury, postpartum hemorrhage, third- and fourth-degree laceration, or episiotomies [28]. Draycott et al. published on a mandatory shoulder dystocia training course that was implemented in the UK as part of the SaFe study beginning in 2000 and showed that, though there was no decrease in shoulder dystocia, there were improved neonatal outcomes with brachial plexus injury rates dropping from 9.3% to 2.3% [29].

Other obstetric emergencies in which team training and simulation are often utilized are postpartum hemorrhage, emergency cesarean section, and eclampsia due to requirements of a multidisciplinary team and a rapid response [30]. Fransen et al. evaluated the effectiveness of a one-day simulation-based team training that incorporated teamwork training in the context of clinical training utilizing both high-fidelity simulation and team training. They utilized the traditional hallmarks of teamwork training including leadership and role clarity, distribution of workload, situational awareness, and directed communication and also utilized SBAR (situation, background, assessment, and recommendation) for their handovers between teams. Participants assigned to training performed specific scenarios of increasing difficulty throughout the day: shoulder dystocia, eclampsia, umbilical cord prolapse, postpartum hemorrhage, and resuscitation of a pregnant woman. They found the composite outcome of obstetric complications did not differ significantly between groups that were trained versus those who were not. Team training, however, did show a reduction in trauma due to shoulder dystocia and increased invasive treatment for severe postpartum hemorrhage [31]. Egenberg et al. published on the use of interprofessional team training during postpartum hemorrhage and showed, after interprofessional training, that there was a significant reduction in the amount of total blood products given. It was hypothesized this was due to improved awareness and the following of hemorrhage protocols on the unite [32].

Patient safety in obstetrics still poses a major public health concern in the USA and internationally due to high rates of maternal and neonatal morbidity and mortality [33]. Simulation and team training provide much needed skills acquisition, team communication, and provider comfort with obstetric emergencies but fail to consistently show an improvement in clinical outcomes. Despite the lack of consistency of evidence on patient safety and simulation in obstetrics, the evidence surrounding improved communication would lend us to believe that safety may improve over time due to the benefits from teams working more consistently together. Standardizing protocols and simulation training for obstetric providers may improve clinical outcomes and patient safety in the long term, but more research is needed and protocols need to be validated.

Gynecology and gynecologic surgery is another area of focus for research on the use of simulation strategies to improve patient safety. Prior to discussing simulation's effects on safety in gynecologic surgery, it is important to discuss what are thought to be the key causes of errors during gynecologic surgery. From a liability perspective, patient harm has been linked to surgeon incompetence, inexperience, and lack of technical skills. Parker published a video review of surgical errors in 2010 and described the causes of errors during laparoscopic surgery. These were classified as visual errors or errors of inexperience. Visual errors are due to problems of visual perception and processing and may be caused by "tunnel vision" or the imprinting of information of the brain that then excludes other contradictory information. Errors of inexperience are due to a lack of experience in a particular procedure. He describes two methods of thinking in cognitive science: deliberate or knowledge-based and instinctive or unconscious processing [34]. It is thought that with increased experience, knowledge-based cognitive behaviors can become more instinctual and, therefore, potentially safer. This would lead us to believe that simulation, by playing a role in developing competence, with repetition may lead to instinctual skills that would be useful in the operating room.

How does simulation impact surgical expertise? It is intuitive that to achieve expertise, both repetitive practice and actual experience are necessary components to high-level performance. Long gone are the former mantras of "see one, do one, teach one." It has been described in both medical and nonmedical fields that it is necessary to have 5000 or more hours of deliberate learning and practice to become an expert or as long as

10 years of intense experience to achieve a high level of competency [35]. To put that into practical real-life terms, for a surgeon performing two hysterectomies a week at 3 h per procedure, they would be getting approximately 24 h of intense real-life experience per month or 288 h per year. At this rate, it would require almost 20 years to become an expert, and, in gynecologic surgery, this surgeon would be considered "high volume." It is also important to note, however, that practice over time likely has more beneficial effects than focused and lengthy practice at one give time; for example, daily practice of a technical skill such as laparoscopic suturing during fellowship training for 1 h per day for 10 days would likely be more beneficial than a 1 day, 10 h, continuing medical education course that attempts to teach and practice all aspects of the same skill [36]. Given the lack of time and the decreased volume experienced by individual surgeons, extended simulation may have a role in trying to achieve the number of hours required to reach "expert levels."

With the implementation of duty hour restrictions and the expansion of technologies and surgical procedures performed, training programs for surgical subspecialties are relying more heavily on simulation-based education [37]. General surgery programs are now requiring the successful completion of Fundamentals of Laparoscopic Surgery and Fundamentals of Endoscopic Surgery. These training programs have demonstrated clinical correlations between scores on simulation assessments and technical skills in the operating room [38, 39]. Unfortunately, there is a paucity of evidence regarding how these skills impact patient safety in terms of patient outcomes. But this lack of evidence has not stemmed the use of FLS for graduation from residency, hospital certification, and privileging and, even, is required training for malpractice coverage [40].

In addition to individual training, simulation has been used in gynecologic surgery in the form of team training similar to obstetrics. Robotic surgery, in particular, significantly lends itself to team training due to the complexity of the setup and the equipment. Schiff et al. published on the quality of communications in robotic surgery by surveying all members of the operating room team after procedures and found that those cases that communication was reported as poor showed a greater estimated blood loss and longer operating time. They concluded these outcomes were due to poor communication and identified team training as a potential way to improve these outcomes [41]. Team training programs have become more widespread in a variety of surgical subspecialties and allow for the entire surgical team to work in better cohesion by training specifically to that goal. Though the evidence is limited, it is inherent that a better communicating team would likely lead to improved outcomes [42].

Mandatory training and implementation of new protocols is another arena of simulation that has limited evidence showing benefit in gynecology. Most promising, however, recently, was a publication out of the University of Michigan utilizing a training/simulation program for the implementation of a universal cystoscopy program at the time of hysteroscopy. Their evidence showed increased utilization of cystoscopy after training and decreased rates of delayed injury to the ureter [43].

In 2008, the WHO, in coordination with the Safe Surgery Saves Lives Program, instituted a Safe Surgery checklist with 19 categories that includes the sign-in, time-out, and sign-out that is now performed as a standard in many operating rooms. Haynes et al. utilized this checklist to perform a prospective pre- and posttest intervention and showed a significant decrease in postoperative complications and deaths, most of which were due to surgical site infection and related to dosing or preoperative antibiotics [44]. The Society of Gastrointestinal and Endoscopic Surgeons (SAGES) has now modified this checklist for laparoscopic surgery and included a guide to help cope with equipment issues in hopes of improving quality, efficiency, and communication [45]. Checklists are frequently described in the simulation literature as tools to standardize care and create protocols where previously none existed. The use of checklists allows a better team approach to a patient in the surgical setting.

Conclusions

The implementation of a simulation program for obstetrics and gynecology will improve team communication, improve error reporting, and likely have a beneficial impact on long-term patient safety in your organization. Utilizing the tools in this book will help individuals develop simulation programs within their institutions, but it is important to address the culture of safety in addition to addressing the needs for new skill acquisition and maintenance of skills. The culture of safety, to report errors, prevent errors, and maintain skills, needs to arise from a top-down approach. It is important, first, that practice and hospital administrations are involved to ensure that blame-free reporting occurs, and it is widely known in the organization that error reporting and team training are expected or required. It then falls to clinical care teams to implement these cultural changes which may only be done with mutual trust between administration, physicians, nurses, and staff. Simulation is an important part of training and maintenance of technical skills in obstetrics and gynecology and will continue to be studied to show improved patient outcomes and patient safety.

References

1. Vincent C. In: Vincent C, editor. Patient safety. Chichester: John Wiley and Sons; 2010.
2. Kohn LT, Corrigan JM, Donaldson MS, editors. To err is human: building a safer health system, I.o. Medicine, Editor. Washington, DC: National Academy Press; 1999.
3. Patient Safety. http://www.who.int/patientsafety/about/en/. Accessed 2017.
4. Free from harm accelerating patient safety improvement fifteen years after to err is human. Report of an expert panel convened by the National Patient Safety Foundation; 2015. National Patient Safety Foundation: www.npsf.org/resource/resmgr/PDF/Free_from_Harm.pdf.
5. Emanuel L, Berwick D, Conway J, Combes J, Hatlie M, Leape L, et al. What exactly is patient safety? In advances in patient safety: new directions and alternative approaches. AHRQ; 2008. https://www.ncbi.nlm.nih.gov/books/NBK43629.
6. Gluck PA. Patient safety: some progress and many challenges. Obstet Gynecol. 2012;120(5):1149–59.
7. Gluck PA. Medical error theory. Obstet Gynecol Clin North Am. 2008;35:11–7.
8. Patient safety primer, safety culture. U.D.o.H.a.H. Services, editor. Agency for Healthcare Research and Quality; 2016. https://psnet.ahrq.gov/primers/primer/5/safety-culture.
9. Sheth S, McCarthy E, Kipps AK, et al. Changes in efficiency and safety culture after the integration of an I-PASS supported handoff process. Pediatrics. 2016;137(2):e20150166.
10. Commission TJ. The essential role of leadership in developing a safety culture, D.o.C.C. cations, editor; 2017. pp. 1–8.
11. Morello RT, Lowthian JA, Barker AL, et al. Strategies for improving patient safety culture in hospital: a systematic review. BMJ Qual Saf. 2013;22:11–8.
12. Abuhamad A, Grobman W. Patient safety and medical liability. Obstet Gynecol. 2010;116(3):570–7.
13. Reason JT. Managing the risks of organizational accidents. Aldershot: Ashgate Publishing; 1997.
14. Helmreich RL. On error management: lessons from aviation. BMJ. 2000;320:781–5.
15. Penney G, Brace V. Near miss audit in obstetrics. Curr Opin Obstet Gynecol. 2007;19:145–50.
16. Fox MD, Bump GM, Butler GA, Chen LW, Buchert AR. Making residents part of the safety culture: improving error reporting and reducing harms. J Patient Saf. 2017. https://doi.org/10.1097/PTS.0000000000000344. [Epub ahead of print].
17. Rall M, Gaba D. Human performance and patient safety. In: Miller RD, editor. Miller's anesthesia. Philadelphia: Elsevier Churchill Livingstone; 2005.
18. Haller G, Garnerin P, Morales M. Effect of crew resource management training in a multidisciplinary obstetrical setting. Int J Qual Health Care. 2008;20(4):254–63.
19. Pettker CM, Thung S, Raab CA, et al. A comprehensive obstetrics patient safety program improves safety climate and culture. Am J Obstet Gynecol. 2011;204(3):e1–216.
20. Mancuso MP, Dziadkowiec O, Kleiner C, Halverson-Carpenter K, Link T, Barry J. Crew resource management for obstetric and neonatal teams to improve communication during cesarean births. J Obstet Gynecol Neonatal Nurs. 2016;45(4):502–14.
21. Nielsen PE, Goldman MB, Mann S, et al. Effects of teamwork training on adverse outcomes and process of care in labor and delivery. Obstet Gynecol. 2007;109:48–55.
22. Nielsen PE, Mann S. Team function in obstetrics to reduce errors and improve outcomes. Obstet Gynecol Clin North Am. 2008;35:81–95.
23. Phipps MG, Lindquist D, McConaughey E, et al. Outcomes from a labor delivery team training program with simulation component. AJOG. 2012;206(1):3–9.
24. Grobman WA. Shoulder dystocia: simulation and a team centered protocol. Semin Perinatol. 2014;38(4):205–9.
25. Deering S, Poggi S, Macedonia C, Gherman R, Satin AJ. Improving residency competency in the manage-

ment of shoulder dystocia with simulation training. Obstet Gynecol. 2004;103(6):1224–8.

26. Goffman D, Heo H, Pardanani S, Merkatz IR, Bernstein PS. Improving shoulder dystocia management among resident and attending physicians using simulation. Obstet Gynecol. 2008;112(6):1284–7.

27. Grobman WA, Miller D, Burke C, Hornbogen A, Tam K, Costello R. Outcomes associated with introduction of a shoulder dystocia protocol. Am J Obstet Gynecol. 2011;205:513–7.

28. Kim T, Vogel RI, Mackenthun SM, Das K. Rigorous simulation training protocol does not improve maternal and neonatal outcomes from shoulder dystocia. Obstet Gynecol. 2016;127(Suppl 1):3S.

29. Draycott T, Crofts J, Ash J, Wilson L, Yard E, Sibanda T, Whitelaw A. Improving neonatal outcome through practical shoulder dystocia training. Obstet Gynecol. 2008;112(1):14–20.

30. Clark EA, Fisher J, Arafeh J, Druzin M. Team training/simulation. Clin Obstet Gynecol. 2010;53(1):265–77.

31. Fransen AF, van de Ven J, Schuit E, van Tetering AC, Mol BW, Oei SG. Simulation-based team training for multiprofessional obstetric care teams to improve patient outcome: a multicenter, cluster randomised controlled trial. BJOG. 2016;124(4):1471–528.

32. Egenberg S, Øian P, Eggebø TM, Arsenovic MG, Bru LE. Changes in selfefficacy, collective efficacy and patient outcome following interprofessional simulation training on postpartum haemorrhage. J Clin Nurs. 2017;26(19–20):3174–87.https://doi.org/10.1111/jocn.13666. Epub 2017 Mar 12.

33. Buchmann EJ, Stones W, Thomas N. Preventing deaths from complications of labor and delivery. Best Pract Res. 2016;36:103–15.

34. Parker WH. Understanding errors during laparoscopic surgery. Obstet Gynecol Clin. 2010;37(3):437–49.

35. Ericsson KA. Deliberate practice and acquisition of and maintenance of expert performance in medicine and related domains. Acad Med. 2004;79:S70–81.

36. Parker WH, Johns A, Hellige J. Avoiding complications of laparoscopic surgery: lessons from cognitive science and crew resource management. J Minim Invasive Gynecol. 2007;14:379–88.

37. Schwab B, Hungness E, Barsness KA, McGaghie WC. The role of simulation in surgical education. J Laparoendosc Adv Surg Tech A. 2017;27(5):450–4. https://doi.org/10.1089/lap.2016.0644. Epub 2017 Jan 24.

38. Feldman LS, Hagarty S, Ghitulescu G, et al. Relationship between objective assessment of technical skills and subjective in training evaluations in surgical residents. J Am Coll Surg. 2004;198:105–10.

39. Sroka G, Feldman L, Vassiliou MC. Fundamentals of laparoscopic surgery simulator training to proficiency improves laparoscopic performance in the operating room- a randomized control trial. Am J Surg. 2010;199:115–20.

40. Derevianko AY, Schwaitzberg SD, Tsuda S, Barrios L, Brooks DC, Callery MP, Fobert D, Irias N, Rattner DW, Jones DB. Malpractice carrier underwrites fundamentals of laparoscopic surgery training and testing: a benchmark of patient safety. Surg Endosc. 2010;24(3):616–23.

41. Schiff L, Tsafrir Z, Aoun J, Taylor A, Theoharis E, Eisenstein D. Quality of communication in robotic surgery and surgical outcomes. JSLS. 2016;20(3):e2016.00026.

42. Liberman D, Trinh QD, Jeldres C, Valiquette L, Zorn KC. Training and outcome monitoring in robotic urologic surgery. Urology. 2011;9(1):17–22.

43. Chi AM, Curran DS, Morgan DM, Fenner DE, Swenson CW. Universal cystoscopy after benign hysterectomy: examining the effects of an institutional policy. Obstet Gynecol. 2016;127(2):369–75.

44. Haynes AB, Weiser TG, Berry WR. A surgical safety checklist to reduce morbidity and mortality in a global population. N Engl J Med. 2009;360:491–9.

45. Varela E, Michael Brunt L. SAGES laparoscopic surgery checklist. In: Tichansky MJ, David S, Jones DB, editors. The SAGES manual of quality, outcomes and patient safety. New York: Springer Science and Business Media; 2012.

The Why, Who, What, and Where to Implement a Simulation Program in Obstetrics and Gynecology

Kay Daniels

Introduction

In this chapter we will provide you with a practical approach to initiating or expanding an obstetric and gynecologic simulation program. The chapter will be divided into the "Why, who, what, and where" of implementation of a simulation program.

This chapter can by no means cover all the various possibilities for the use of simulation but reflects the author's experience and observations. Talking to others who have gone thru this process is invaluable, and actually taking the time to visit and observe in person other simulation programs is time well spent.

> **Key Learning Points**
> - Implementation of a simulation program should always begin with a focus on why it is needed and who is to be trained.
> - Curriculum will be formatted to focus on the learning objectives, and equipment should not be purchased until these are determined.
> - Simulation can be done both in a simulation center and in situ depending on the goals of training and facilities available.

The first question that must be answered is:

Why: Why Do You Want to Implement a Simulation Program in Your Institution?

There are a variety of answers depending on your institution. As this is a crucial step, take the time to really consider what is (are) the goal(s) for your program.

Here are some considerations.

Residency Training

The July 2016 requirements from the Accreditation Council for Graduate Medical Education (ACGME) for obstetrics and gynecol-

K. Daniels (✉)
Department of Obstetrics and Gynecology, Stanford
Health Care, Palo Alto, CA, USA
e-mail: kdaniels@stanford.ed

© Springer International Publishing AG, part of Springer Nature 2019
S. Deering et al. (eds.), *Comprehensive Healthcare Simulation: Obstetrics and Gynecology*,
Comprehensive Healthcare Simulation, https://doi.org/10.1007/978-3-319-98995-2_9

ogy state "Acceptable simulation includes a range of options from low to high fidelity. The Review Committee does not expect each program to have a simulation center; however, incorporation of simulation in residency education is required" [1]. With this in mind, many residency programs are starting or broadening their simulation programs. The use of simulation for residency training offers a variety of options including but not limited to:

- Simulation task training to introduce new skills that are better perfected on a mannequin than in a live person, such as laparoscopic technique or shoulder dystocia maneuvers
- Improving resident performance in often seen events such as postpartum hemorrhage (PPH), stat cesarean deliveries, and severe preeclampsia
- The opportunity to expose residents to rare events that they may not have a chance to experience in their 4 years of residency, for example, maternal cardiac arrest and vaginal breech.

Team Training of Labor and Delivery or Postpartum/Antepartum Units

In 2004 the Joint Commission released a sentinel event alert titled *Preventing infant death and injury during delivery* that stated

"Communication issues topped the list of identified root causes (72 percent)."

The Joint Commission went on to recommend that organizations:

1. "Conduct team training in perinatal areas to teach staff to work together and communicate more effectively
2. For high risk events such as shoulder dystocia, emergency cesarean delivery, maternal hemorrhage, and neonatal resuscitation conduct clinical drills to help staff prepare for when such events actually occur and conduct debriefings to evaluate team performance and identify areas for improvement" [2].

Following the release of this sentinel event, attention was directed toward the development of training of teams to reduce these communication errors and improve outcomes. This led to the

adaptation of crew resource management (CRM) from the aviation field and development by the military of TeamStepps [3, 4]. Use of simulation is the perfect setting to introduce, reinforce, and practice effective team performance.

Simulation can be a powerful tool to assist in identifying the causes of and lowering of malpractice cases. Data suggests that programs with active simulation programs have been able to decrease their malpractice exposure [5, 6].

Uncovering System Errors on Your Unit/ Readying a New Unit for Patient Care/ Planning for a Complicated Procedure

Simulation can be used either to identify preexisting system errors in your unit [7] or to explore the potential system errors in a new unit before opening for patient care. When the Women and Infants Hospital in Rhode Island opened a new NICU, it was fivefold larger than their previous unit and extended over two floors. To accomplish a successful transfer, simulation sessions were scheduled and made possible the correction of problems before the patient move-in date. This endeavor "substantially elevated the perception of the value of simulation within the institution" [8].

In centers that have procedures that require multiple teams of various disciplines to participate, the opportunity to do a "dress rehearsal" can correct vulnerable areas beforehand. As reported by August et al., the use of simulation to rehearse a rare and difficult surgical procedure EXIT to ECMO was successful because simulation enabled the interdisciplinary teams (MFM, pediatric surgeon, anesthesiologist, pediatric cardiology, nursing and pediatric perfusion specialists) to identify and correct potential problems before the surgery [9].

These uses of simulation can produce the most concrete examples of the value of simulation and aid to garner support from both the staff and hospital administration.

Nursing Education

Simulation drills are a highly effective modality to introduce new policies or standard algorithms to the unit. New nurses to the unit or travelers are especially important to acquaint in a simulation fashion to the rapid workflow of an acute unit such as labor and delivery [10, 11].

Once the *WHY* has been answered, the *WHO* can now be identified. The *WHO* is multilayered. Who are your learners, who will be your simulation team, and who in administration will be supporting your program?

Who (Learners)

Residency Training

Introduction of simulation for residency training should start early in the 4-year curriculum. Many institutions have put in place with great success "intern boot camp." This intensive education program given at the start of intern year has been invaluable for allowing the interns to come to the ward prepared and ready to be truly helpful members of the team. Simulation is incorporated in many of these programs and in Israel; they now have a national mandate for all programs to provide a simulation-based pre-internship workshop [12, 13].

Although the intern boot camp is most often done as a resident-only training, an effort should be made later in residency not to remain in the silo of resident-only training. Advancing the resident simulation experience to include multidisciplinary or intraprofessional team training is crucial.

Team Training Multidisciplinary or intraprofessional simulation training is a more complicated and time-consuming endeavor, yet the rewards of improving the entire team's performance cannot be understated. Team training should be envisioned as including not only all medical providers but all personnel who work on the unit – scrub techs, clerks, etc.

Barriers to having all disciplines present are numerous. Possible solutions to personnel attendance include:

- MD/DO/CNM attendance – various institutions have successfully involved their attending providers using the following approaches:
  - Providing financial compensation for participation.
  - Participants receive discount on the malpractice premiums for yearly participation.

- Providing MOC 4 or CME credit for participation.
- Require provider attendance to maintain hospital privileges.
- Resident attendance.
  - Resident involvement can be done as a mandatory attendance during their protected teaching time.
  - To maximize learning, each simulation should include no more than three residents at a time. This will allow each resident to take an active role and be in the "hot seat" as the primary responder.
- Nurse Participation.
  - Require RN attendance
  - Providing CEU credit
  - Transitioning the present nursing education program to be a simulation-based education program

Who (Simulation Team Members)

Residency Training

Providing resident-only simulation training will be easy to schedule as it can be done during resident protected teaching time. Your faculty should include not only the core simulation team but also specific content experts, for example, when teaching fundamentals in laparoscopic surgery (FLS), enlist your minimal invasive surgery (MIS/MIGS) faculty as additional faculty trainers.

Team Training

When the goal is team training, both the planning sessions and the simulation sessions can be a challenge to schedule but worth the effort. Ensure that a representative from each discipline who works on the unit (OB, anesthesia, nursing, OR staff, pediatrics, nurse educator/management) is involved with the discussion and decision of the scenario chosen. Allowing creation of the learning objectives to be done jointly will ensure that each discipline has relevant teaching points for their specialty. When possible, have a member from each discipline available for the debriefing process providing subject matter expertise. Examples of learning objectives created for full team simulation scenario are listed in Table 9.1.

Table 9.1 Example clinical question, learning objectives, and metric for obstetric simulation

Clinical question:
What are the tasks required of each subspecialty for timely, efficient, and safe transfer of a patient from the labor room to the operating room for a stat cesarean delivery?
Nursing learning objectives:
Demonstrate verbal acknowledgment of obstetrician's decision for stat cesarean
Demonstrate clear communication to charge nurse about stat cesarean so they can notify anesthesiologist of emergency and have technicians prepare operating room
Demonstrate rapid preparation of patient lines (fetal monitors, intravenous lines, Foley catheter, epidural catheter, etc.) and physically transfer patient without delay
Obstetrics learning objectives:
Demonstrate clear communication of decision for stat cesarean
Demonstrate compassionate communication with family member without delaying transfer
Assist bedside nurse with physical transport to operating room
Anesthesia learning objectives:
Evaluate patient stability and support airway, breathing, and circulation as needed for transport
Demonstrate rapid preparation of operating room for stat cesarean including stat general anesthesia medications and airway management equipment or stat spinal if appropriate
Utilize all available resources including other anesthesiologists and anesthesia technician
Technician learning objectives:
Anesthesia technician demonstrates rapid preparation of operating room including checking emergency and advanced airway equipment and readiness to assist anesthesiologist with moving patient onto table, attaching monitors, and starting preoxygenation or other tasks as required
Operating room technician demonstrates rapid preparation of operating room equipment
Team learning objective:
Team demonstrates efficient, rapid, and safe transfer of patient from labor room to operating room for stat cesarean
Metrics:
How many seconds elapse between decision for stat cesarean and arrival in operating room?
What barriers exist and how long of a delay do they cause when transferring patient from labor room to operating room for stat cesarean?

Reprinted with permission from Wolters Kluwer Inc. Austin et al. [5]

Uncovering System Errors on Your Unit/Readying a New Unit for Patient Care/Planning for a Complicated Procedure This will be of the greatest benefit if all relevant team members are present. This may include nonmedical personnel – clerks who make the emergency call or off-unit personnel such as the blood bank or the hospital code team if they are part of the simulation scenario.

Who (Engaging the Institution)

Garnering long-term support for simulation program requires an appreciation for the institutions' priorities. The following parties have a vested interest in the simulation program for distinct reasons and should be engaged early in the planning process.

Nursing Administration

The priority for nursing will often be nurse education and employee satisfaction. Most hospitals have active nursing education departments. Simulation programs should actively engage the yearly learning objectives of the hospital's nursing administration as part of the scenario. Ensuring that a nursing educator or manager is at the planning meeting will facilitate this goal.

Risk Management

Decreasing medical claims through improved clinical practice and patient-provider communication is one of the major priorities of risk management. Invite a representative from risk management to the simulation debriefing and allow them to educate your providers on proper documentation and optimal communication techniques with patients when untoward events have occurred. Reviewing active or past malpractice cases, root cause analysis (RCA), or sentinel events, risk management can identify needed areas for improvement specific for your organization. These issues can then be incorporated into the simulation scenario.

Patient Safety/Quality Improvement Committee

Identification and correction of system errors are a crucial goal of all QI programs. Simulation is an excellent methodology to uncover system errors in a very tangible way. Having video to show a suboptimal workflow or a glaring system error is a powerful driver for change. Spending time in the debriefing sessions to exclusively discuss system errors as seen by the frontline providers is invaluable. To maximize effectiveness, a system must be in place to engage the QI committee so that the changes uncovered in simulation can be addressed and corrected (Table 9.2).

What (Curriculum/Equipment)

What you will be simulating depends on your goals as previously determined.

Residency Training

If the goal is primarily residency training of procedures and techniques, there are many tools at your disposal for task training [14].

Team Training

Determining the curriculum can be accomplished by gathering local data: sentinel events RCAs/near misses. Also including staff input as what issues they can identify on the unit can allow you to create a tailored library of scenarios that can be

used to ensure the teams are better prepared for the next such event. If local data is not available, using national data for malpractice suits can be used effectively.

Equipment

What equipment is needed for the simulation will be determined by two factors, the learning objectives of the scenario and the site of the simulation. For example, if one of the learning objectives is to highlight teamwork, communication, and concerns when performing general anesthesia, having a full-body model would be crucial to allow anesthesia to perform intubation.

The site of the scenario will also be a determining factor for the equipment used. If the course is performed in a simulation lab, heavy computer-driven full-body mannequins that do not need to be moved can be used. However, if the simulation site is labor and delivery, light-weight noncomputer-run mannequins or task-training models with standardized patients that are easily movable are best and can easily be adapted.

Uncovering System Errors on Your Unit/ Readying a New Unit for Patient Care/ Planning for a Complicated Procedure

Curriculum and equipment are dependent on the stated goal. Simulation has the potential both to uncover present latent system errors and to identify potential difficulties. Using simulation allows

Table 9.2 System error and corrections

Author	Latent error	Solution
Preston et al. [7]	Inefficient call system	Repositioning of call bells (i.e., NICU call bell at head infant warmer (not at the head of mother's bed)
personal communication	Inefficient access to uterotonics	"Postpartum hemorrhage kit" was developed by pharmacy services, which included methylergonovine, carboprost, and misoprostol. All three medications were then placed in the refrigerator in an insulated box
Lipman et al. [15]	Inefficient move to the OR in a stat cd	Change in process for patient movement including disconnecting IVs at proximal port, pumps made available in each OR, transporting on the LDR bed, not transferring to a gurney
Hamman et al. [17]	Delay in calling teams for urgent case	Multiple solutions implemented including specific code page and call back number

you to determine the optimal crisis management for your unit.

During a crisis, the usual routine cannot be examined, nor can there be a randomized trial during an emergency due to ethical and logistic restraints. Yet using simulation to create and review the process can be revealing. Lipman et al. performed a simulation study that examined where was the best location to perform a perimortem cesarean delivery on their unit. Teams were given the simulation of a maternal code in the LDR and were randomized to either perform the cesarean delivery in the OR or in the LDR. All teams were aware of the desired delivery within 5 min of the arrest. The simulations were timed, and the team discussed and analyzed the pros and cons of each location in the debriefing. Despite the lack of room in the LDR for all the necessary staff (NICU, code team, surgeons), the effects of moving to the OR – which was only across the hall – revealed that providers performed suboptimal CPR when moving to the OR and there was a consistent delay in actual delivery with the median times of 7:53 min with the move to the OR in contrast to the median time of delivery of 4:25 min if performed in the LDR. Therefore, the simulation allowed that OB unit to agree that any perimortem delivery should be done in the LDR [15].

Where: Simulation Lab Versus In Situ Versus Classroom Versus Tabletop

The choice of where to do the simulation is dependent on:

1. Goal of the simulation
2. Time allotted for the participants
3. Availability of the site

Simulation labs offer the opportunity to have undisturbed time away from the unit. Simulation centers are the optimal site to learn new information that require in-depth discussion – i.e., ACLS or NRP – or tasks that are time intensive for cleanup such as demonstrating quantitative blood loss. The limitations of simulation center include the time needed to travel to the center and the lack of verisimilitude of the environment, which makes it difficult for some participants to optimize their learning. In addition, system errors cannot be identified.

In situ or labor and delivery simulations are at the vicissitudes of the workload of the unit, and the potential for not having a room available is very real. However, working in the real environment allows participants to more easily incorporate what they learn in simulation into their daily routine. System error identification is an easy by-product of in situ drills. To mitigate the consequence of not being able to do an in situ simulation, an alternative spot close to the unit should be identified as a backup site and equipment to turn a waiting room or classroom into an "OR" available.

Classrooms can easily be used for task-training simulations and tabletop or "talking simulations." Tabletop simulations allow an opportunity to discuss complex patient scenarios and talking thru what the providers would do allowing for valuable educational moments.

Other Considerations Are

Creation of a Safe Zone When Doing Simulation

It is paramount for learning that your participants feel secure in the knowledge that they will not be judged during the simulation and that no reporting of their performance is planned. Rudolph et al. explain that creating a safe environment for simulation and debriefing "creates a setting where learners can practice new or familiar skills without the burden of feeling that they will be shamed, humiliated, or belittled" [16]. There are a variety of ways to accomplish this important goal including a prebriefing that includes setting expectations and assuring confidentiality you can also consider having all participants sign a confidentiality form prior to participating and reiterating that "what happens in simulation, stays in simulation." This will all help to maximize learning.

Do You Want to Record and Use Video During the Debriefing?

Video playback can be a compelling teaching tool. Learners can more easily see their effectiveness as communicators. Viewing team skills with the use of video playback allows a more realistic assessment of performance. However, for some learners, video can be a distracting and even a disquieting experience. Learners must be reassured that the video will be kept confidential or even destroyed after the viewing. Video playback should be used judiciously and wisely.

Is There Time to Offer a Task-Training Portion Before the Full Simulation?

Combining a short presimulation period of task training, i.e., learning how to do a B-Lynch or place a uterine tamponade balloon before a full team training for postpartum hemorrhage, allows the participants to practice a skill before using it in a full simulation. This format can be a powerful learning experience.

Should the "In Situ" Simulations Be Announced or Unannounced?

Although "mock codes" have been used for years on medical wards and unannounced drills guarantee medical personnel are present to participate, starting a new simulation program with unannounced codes may create resistance. Introducing simulation initially in a relaxed planned format will have better long-term acceptance. Unannounced drills if desired can be introduced in the future.

Summary

In summary, a well-planned and thoughtful introduction will allow simulation to become an integral and valued component of a comprehensive patient safety program. Begin with defining *why* you are embarking on a simulation program. Is it for residency training only, team training, or improving the workflow on your unit? Why is followed by the *who, what, and where*. *Who* will

be your learners, and who do you need on your simulation team. Understanding *who* are the stakeholders and including them early in the planning are crucial for sustainability of the program. *What* refers to the curriculum and the equipment needed to accomplish your learning goals. Customizing your program for the unique gaps experienced in your institution will create buy-in from your learners and team members. Curriculum should include the concept of a safe zone allowing learners to practice difficult and new skills without judgment. *Where* can vary between a simulation lab, "in situ" on the ward, and a classroom for a tabletop simulation. "In situ" setting for simulation offers the benefit of reviewing the workflow of the unit allowing latent system errors to be revealed. Simulation is of proven benefit and should be incorporated for teaching, team training, and improving care delivered in any institution.

References

1. http://www.acgme.org/Portals/0/PDFs/FAQ/220_obstetrics_and_gynecology_FAQspdf. Accessed 2 Jan 2017.
2. http://www.jointcommission.org/sentinel_event_alert_issue_30_preventing_infant_death_and_injury_during_delivery/. Accessed 2 Jan 2017.
3. https://www.ahrq.gov/teamstepps/index.html. Accessed 2 Jan 2017.
4. Nielsen P, Mann S. Team function in obstetrics to reduce errors and improve outcomes. Obstet Gynecol Clin N Am. 2008;35:81–95.
5. Austin N, Goldhaber-Fiebert S, Daniels K, Arafeh J, Grenon V, Welle D, Lipman S. Building comprehensive strategies for obstetric simulation drills and communication. Anesth-Analg. 2016;123(5):1–10.
6. Gee D. Using simulation to decrease medical liability. https://www.facs.org/~/media/files/education/aei/presentation/value%20panel_01%20gee.ashx. Accessed 18 Feb 2017.
7. Preston P, Lopez C, Corbett N. How to integrate findings from simulation exercises to improve obstetric care in the institution. Semin Perinatol. 2011;35:84–8.
8. Bender J. In situ simulation for system testing in newly constructed perinatal facilities. Semin Perinatol. 2011;35:80–3.
9. Auguste T, Boswick A, Loyd M, Battista A. The simulation of an ex utero intrapartum procedure to extracorporeal membrane oxygenation. J Pediatr Surg. 2011;46:395–8.

10. Olejniczak E, Schmidt N, Brown J. Simulation as an orientation strategy for new nurse graduates: an integrative review of the evidence. Simul Healthc. 2010;5:52–7.

11. Hargreave L, Nichols A, Shanks S, Halamak L. A handoff report card for general nursing orientation. J Nurs Adm. 2010;40(10):424–31.

12. Krajewski A, Filppa D, Staff I, Singh R, Kirton O. Implementation of an intern boot camp curriculum to address clinical competencies under the new accreditation Council for Graduate Medical Education supervision requirements and duty hour restrictions. JAMA Surg. 2013;148(8):727–32.

13. Minha S, Shefet D, Sagi D, Berkenstadt H, Zvi A. "See one, Sim one, do one " a national pre-Internship boot-camp to ensure a safer "student to doctor" transition. PLoS One. 2016;11(3):e0150122.

14. http://www.acog.org/About-ACOG/ACOG-Departments/Simulations-Consortium/Simulations-Consortium-Tool-Kit.

15. Lipman S, Daniels K, Cohen SE, Carvalho B. Labor room setting compared with the operating room for simulated perimortem cesarean delivery. Obstet Gynecol. 2011;118(5):1090–4.

16. Rudolph J, Raemer D, Simon R. Establishing a safe container for learning in simulation the role of the Presimulation briefing. Simul Healthc. 2014;9(6):339–49.

17. Hamman W, Beaudin-Seiler B, Beaubien J, Gullickson A, Gross A, Orizondo-Korotko K, et al. Using in situ simulation to identify and resolve latent environment threats to patient safety: case study involving a labor and delivery ward. J Patient Saf. 2009;5(3):184–7.

Part II

Simulation Modalities and Technologies in Obstetrics and Gynecology Simulation

Standardized Patients and Gynecological Teaching Associates

Lou Clark, Chelsea Weaks, Renee M. Dorsey, Vanessa Strickland, and Shirley McAdam

Introduction

Standardized patients (SPs) are people recruited, hired, and trained to portray patients by SP Educators in order to support health-care trainees through formative and summative educational activities designed to develop clinical skills [1, 2]. SP Educators hail from a variety of disciplines and support trainees by using their diverse professional backgrounds as health-care practitioners, teachers, trainers, communication experts, and also theatre artists to coach SPs to authentically portray patients. SPs most typically "…portray common clinical complaints in a simulated medical environment" [3, p., 196]. A significant benefit of the simulated environment is minimal risk to the learners and SPs, with no risk to patients seen in hospitals. Other advantages of employing SPs include their ability to repeat the same role again and again for multiple learners, their capacity to portray a number of clinical cases simulating patient complaints that may not be readily available among patients in clinic, the fact that they may be trained to provide constructive feedback, and the fact they can provide learners with written and verbal feedback on clinical communication skills [4].

Since the 1960s when Dr. Howard Barrows [5] first implemented SPs with his neurology residents at Los Angeles County Hospital, the use of human simulation has grown to the point where most US medical schools (and many abroad) as well as numerous allied health professions have developed comprehensive SP programs. While SPs are most commonly known for portraying clinical complaints scripted in standardized patient case scenarios, their use has expanded to include a variety of roles such as physical exam teaching associates (used to teach beginning medical students foundational elements of the physical exam) and case observers, (used for quality assurance to watch and assess as other SPs perform with learners).

The obstetrics and gynecology (OB/GYN) specialties are a good example of how SPs work routinely with faculty across the United States in service of medical student and advanced learner

L. Clark (✉) · R. M. Dorsey · V. Strickland
Uniformed Services University of the Health Sciences, Val G. Hemming Simulation Center, Silver Spring, MD, USA
e-mail: Louise.Clark@simcen.usuhs.edu;
Renee.Dorsey.ctr@simcen.usuhs.edu;
Vanssa.Strickland.ctr@simcen.usuhs.edu

C. Weaks
Gynecological Teaching Associate Program, School – Eastern Virginia Medical School, Sentara Center for Simulation and Immersive Learning, Norfolk, VA, USA
e-mail: Smith002@EVMS.EDU

S. McAdam
Clinical Simulation Laboratory at the University of Vermont, Burlington, VT, USA
e-mail: shirley.mcadam@med.uvm.edu

© Springer International Publishing AG, part of Springer Nature 2019   97
S. Deering et al. (eds.), *Comprehensive Healthcare Simulation: Obstetrics and Gynecology*,
Comprehensive Healthcare Simulation, https://doi.org/10.1007/978-3-319-98995-2_10

Key Learning Points
- Understand the evolution of actual patients to SPs and GTAs in OB/GYN simulation activities and supporting evidence for the use of GTAs in medical education.
- Be able to explain best practices for working with SPs and GTAs in formative and summative sessions.
- Gain practical information for recruiting, hiring, and training SPs.

instruction. SPs are used in OB/GYN simulation activities for case portrayals and in hybrid simulations with mannequins and partial task trainers. However unlike these simulation modalities, when SPs known as gynecological teaching associates (GTAs) work, there is risk involved as they are teaching invasive exams including the speculum, bimanual, and rectal exams to learners using their own bodies. So, it is of the utmost importance that faculty and trainees collaborate with SP Educators and GTAs to create safe, intentional, and respectful learning environments. This chapter focuses on the development, role, and best practices for working with GTAs and SPs receiving invasive exams, best practices for training SPs, and logistical information relevant to working with SPs such as recruitment and cost.

The Development of GTA Programs

Before the use of GTAs – highly trained women as a tool for pelvic exam instruction – a common setting for a student to perform their first exam was in a room with a clinical patient and an instructor. In this setting, exam instruction often followed the framework of demonstration by faculty followed immediately by performance of the exam by the student [6, 7]. This was described in detail by Dr. Robert Kretzschmar, one of the first physicians to begin the development of pelvic exam instruction. He described this standard as a "triangular setting" where the patient was exploited by nature of the learning environment [6, p., 367]. The interaction between student and faculty was hindered by the necessity of having the patient present; however the patient's needs were also not being met since the student's exam did not impact their care and limited their ability to communicate with their provider [6, 8]. Holzman, Singleton, Holmes, and Maatsch [9] also describe this situation when noting "The learner and the instructor are apt to focus upon the technical aspects of the examination and overlook the needs of the patient" (p. 124).

Perlmutter and Friedman [10] reflected on the need for a change in the teaching model when they discussed the dilemma of whether to use clinic patients. They noted that "Issues of patients' rights (especially women's rights), informed consent, diminishing ward services, and social constraints…" (p. 163) suggested a different approach may need to be taken. Additionally, the anxiety of the learning situation for both the patient and the student was identified as an inherent negative aspect of using patients from the clinic [11].

The use of clinical patients presents an additional challenge in regard to incorporation of technical and communication skills simultaneously. While there was variety in the reported incentives for change across the literature, one of the most commonly identified concerns was communication with the patient [6, 12, 13]. To address this wide range of challenges, programs began developing alternatives to using patients for the initial pelvic exam instruction. These program alternatives have become an accepted part of undergraduate medical education and continue to develop as more research reinforces their effectiveness.

Employing GTAs to Teach the Pelvic Exam Is Advised

Over the course of the last 50 years, alongside the development of standardized patient methodology, the development of GTA instruction has evolved despite some common misconceptions of their roles. The use of highly trained women who can provide feedback and refinement on exam technique as well as effective communication strategies is no longer a new phenomenon. GTA methodology is rooted in educational theory and practice and uses defensible strategies to engage the learners throughout a structured session while retaining a relatively low stress environment. There are a large variety of techniques and frameworks that are utilized for instruction of the exam, and each has its own benefits that align with many of the identified challenges with the previous use of clinical patients in the hospital.

The initial steps to address the challenges surrounding clinical patient usage allowed the implementation of educational theory that led to the current-day GTA programs. While there are a variety of instructional approaches that were attempted, the current standard in the United States is the use of GTAs for pelvic exam instruction [14]. There are multiple designs for the instructional session composition, but the major approaches are structured to include one or two GTA instructors leading small group sessions without faculty being directly involved in each session. Other structures of note that are still in use today use GTAs in addition to faculty instruction in small group settings or use live models to allow for faculty demonstration of the exam in larger groups.

Even in the early research it was noted that the skills the students gained from sessions with GTAs had benefits when compared to instruction by a gynecologist. The cognitive scores of the students instructed by physicians and GTAs were nearly identical; however, the GTA-trained students scored significantly better in psychomotor and interpersonal skills [9]. Similar findings are present throughout the literature, reiterating the efficiency of the communication training during a GTA session when compared to a session with physician faculty or mannequin instruction [15–17]. With these repeated results, it is a commonly accepted benefit of GTA training that the communication skills that are essential to a strong doctor-patient relationship are started in tandem with technical skill acquisition.

Evidence

Recommendations for Undergraduate Medical Education Curricula and Training

Undergraduate medical education is a topic of vast discussion when considering professional organizations. The use of GTAs for pelvic exam instruction is somewhat of an outlier, in that the direct statements regarding their use are limited. When making the overarching recommendations for medical education for this area, the AAMC [18] recommended repeated practice with constructive feedback to refine clinical skills, which requires the inclusion of "a trained observer, such as a supervising physician or an experienced patient" (p.7). They also specifically identify the ability to engage and communicate with the patient as a critical competency. While there is no statement in the recommendations directly addressing the method of instructing the pelvic exam, the mention of constructive feedback parallels the concerns that were initially addressed by the design of GTA instruction. Additionally, this recommendation supports the use of standardized patients, which were the basic framework of the GTA design. The mention of trained observers as well as the focus on feedback and refinement suggests the use of GTA instruction meets these recommendations for overall undergraduate medical education.

The Association of Professors of Gynecology and Obstetrics (APGO), specifically the Undergraduate Medical Education Committee (UMEC), released a clinical skills curriculum opinion in 2008 [19]. This opinion defines four frameworks for pelvic exam instruction, investigates the data, and ranks them based upon the available research. The differences between these four student practice options were described in detail, but ultimately the GTA was identified as the method of choice "followed by computerized plastic pelvic models, live models and non-computerized plastic models" (p.9). The statement went on to say that the use of clinic patients as the initial examination training was not advised without, at minimum, practice on a non-computerized model if the other design methods were not available. The benefits highlighted were the ability of GTAs to provide timely feedback, the lack of ethical concerns, and the fact that faculty are not required to be present during the instruction. The cost of physician instruction was mentioned as well, as if to reiterate the benefits inherent in this methodology. Finally, it was reinforced that it is essential that students practice the hands-on skills while receiving feedback and specifically that simply lecturing and providing a film are not adequate instructional practices when used alone.

The basic framework suggested by the UMEC in regard to the best practice design of a pelvic exam teaching session includes an introductory instruction followed by a demonstration of the exam by an instructor and then supervised practice with the technique [20]. The preliminary instruction offered the inclusion of one or more of the following: lecture, video, reading materials, PowerPoint presentation, and class discussion. The supervised practice had a broad range of options for methodologies including hospital patients, plastic pelvic models, live models, and gynecology teaching associates.

An important distinction to make when discussing the use of clinic patients in medical educational overall is that clinic patients are still commonly used in clerkship experiences. In the OB/GYN clerkships, many US medical schools use clinic patients for opportunistic practice and training after the initial instructional experience [14].

Effectiveness of GTAs for Training Undergraduate Medical Students

Several recent studies demonstrate the effectiveness of using GTAs in the undergraduate medical school curriculum [21–23]. A trend highlighted is the tendency of early learner anxiety around performing the pelvic exam and that working with GTAs is shown to improve student confidence as well as technical skill [22]. Introducing GTAs early in the undergraduate medical curriculum in support of initial learner experiences of

performing the pelvic exam and then at the start of the OB/GYN clerkship rotation as refresher training has been shown to be effective for combatting learner anxiety and also for technical skills development [24].

Implementing SPs and GTAs in OB/GYN Simulation Activities

The goal of this chapter section is to share the best practices and expert advice on working with SPs and GTAs when implementing OB/GYN simulation activities. Topics addressed in this section include curriculum development, recruiting SPs and GTAs, costs and resources, SP and GTA training, faculty involvement, and formative and summative sessions with GTAs and SPs.

Curriculum Development

Curriculum development involving SPs should be approached as a collaborative process. Subject matter experts (SMEs), in this case OB/GYN faculty members, bring their knowledge to the table and SP Educators work with them to create simulation events that accurately teach (formative events) or assess (summative events) learner skills [24]. When designing new curriculum or revising existing curriculum, we recommend that SMEs and an SP Educator have an initial meeting (ideally face to face) in which the SMEs clearly identify the following:

- Educational goals and objectives
- Guiding educational or professional milestones related to the goals and objectives
- Number of participating learners and faculty
- Desired length of session
- Demographics including age, gender, and specific physical characteristics or hiring requirements for SPs or GTAs

During this meeting, the SP Educator may ask follow-up questions that pertain to the educational goals and objectives, learner level, or other related topics. Based on this additional information, SP Educators may suggest options for SP case scenario development, an SP or GTA training schedule/protocol, development of assessment tools (for summative activities), options for providing constructive feedback (for formative activities), and overall event logistics.

The initial meeting should conclude with the SMEs and SP Educator agreeing to a series of tasks and who is responsible for the completion of each task. See Table 10.1 for a sample checklist of tasks.

Once the tasks and responsibilities are assigned, it is important to choose a date for the simulation activity, and then review your timeline backwards from the event date. Ideally, we recommend planning for new events start 1 year in advance of the event date and no later than 6 months in advance of the date. This is crucial as each part of the process that follows builds on the next, and the educational impact as well as optimal cost-effectiveness of simulation events is directly correlated to preparation.

When SP case scenarios and accompanying evaluation tools (i.e., checklists) – such as those used in Objective Structured Clinical Examinations (OSCEs) – are needed, we recommend the SMEs and SP Educator have a follow-up development meeting. During this meeting, faculty will build on educational goals and objectives by identifying a specific patient case(s) SPs will portray during the simulation event. It is often useful for faculty to model SP case scenarios after patients they have seen in hospitals or outpatient clinics. During this meeting the SMEs should provide all of the medical information relevant for SPs to accurately portray the case (i.e., chief complaint, relevant social history, history of present illness, medical history, physical signs and symptoms, and communication style preferences). The SP Educator will contribute by anticipating question SPs will ask with the goal of making the case as complete as possible prior to the training session. A sample case scenario with assessment materials used in our OSCE for medical students following their OB/GYN clerkship is included in this chapter for your reference. It is important for faculty to keep in mind that SPs want to get a picture of this patient as a whole person – not just a patient with a medical problem – so content that may seem superfluous such as hobbies, underlying memories or physical experiences associated with medical care, or a reason for seeking medical care today (as opposed to yesterday) supports SPs in creating authentic portrayals [25]. The ability of SPs to create authentic portrayals directly contributes to the ability of learners to be present and invested in simulation activities.

When creating new SP cases, we also recommend rehearsing the scenario, prior to using it with learners. Ideally, the SME author will recruit a peer who does not know the case to play the learner and role-play it with the SP Educator. Following the rehearsal, the SME should score any assessment tools designed for faculty observers, and the SP Educator should score any assessment tools designed to be scored by SPs. Based on the rehearsal, the SME and SP Educator can make needed modifications to the case scenario and assessment tools prior to the SP training session.

Recruiting SPs and GTAs

One of the most critical components of implementing a program that includes SPs and GTAs is finding qualified personnel who have experience in this area and are good candidates to be trained. We have found that one of the best ways to recruit for both of these roles is by word of mouth from current employees. However, for those developing new programs, we recommend reaching out to established programs in your region for guidance and advice. The Association of Standardized

Table 10.1 Sample checklist of tasks

Task/planning	Person responsible
SP/GTA recruitment	
Faculty recruitment	
SP case scenario development	
Assessment tool development	

Logistical plans:
  Duration of each SP encounter
  duration for overall day/event	

Patient Educators website (http://www.aspeducators.org/) is a valuable resource for identifying programs in your region [26]. Established programs in your area may provide region-specific suggestions including contacts for theater/actor list serves where you may advertise, home school programs especially helpful for recruiting adults from mid-20s to mid-40s and adolescents, retirement communities, and small business owners. Since most SP work is on-call – meaning part-time with no guarantee of a fixed schedule or certain hours – it is optimal to recruit from communities in which people have flexible schedules.

It should also be expected that recruiting GTAs and/or SPs willing to participate in invasive exams is often more difficult. For this reason, plenty of lead time must be allowed for the recruitment, hiring, and training process. Additionally, supervising faculty course directors must make their training goals, objectives, and needs clear as soon as possible to the SP Educator – ideally up to 6 months in advance for sensitive exams (and preferably for patient case scenarios as well). At our institutions, our SP Educator teams implement more than 250 events per year utilizing SPs, so faculty should plan for lead time and realize that their event is likely one of many in progress – all of which must be cast, scheduled, and trained.

When considering recruitment efforts for all SPs but especially for GTAs, one should consider the applicants' motivations. We have found GTAs are motivated to do this work for several reasons including a love of teaching and comfort with using one's body to teach others; a desire to help train future clinicians having had poor past experiences with clinicians during which they felt disregarded, condescended, and uncared for; and being empowered by the ability to give learners a safe space for trial and error. Other reported GTA motivations include interest in promoting women's health and the altruistic nature of the work [27]. It is important to demystify what drives women to become GTAs for two reasons: first, because there has long been a stigma around morality and GTA work which continues to a lesser degree today [28] and second, and more practically, because it may assist faculty and SP Educators in recruiting the most motivated, qualified GTA employees.

Finally, we recommend using a GTA recruitment guide and have included a template in this chapter. In addition to motivation for seeking work, we assess applicants for general qualities successful GTAs possess including abilities to lead in a facilitative manner, creating a safe learning environment, teach confidently but calmly under pressure, collaborate with others, be reliable, and maintain a positive body image. Additional essential screening items assess communication skills and physical characteristics and concerns. Successful recruitment of SPs and GTAs leads to lower attrition of employees, allowing for effective resource management and cost-effectiveness in relation to SP training (Fig. 10.1).

Costs and Resources

Overall, research supports that using GTAs rather than faculty is a cost-saving measure, in addition to being as – if not more – effective in training learners on how to perform a pelvic exam [9, 17, 29]. However, starting and maintaining an SP or GTA program requires funding and resources. Potential primary costs to consider include one or more full-time SP Educators or a GTA trainer to oversee your program, space needed (if not already provided), and funding for SP and GTA pay. In the United States GTA pay varies depending on region and based on the authors' experience may run anywhere from $40 to $75 per hour per GTA for teaching sessions in major metropolitan areas. Full-time SP Educator salaries are also variable, especially depending on region of the country. To determine a competitive and fair salary, we recommend consulting board members of the Association of Standardized Patient Educators [26]. Secondary costs would include supplies such as disposable speculums and other consumables, any facilities costs, and training time.

a

GTA Recruitment Guide

Date: _____   Applicant: _____

Interviewer: _____   Applicant Supplied Resume: ☐ Yes ☐ No

General GTA Characteristics

Applicants were assessed on their ability to:	Yes	No
Lead in a facilitative manner		
Create a safe learning environment		
Teach with a calm, confident demeanor		
Collaborate with trainers, learners, and other GTAs		
Be prompt, reliable, and consistent		
Express a positive body image		
Comments:		

Applicants were asked to:	Yes	No
Discuss motivation for their interest in the work		
Describe medical experience related to women's health issues		
NOTE: Applicant should consider the potential impact of past clinical or sexual history on GTA work.		
Comments:		

Communication Skills

Applicants were assessed on their ability to:	Yes	No
Give positive and constructive verbal feedback		
Give clear instructions		
Listen well and take instruction		
Reassure nervous learners		

By Renée Dorsey, Scheduling & Recruitment Manger
Val G. Hemming Simulation Center
Uniformed Services University of the Health Sciences

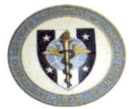

Fig. 10.1 (**a**, **b**). GTA Recruitment Guide. (Reproduced with permission of Uniformed Services University of the Health Sciences)

b

Comments:

Physical Characteristics and Concerns

Applicants were asked if they had:	Yes	No
Uterus		
Cervix		
Ovaries		
Breasts		
Applicants were asked if they have any concerns with sensitivity or pain:	Yes	No
During pelvic exams		
During breast exams		
Comments:		

By Renée Dorsey, Scheduling & Recruitment Manger
Val G. Hemming Simulation Center
Uniformed Services University of the Health Sciences

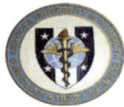

Fig. 10.1 (continued)

Training SPs and GTAs

Training for new recruits may include time with a GTA or SP Educator or faculty member prior to teaching students. In many cases, the training of new GTAs is done by established GTAs, and the two work together as a team. SP training for case scenarios is most often led by SP Educators and generally occurs a few days prior to the event, so that SPs can digest and memorize material. For formative activities same-day training is usually sufficient while summative encounters may require additional practice sessions to ensure they are reliable and reproducible.

SP case training is a collaborative process that is best done in a facilitative style. The training environment should be one in which participants feel comfortable to ask questions, raise issues around any confusing material, come to consensus as to how to portray the patient character, and reach inter-rater reliability for assessing learners. This is essential as the training process for SP case scenarios is, at its best, an extension of the case writing process because the dialogue in the training process has a direct impact on case development, portrayal, and learner assessment. We do recommend, especially for new cases, that faculty attend these sessions to clarify material as well as demonstrate physical exam maneuvers. This is best done with faculty visiting in the second half of the training in order to give the SP Educator and SPs time to review the case and assessment materials, so they may identify any issues that require clarification. It also prevents surprises on the day of the event.

GTA Training

There are many methods of training new GTAs, so there is not one absolute correct way. However, training new GTAs generally takes multiple sessions over the course of several weeks and averages between 8 and 30 hours. GTA training most often involves the trainees being coached by seasoned GTAs and/or a GTA program coordinator who is a member of the SP Educator team. This training technique serves as a model, as GTAs often work in pairs during teaching sessions with medical students. The paired GTA teaching approach has several advantages, some of these include a built-in chaperone and the ability to observe and then move into the teaching role when confident and comfortable to do so. Paired teams of GTAs may also rotate as to who is being examined so neither will receive too many exams, and learners experience multiple teaching styles as well as anatomies. Siwe et al. [30] discuss the resources involved in training and employing GTAs in relation to the benefits and explain that "this model is costly, takes time and effort to sustain, but is worthwhile as it creates a relaxed and interactive setting that promotes students' confidence and competence" (p. 217). Other GTA training components may include anatomy and physiology review; technique training on the breast, abdominal, and pelvic exams; lectures; films; communication skills training; and training with the program coordinator and students. [6, 17, 31]. A sample GTA training plan is included in this chapter for your reference (Fig. 10.2).

In addition to training for new GTAs, many SP programs also have training for cases in which SPs who are not necessarily GTAs receive pelvic examinations as part of assessment events. While this does not require as extensive level of training as GTA training (because these SPs will not be teaching the exams – rather receiving them only), the training for these events should be noted as well. These cases tend to have many logistics associated with them involving supplies needed for the pelvic exam, room setup, universal precautions/ hygiene issues, and chaperones. We have found it helpful to use light source handles that are compatible with disposable, plastic speculums. The light

sources (as opposed to stand-up lamps to the side of the exam table) offer learners a better view for the pelvic examination. Using disposable speculums reassures SPs that the highest standards of hygiene are being followed for their safety. It is important to review all of these logistics carefully with the SPs so – if need be – they can advocate for themselves during an encounter with a learner. For example, if the learner does not glove properly or wash their hands, SPs should feel empowered to direct them to do so prior to doing an invasive exam. It is essential that SPs feel confident and comfortable with the many logistics associated with pelvic examinations occurring as part of assessment events, as this contributes to positive experiences for all involved as well as minimizes the risk of injury to the SPs.

Faculty Involvement

In addition to reinforcing personal privacy, we recommend that faculty partner with SPs and GTAs to ensure their safety and adherence to universal precautions during simulation events. While the pelvic exam is not a completely sterile exam, there are precautions SPs and faculty can uphold. Students should use proper gloving techniques to ensure the well-being and comfort of the patients. Additionally, faculty can reinforce proper insertion and removal techniques for the speculum exam with students. Especially important to emphasize with students is that once they insert the speculum, they should not adjust it up or down (only forward and back) as this causes discomfort and pain. When removing the speculum to avoid causing pain, students should not close the speculum too early as this pinches the cervix and also not to remove the speculum in the completely open position. While the exam is meant for education, these common initial errors are uncomfortable and care must be taken to ensure they do not occur. GTAs have also provided feedback that they are more comfortable when the external exam of the labia is done with two fingers and minimal touch. At our simulation center, the OB/GYN clerkship director holds a practice session with task trainer models, so stu-

a

GTA CORE TRAINING – EXAM 101

Key to terms
NGTA – New GTA in training
Trainer – Either head trainer or adjunct trainer
Learner – The role of the student during an actual GTA session

SESSION OBJECTIVE	Day 1- Orientation
Role of the GTA	• Manual orientation
Overview of GYN exam	• Introduction to Learner levels • Introduction of Anatomy terms
Introduction to Female Anatomy/Landmark	• Manual anatomy/diagram review • Vocabulary and Glossary discussion
Questions Frequently Asked by NGTAs	• Meet and Greet with GTAs
SESSION OBJECTIVE	Day 2- Intro and External
Room Preparation/Sanitation	• Demonstration in exam room • Sanitation/OSHA Precautions • Discussion and room preparation
Introduction section	• Review of GTA Training section for Introduction • Directed Observation and Discussion
External Structure Exam section	• Directed Observation and Discussion
Dual Instructor Session for Introduction and External Exam Module	• Each NGTA gets multiple opportunities as both learner and instructor
SESSION OBJECTIVE	Day 3- Speculum
Review of Introduction and External Exam Sections	• Practice speaking aloud without guidance if possible – Introduction and External Exam

Developed at Eastern Virginia Medical School by Chelsea Smith, M.Ed., Gynecological Teaching Associate Trainer

Fig. 10.2 (**a–d**). GTA training schedule. (Reproduced with permission of Sentara Center for Simulation & Immersive Learning, Eastern Virginia Medical School)

b

Room set up and break down procedure practice	• Use of pictures for setup
Manual and Speculum Review and Speculum 101	• Review of manual section • Practice handling the speculum
Dual Instructor Session for Speculum Exam Module	• Each NGTA gets multiple opportunities as both learner and instructor
SESSION OBJECTIVE	**Day 4- Bimanual**
Demo supply usage	• Review of manual section for Pap and Uterus model usage • Practice explaining these sections with supplies/demos
Technique Practice	• Each instructor talking through the sections they need to practice – practice combining External and Speculum
Bimanual Video Review	• Review of GTA Training section for Bimanual • Directed Observation and Discussion
Dual Instructor Session for Bimanual Exam Module	• Each NGTA on table • Ideally each NGTA gets multiple opportunities as both learner and instructor
SESSION OBJECTIVE	**Day 5- Rectovaginal**
Technique Practice	• Practice aloud without guidance if possible • NGTA on table practicing sections
Rectovaginal Review	• Review of GTA Training section for Rectovaginal • Directed Observation and Discussion

Developed at Eastern Virginia Medical School by Chelsea Smith, M.Ed., Gynecological Teaching Associate Trainer

Fig. 10.2 (continued)

c

Dual Instructor Rectovaginal Exam	• Each NGTA on table • Ideally each NGTA gets multiple opportunities as both learner and instructor
Pelvic Exam Summary	• Review of Overall Exam
SESSION OBJECTIVE	*Day 6 (Ideally beginning second week)* *Dry Run Practice*
Recap of First Week	• This includes questions that may have come up since last meeting
Exam Closure/Patient Education	• Closure and safety • Discussion of facilitation style • Safety discussion – injury protocol
Full Exam Practice	• "Stumble through" – no coaching • NGTA1 on table, NGTA2 as learner, trainer as learner as needed
Group Feedback	• Standardization of techniques • Group challenges for learners • Self Assessment
GTA Full Teaching Session	• "Stumble through" – no coaching • NGTA2 on table, NGTA1 as learner, trainer as learner as needed
Group Feedback	• Standardization of techniques • Group challenges for learners • Self Assessment
Debrief	• Includes discussion of timing for each NGTA
SESSION OBJECTIVE	*Day 7- Debrief and Breast Exam*

Developed at Eastern Virginia Medical School by Chelsea Smith, M.Ed., Gynecological Teaching Associate Trainer

Fig. 10.2 (continued)

dents can rehearse the pelvic exam prior to working with SPs during the OSCE later that week. An SP is present at these practice sessions, so she can offer coaching on communication skills from the patient perspective. (In ours and most SP programs, new employees are trained on how to provide constructive written and verbal feedback on learner communication skills.) The majority of discomfort and injury that occurs for GTAs and SPs happens when students use a harder touch than necessary on the external labia exam or improper speculum insertion or removal techniques during the pelvic exam. Faculty can be especially helpful in safeguarding against SP discomfort if they are acting as chaperones during assessments.

It is also highly recommended that faculty who are working with the students have an opportunity to, at a minimum, sit down with the SP Educator or trainer who oversees the GTAs prior to training or event sessions. This allows the faculty to get a better understanding of what the learners will face when going through the sessions, as well as to ask questions and engage the educator to ensure all of the program's goals and expectations are being met. Additionally, this enables SPs and GTAs to share any personal circumstances of which faculty and students should be made aware (i.e. piercings, if the woman has her period, whether or not it is difficult to see her cervix) and to check as regards appropriateness of speculum size.

d

Recap of Day Six	• Review and debrief pelvic exam • Safety techniques and injury protocol
Teaching Techniques and Special Considerations of Pelvic Exam	• Special considerations/techniques • May include troubleshooting Speculum
Breast Exam Review	• Directed Observation and Discussion
Dual Instructor Breast Exam	• Each NGTA on table • Ideally each NGTA gets multiple opportunities as both learner and instructor
SESSION OBJECTIVE	*Day 8 – Practice of full integrated exam*
Recap of Day Seven	• Answer Breast Exam Questions
Practice Breast Exam	• Practice aloud without guidance • NGTA on table practicing Breast Exam
Full Exam Practice	• Breast and Pelvic Combined • Let NGTA run as if a normal session
Group Feedback	Provided by the Learners and Trainer
SESSION OBJECTIVE	Final Check-off (Scheduled Solo Assessment)
Full Session - Trainer	Final Check –off of complete examination

Developed at Eastern Virginia Medical School by Chelsea Smith, M.Ed., Gynecological Teaching Associate Trainer

Fig. 10.2 (continued)

When preparing students to participate in GTA formative sessions, we also recommend faculty first observe a session so they have a full understanding of what happens in the room. Following this experience, it is helpful for faculty and SP Educators or GTA trainers to collaborate on an orientation for students that emphasizes communication skills in addition to physical exam skills. Many students are unaware of the expectations and structure of the sessions and this alone can create unnecessary anxiety and concern. Some articles suggest that lowering anxiety can overall aid in the student's knowledge retention and state that they are coming away from the sessions with competency in the skills [10]. Conversely, some research stated that anxiety was a benefit as it increased the learner's motivation and androgenic response [13]. In either case, research shows that students receiving orienta-tion from faculty members are better able to inte-grate information presented into successfully performing invasive exams [6, 32]. Additionally, some students will come to this training exercise having had bad past experiences as patients or with women's health. It is important faculty invite students to approach them with individual concerns privately so issues may be addressed before the simulation event.

Along with providing an inclusive team-based introduction and clear orientation, it is imperative that faculty provide constructive feedback to learners and validate SP and GTA feedback. Having the SP or GTA and faculty members work as a team to support the learner yields optimal results. When faculty dismiss or undermine SP or GTA feedback, negative ramifications include learners being confused or discounting on the feedback.

Formative and Summative Sessions with GTAs and SPs

As mentioned earlier in this chapter, GTAs are more often used for formative, teaching sessions while SPs may be employed for assessments – to undergo breast and or pelvic examinations – most often occurring at the end of the OB/GYN clerkship rotation for medical students. The distinction of formative or summative is significant as each has different educational objectives and therefore necessitates discrete skills and logistics.

Formative teaching sessions are most often led by GTAs who are providing instruction using their own body or that of a teaching partner. In order to do this, GTAs have been trained in elements described earlier in this chapter and in many cases often perform the exam on another GTA prior to teaching students. So, GTAs train medical students to complete the full well-woman exam because they have performed it themselves and learned the supporting anatomy and physiology didactic information. GTAs are also able to instruct learners on communication preferences from the patient perspective.

We recommend that the formative GTA sessions begin with a discussion on language, communication, and speculum use between the GTAs and students – prior to the demonstration. Next, we suggest that one GTA demonstrate the exam on the other. She should begin outside of the exam room and role-play the encounter just as if she were the provider in order to model the best practices for communication skills throughout the session from start to finish. After the demonstration, students should take turns performing the encounter including introduction, exam, and conclusion. GTAs should rotate who is being examined and who is observing. As this is a formative session, either of the GTAs may stop the encounter at any point to coach and ask questions or for safety purposes. The students should watch and learn from each encounter even if they are not the ones performing the exam. We suggest two GTAs are paired with no more than four students for this type of session which should generally last about 2 hours, and each GTA will have received two pelvic exams. The number of pelvic exams per GTA per session is variable, but our general recommendation is eight or less pelvic exams per GTA per day. This style of formative session is often held once during the pre-clerkship curriculum and then as a refresher for students as refresher training at the beginning of their OB/GYN clerkship year.

Assessment days or testing days often raise the level of tension for both students and SPs. For this reason and also to minimize risk of discomfort or injury to the SP, we recommend women receive fewer pelvic exams than in a teaching session – ideally no more than six over the course of a single daylong event. SPs must also have time between these encounters to properly clean themselves and rest (this time is built in with the formative sessions because the GTA pairs rotate in terms of who is receiving the exam). SPs are more prone to anxiety on assessment days than when they work as GTAs teaching students in formative sessions. In the teaching role, GTAs feel more empowered, as compared to assessment days when students direct the encounter and pelvic exam. GTAs who work on assessment days as SPs can also anticipate student errors that may cause them discomfort because of their increased knowledge of the well-woman exam. Rather than being able to correct them as they would in teaching sessions, SPs are usually directed to clearly express pain verbally and nonverbally. Therefore, it is important that SPs receiving pelvic exams in assessment situations be supported in expressing pain to learners and validated if they need to tell the student to stop the exam. Faculty should provide support if such an instance occurs by stepping in and concluding the encounter – particularly if the speculum must be removed. Then, the SP or faculty should bring any issue that involves discomfort or injury to the attention of the SP Educator.

Perhaps our strongest recommendation for the successful implementation of simulation events of any type is for faculty and SP Educators to work together early and often. This is done by first identifying learning goals and objectives and then collaborating together – the faculty bringing the context expertise and the SP Educator bringing the simulation expertise – to create optimal events for learners giving special care to the safety and emotional well-being of all participants.

Conclusion

SP and GTA methodology – rooted in more than 50 years of educational theory and practice – demonstrates that this methodology has been developed and tested over time. SPs and GTAs are valuable assets for OB/GYN practitioners seeking to engage trainees in simulation events. In order to implement successful, cost-effective learning activities with SPs and GTAs, our recommendation is to begin by setting educational objectives and work far in advance of event dates. This will ensure plenty of time for scenario development and faculty recruitment and for providing the focused training required when working with SPs and GTAs.

Please see the end of this chapter for sample case scenario.

Acknowledgements Special thanks to Robin Nicholson and Emily Sucher for providing insights from their perspectives as standardized patients.

Annie Gibson

Date(s) and content revised: Revision 4/11/17 by Vanessa Strickland; changed format

Case author and date written: Andrea Creel, MSW, Katarina Shvartsman, MD, updated by Vanessa Strickland, 2017

Case objective(s) for students: Understand risk factors, mechanism of transmission, and treatment for chlamydia infections. Demonstrate clear communication skills and be able to explain the diagnosis, treatment, and follow-up plans to a standardized patient.

Differential diagnosis: Chlamydia

Presenting complaint/opening statement): "I got a call from the clinic nurse to come back in after my visit 3 weeks ago. I also decided that I should get some birth control because I don't want to get pregnant."

Appropriate examinee level as written: OB/GYN Clerkship Assessment

Patient demographics:

Age range: 21 (20s)
Gender: Female
Ethnicity: Any
Height/Weight: Normal

Medical setting/location: OB/GYN Office
Patient clothing: Street clothes
Is there a gown required during encounter? No
Is there a door sign with this case? Yes, CAE Pre-encounter

Presenting Situation

Patient Information

Name: Annie Gibson
Setting: Gynecology Clinic

Annie Gibson is a 21-year-old college student (LMP 1 week ago) who has come to the gynecology clinic to follow up on recent test results.

She was seen 3 weeks ago by your colleague in the clinic and underwent a pelvic examination, breast exam, Pap smear, and testing for gonorrhea and *Chlamydia*. Her pelvic and breast exams were reported as normal and her Pap smear was normal.

Her test for *Chlamydia* is positive and she received a phone call from your clinic to return for an appointment to discuss her lab results. She is also requesting something for birth control.

Student Instructions

Tasks:
Take an appropriate history.

Discuss her test results. Provide counseling and information.

Counsel her on options for contraception, prevention of sexually transmitted infections, and any follow-up needed.

Discuss any additional studies you recommend at this time.

Time Limit: 20 Minutes

You have 20 minutes with Ms. Gibson.

You will hear a 2 minute warning prior to the end of the 20 minutes with the patient.

Then you will have 10 minutes to complete a post-encounter exercise.

After you have completed the post-encounter exercise,

you may return to the room for feedback as time allows.

Trainer Notes – Annie Gibson Case
Trainer: Vanessa Strickland
Date: Training date April 4th, 2017 for 4/20/17
Activity: 3rd year OB/GYN OSCE/Clerkship

Describe any changes (e.g., specific case information or relevant past medical history) to the checklist: Printed out copies of updated information regarding STIs (*Chlamydia* specifically) and contraceptive options to assist in verifying accuracy of information presented by learners.

Resources:

CDC – https://www.cdc.gov/std/healthcomm/fact_sheets.htm

Reproductive Access.Org – http://www.reproductiveaccess.org/resources/

Describe any changes in or clarification to case details and why: Need to course director for clarification on how many specifics the learners need to ask about regarding the characteristics of the patient's period.

Describe any changes in the door sign:

Describe adjustments or changes in SP portrayal (e.g., affect, verbal or non-verbal cues):

Describe changes in information/responses given by SPs (e.g., medication cards, findings cards, ways of answering open- and close-ended questions):

Describe any new training tools/aids/techniques used (e.g., relevant Mind Map, timelines, previous encounters reviewed):

Describe props and how used:

Describe any pressing issues for immediate or future changes (e.g., new questions to checklists):

Describe any problems/difficulties to bring to debrief/SPOT meeting for resolution (e.g., student issues from debrief, awkward case moments):

Patient name:	Annie Gibson
Clothing:	Street clothes
Reason for visit:	STI test results
Opening statement:	*"I got a call from the clinic nurse to come back in after my visit 3 weeks ago. I also decided that I should get some birth control because I don't want to get pregnant"*
Social history:	**Age/work/basic background:** 21-year-old college student at Montgomery College. You work at Claire's at Montgomery Mall
	Current Living Situation: You live with your mother and father. You are a military dependent because your father is active duty military (Army Sergeant). You have a younger sister [11] and a 15-year-old brother. Your father works long hours as a supply clerk and is often gone from home. Your Mom works part-time. You have a strained but tolerable relationship with your mother and a distant relationship with your father. When you thought you were pregnant once, you told your mother about being sexually active, and you and she had an argument and a shouting match about it. Your mother doesn't know you are at the clinic today. Your mother wants you to stop seeing your boyfriend

Communication	**Your stated reason/motivation for visit today:** You received a phone call from your clinic to return for an appointment to discuss your lab results and you were interested in discussing birth control. Your test for *Chlamydia* is positive, but you are not aware of the result until the student informs you during the encounter
	Affect: When the encounter first starts, you are apprehensive and nervous because you don't know what to expect. After you receive the results of your test for *Chlamydia*, you are shocked, a little angry, and embarrassed
	You are generally agreeable and interested in knowing more about different birth control options. Don't insert questions at random. You will be primarily listening, letting the student take the lead in the interview. If the student asks you if you've decided on a birth control option, you should decisively say: "I think I want that IUD like my friend." It doesn't matter if they/you choose the Mirena or Skyla IUD (different brands of hormonal IUDs). Allow the student to initiate an end to the encounter
	Because you have *Chlamydia*, the doctor will not be able to insert an IUD today, so they should advise you to make an appointment to come back for a repeat gonorrhea and chlamydia test. *However*, they should advise you on some form of intermediary birth control option (known as "interval birth control") until you are able to get an IUD (i.e., they shouldn't have you leave the office with no birth control plan in place). If they advise you to use condoms until you can get the IUD inserted, you should bring up your concerns about your boyfriend not wanting to use condoms and your fear of losing him if you insist on them. And you are afraid that if you refuse sex (i.e., abstinence) he will definitely dump you
	If they advise you to use the patch, pill, ring, etc. temporarily until you can get an IUD you are agreeable as long as they reassure you that after the waiting period (either 3 months or until infection is cleared) you can get the IUD inserted as a more long-term birth control method since that is your preference
	If the student does not bring up the IUD as a birth control option, then at the end of the encounter, you should say, "I know you didn't mention it, but I think I want the IUD like my friend." If you are told that you cannot have an IUD due to contraindications, you should state: "I guess I'll go home and think about it some more then"
History of present illness:	*None*
	If asked, you have no any vaginal or urinary problems (burning, itching, discharge or pain). You have not had pain with sex
Past medical history:	*None*
	"I have no current medical problems"
	"I have never had any sexually transmitted infections"
Menstrual history:	Your periods began at age 13. They were irregular for about a year coming every 2 or 3 months. Now, they come every 4 weeks (approx. 28 days). Your flow is medium for about 4–5 days. You have some mild cramps that are not really a problem. Occasionally, around exam time or when you are very stressed out, your periods sometimes come a little early or a little late. If asked how many pads or tampons you go through per day during your period, you respond, "I don't know, maybe 4 or 5? I don't really keep track"
Current medications:	No prescriptions, takes an occasional Motrin for cramping during period, Tylenol for headaches
	"I don't take any prescription medications"
	"I take an occasional Tylenol for a headache"
Allergies:	"I do not have any allergies that I know of"
Social history:	**Activities:** You are a pretty good college student at Montgomery College and you're majoring in business. You're not really sure what you want to do after you graduate and are feeling a little worried about it. You do have a part-time job at the Claire's store at the mall which you like okay
	Sexual History: You have been having sex for 3 years now and have been with your current boyfriend, Mark, for 4 months. Before him, you had two other male partners. You have used condoms in the past with other partners, but your current boyfriend really doesn't like them. You are afraid that if you insist on using them, you will lose him
	You usually have vaginal intercourse and once in a while oral sex. You have never had anal sex. You have never been pregnant and had your first pelvic exam three weeks ago. You have never been sexually abused or raped. The last time you had sex was 2 days ago. Your current boyfriend, Mark, is your only partner in the past 6 months
	You heard a rumor about a month ago that Mark may be having sex with another girl at school, but you haven't talked to him about it. Again, you are afraid that you will lose him as a boyfriend. You like him a lot and don't want to lose him
	Alcohol: You drink about 1–2 beers at parties on the weekends. You like the way the alcohol makes you feel more relaxed and buzzed. You have never been drunk or blacked out due to alcohol consumption
	Drugs: None
	Tobacco: You smoke about ½ pack of cigarettes a day and have been smoking since you were 14. You don't have any intention to quit at this time

Health maintenance practices:	**Immunizations:** If asked whether you received Gardasil vaccine, you respond "I don't think so" **Diet:** You eat a typical "American" diet. Because of your busy schedule at school, you eat out more than you probably should – Chipotle and Panera are your favorites. You do try to watch what you eat, though, and try to have salads every day **Exercise:** You use the gym at school where you walk on the treadmill with your friends a few times a week. You also take a yoga class for credit at school **Physical Checkups:** First pelvic exam (3 weeks ago), up to date with your annual physical. At your well-woman exam, you had a normal pelvic exam, a normal breast exam, Pap smear, and received testing for gonorrhea and *Chlamydia*
Family medical history:	Your parents are alive and well. Your grandparents are alive, one with high blood pressure. You know of no other family health problems. There is no history of liver disease or blood clots in your family
Current knowledge/attitude about *birth control* options:	If asked about your preferences for birth control options, you say: "My friend, Sara, has tried the IUD, but I really don't know what I want" If they ask you a follow-up question about what kind of IUD your friend got (i.e., copper or hormonal), you can respond: "I'm not sure but she says that now her periods are really light now" If asked whether you know how an IUD is placed, you respond: "My friend said they put it up inside and that it was pretty painful" If asked if you would like to hear more about other birth control options, you reply that you are interested in hearing more If the student talks to you about birth control pills, you should respond that you are worried that the pill may make you fat. You should NOT bring up this concern until after they have told you information on the risks/benefits of the pill (i.e., later in the encounter). If they counsel you to use condoms, you should bring up your concern that your boyfriend doesn't like condoms and you are concerned about him breaking up with you if you insist on using them. You don't know much about the other birth control options that are presented to you
Current knowledge/attitude about *STIs*:	You learned something about STIs in a health course when you were in high school. You know that HIV will kill people but that condoms can help prevent HIV, and that gonorrhea and *Chlamydia* can be treated with a medicine. You have heard of herpes, but don't know much about it. You have never had a sexually transmitted infection until you found out today that your test was positive for *Chlamydia*. You are shocked, a little angry, and embarrassed

Student Name:_____

SP Initials:_____

1. Sustains a comfortable and supportive environment for patient to respond to sensitive questions (i.e. non-judgmental approach)
   a. Yes
   b. No

2. Establishes dialogue (i.e. checks for understanding, asks for patient feedback, etc.) when sharing information/counseling patient on Chlamydia infection.
   a. Yes
   b. No

3. Student discusses Chlamydia and pap result:
   [ ] Discusses both results.
   [ ] Discusses only Chlamydia or pap result.
   [ ] Does not discuss test results.

Comment: _____

4. Student explains Chlamydia treatment and risks/sequelae of untreated Chlamydia   [ ]
   Student discusses appropriate treatment for Chlamydia and
   and risks/sequelae of disease. [2]
                  [ ] Student discusses risks/sequelae of disease or treatment of
                       Chlamydia, but not both. [1]
                  [ ] Student does not discuss treatment of Chlamydia or
                       risks/sequelae. [0]

Comment: _____

5. Student offers Gardasil vaccine:
                  [ ] Offers patient Gardasil vaccine series.
                  [ ] Does not offer patient Gardasil.

Comment: _____

6. Student offers additional STI screening and discusses sexually transmitted disease prevention:
                  [ ] Student offers additional screening tests and discusses STI prevention. [2]
                  [ ] Student offers additional screening tests or STI prevention, but not both. [1]
                  [ ] Student does not offer any additional screening or discuss STI prevention. [0]

Comment: _____

7. Student takes a menstrual history (menarche, interval, duration, and flow):
                  [ ] Students takes appropriate menstrual history

                  [ ] Student does not take a menstrual history.

Comment: _____

8. Student takes a sexual history (inquires about sexual activity, history of STIs):
                  [ ] Student asked about both items above.
                  [ ] Student asked about only 1 of the items listed above.
                  [ ] Student didn't take a sexual history.

Comment: _____

9. Student asks about substance abuse (alcohol, tobacco, drugs):
    [ ] Student asked all 3 items listed above.
    [ ] Student asked 1-2 items listed above.
    [ ] Student didn't ask about abuse.

Comment: _____

10. Student initiates discussion of contraceptive options (birth control pills, transdermal (Ortho Evra), Nuva Ring, Nexplanon, Depo-Provera, IUD, condoms, diaphragm, cervical cap, spermicidals, abstinence, emergency contraception)
    [ ] Student discusses at least 6 of the items listed above. [2]
    [ ] Student discusses 1-5 items above. [1]
    [ ] Student didn't discuss contraceptive options. [0]

Comment: _____

11. Student discusses risks/benefits/side effects of at least 3 contraceptive options:
    [ ] Student provides accurate information about at least 3 options.
    [ ] Student provides risks/benefits/side effects, but with some inaccurate
        information or for fewer than 3 contraceptive options.
    [ ] Student does not provide risks/benefits/side effects of any
        contraceptive options.

Comment: _____

12. Student discusses appropriate timing of IUD insertion (after negative repeat test) and interval contraception.
    [ ] Student discusses both appropriate timing of IUD and interval plan [2]
    [ ] Student discusses either appropriate timing of IUD insertion or interval plan, but not
both [1]
    [ ] Student does not discuss either. [0]

Comment: _____

13. ADDITIONAL NOTES AND COMMENTS:

_____
_____
_____
_____
_____

Faculty Checklist (FAC)

Faculty Information Sheet: STI and Contraceptive Counseling Scenario 2017

Annie Gibson is a 21-year-old college student (LMP one week ago) who has come to the gynecology clinic to follow up on recent test results. She is also requesting something for birth control. She was seen 3 weeks ago by your colleague in clinic and underwent a pelvic exam (reported as normal in medical record), Pap smear, and testing for gonorrhea and *Chlamydia*. Her test for *Chlamydia* is positive, and her Pap smear was normal. She received a phone call from the clinic to return for an appointment to discuss her lab results.

The student is to obtain an appropriate history, including social history. The student should counsel the patient about the *Chlamydia* infection and its treatment, prevention of future sexually transmitted infections, and contraceptive options. The student will not perform a pelvic exam.

The student should obtain appropriate tests for other STIs, offer Gardasil vaccine, and should finalize with a plan for contraception. Once completed, the student will leave the room to complete a post-encounter exercise form.

Feedback: As time allows, the student may return to the room after completing the post-encounter exercise for feedback by the faculty and standardized patient. **Please ensure the student has completed their post-encounter form prior to any feedback.**

Checklist: Please complete the faculty checklist for each student; the instructions are straightforward and are printed on the checklist.

Please score the student on each of the areas listed below:

Student Part

Post Encounter (Section 1 of 1)

1. Please list any additional studies you would like to order on this patient:

2. If Ms. Gibson chose an IUD for contraception, would you be able to place it today? Why or why not?

3. What is your plan for management of this patient?

References

1. Howley LD. Standardized patients. In: *The comprehensive textbook of healthcare simulation*. New York: Springer; 2013. p. 173–90.
2. Wallace P. Coaching standardized patients: for use in the assessment of clinical competence. New York: Springer Publishing Company; 2006.
3. van Zanten M, Boulet JR, McKinley D. Using standardized patients to assess the interpersonal skills of physicians: six years' experience with a high-stakes certification examination. Health Commun. 2007;22(3):195–205.
4. Cleland JA, Abe K, Rethans JJ. The use of simulated patients in medical education: AMEE guide no 42. Med Teach. 2009;31(6):477–86.
5. Barrows HS. An overview of the uses of standardized patients for teaching and evaluating clinical skills. AAMC Acad Med. 1993;68(6):443–51.
6. Kretzschmar RM. Evolution of the gynecology teaching associate: an education specialist. Am J Obstet Gynecol. 1978;131(4):367–73.
7. Godkins TR, Duffy D, Greenwood J, Stanhope WD. Utilization of simulated patients to teach the routine pelvic examination. Acad Med. 1974;49(12):1174–8.
8. Billings JA, Stoeckle JD. Pelvic examination instruction and the doctor-patient relationship. Acad Med. 1977;52(10):834–9.
9. Holzman GB, Singleton D, Holmes TF, Maatsch JL. Initial pelvic examination instruction: the effectiveness of three contemporary approaches. Am J Obstet Gynecol. 1977;129(2):124–9.
10. Perlmutter JF, Friedman E. Use of a live mannequin for teaching physical diagnosis in gynecology. J Reprod Med. 1974;12(4):163–4.
11. Wånggren K, Pettersson G, Csemiczky G, Gemzell-Danielsson K. Teaching medical students gynaecological examination using professional patients – evaluation of students' skills and feelings. Med Teach. 2005;27(2):130–5.
12. Pickard S, Baraitser P, Rymer J, Piper J. Comparative study. Br Med J. 2003;327(7428):1389–92.
13. Pugh CM, Obadina ET, Aidoo KA. Fear of causing harm: use of mannequin-based simulation to decrease student anxiety prior to interacting with female teaching associates. Teach Learn Med. 2009;21(2):116–20. https://doi.org/10.1080/10401330902791099.
14. Hunter SA, McLachlan A, Ikeda T, Harrison MJ, Galletly DC. Teaching of the sensitive examinations:

an international survey. Open J Prev Med. 2014; https://doi.org/10.4236/ojpm.2014.41007.

15. Fang WL, Hillard PJ, Lindsay RW, Underwood PB. Evaluation of students' clinical and communication skills in performing a gynecologic examination. Acad Med. 1984;59(9):758–60.

16. Kleinman DE, Hage ML, Hoole AJ, Kowlowitz V. Pelvic examination instruction and experience: a comparison of laywoman-trained and physician-trained students. Acad Med. 1996;71(11):1239–43.

17. Pradhan A, Ebert G, Brug P, Swee D, Ananth CV. Evaluating pelvic examination training: does faculty involvement make a difference? A randomized controlled trial. Teach Learn Med. 2010;22(4):293–7.

18. Association of American Medical Colleges. 2005. Recommendations for clinical skills curricula for undergraduate medical education (Committee opinion 500). Retrieved from https://members.aamc.org/eweb/upload/Recommendations%20for%20Clinical%20Skills%20Curricula%202005.pdf.

19. Hammoud MM, Nuthalapaty FS, Goepfert AR, Casey PM, Emmons S, Espey EL, et al. Association of Professors of Gynecology and Obstetrics undergraduate medical education committee. To the point: medical education review of the role of simulators in surgical training. Am J Obstet Gynecol. 2008;199(4):338–43.

20. American College of Obstetricians and Gynecologists (ACOG). 2014. Professional responsibilities in obstetric-gynecologic medical education and training (Committee opinion number 500). Retrieved from ACOG website: http://www.acog.org/Resources-And-Publications/Committee-Opinions/Committee-on-Ethics/Professional-Responsibilities-in-Obstetric-Gynecologic-Medical-Education-and-Training.

21. Duffy JMN, Chequer S, Braddy A, Mylan S, Royuela A, Zamora J, et al. Educational effectiveness of gynaecological teaching associates: a multi-centre randomised controlled trial. BJOG Int J Obstet Gynaecol. 2016;123:1005–10.

22. Jain S, Fox K, Van den Berg P, Hill A, Nilsen S, Olson G, et al. Simulation training impacts student confidence and knowledge for breast and pelvic examination. Med Sci Educ. 2014;24(1):59–64.

23. Smith PP, Choudhury S, Clark TJ. The effectiveness of gynaecological teaching associates in teaching pelvic examination: a systematic review and meta-analysis. Med Educ. 2015;49(12):1197–206.

24. Hagen U. Respect for acting. Hoboken: John Wiley & Sons; 1973.

25. Association of Standardized Patient Educators (ASPE). n.d. Retrieved April 2, 2017, from http://www.aspeducators.org/.

26. Janjua A, Smith P, Chu J, Raut N, Malick S, Gallos I, et al. The effectiveness of gynaecology teaching associates in teaching pelvic examination to medical students: a randomised controlled trial. Eur J Obstet Gynecol Reprod Biol. 2017;210:58–63.

27. Downing SM, Yudkowsky R. Assessment in health professions education. New York: Routledge; 2009.

28. Janjua A, Burgess L, Clark TJ. A qualitive study of the impact and acceptability of gynaecological teaching associates. MedEdPublish. 2016;5. https://doi.org/10.15694/mep.2016.000128.

29. Undergraduate Medical Education Committee Faculty. 2008. APGO Medical Student Educational Objectives (8th ed.). Retrieved from https://www.apgo.org/educational-resources/basic-clinical-skills/pelvic-exam/.

30. Siwe K, Wijma K, Stjernquist M, Wijma B. Medical students learning the pelvic examination: comparison of outcome in terms of skills between a professional patient and a clinical patient model. Patient Educ Couns. 2007;68(3):211–7.

31. Livingstone RA, Ostrow DN. Professional patient-instructors in the teaching of the pelvic examination. Am J Obstet Gynecol. 1978;132(1):64–7.

32. Seago BL, Ketchum JM, Willett RM. Pelvic examination skills training with genital teaching associates and a pelvic simulator: does sequence matter? Simul Healthc. 2012;7(2):95–101.

Simulation Modalities for Obstetrics and Gynecology

11

Erin Higgins and Tamika C. Auguste

Introduction

Simulation is a key teaching modality used in obstetrics and gynecology (Ob/Gyn) at various levels of training across the country. Obstetrics, in particular, is a field in which emergency situations frequently arise, requiring the cooperation of various players in the healthcare model to deliver high-quality patient care [1]. As such, teamwork training is especially important in this field, as it provides the opportunity for multidisciplinary training and can be used to improve communication between a diverse group of learners. In contrast with teamwork training, skills-based simulation is important for providers to hone procedural skills outside the clinical setting. The simulators used to teach such skills can range from low-fidelity models made with common household items to high-fidelity models sold by various biomedical companies that closely approximate human anatomy.

A diverse group of healthcare providers are involved in providing care in this field, including medical students, residents, nursing staff, advance practice clinicians (e.g., physician assistants, nurse practitioners), and attending physicians. Simulation education in this field thus must endeavor to reach a wide range of learners at differing skill levels. While simulation has been demonstrated to be beneficial to medical education at all levels of training, there are certain considerations that limit the widespread implementation of simulation in Ob/Gyn. Financial constraints are of particular importance, as some simulators can exceed $100,000. Additionally, there may be space limitations at many institutions that restrict the ability of educators to establish and maintain a dedicated space for simulation training. Finally, there is the issue of availability of knowledgeable staff members who are trained in assessment, debriefing, and design and implementation of a simulation curriculum.

In this chapter, we will review the various modalities of simulation in Ob/Gyn. Task and box trainers, while more simplistic in their design, allow the learner to focus on specific skills, while full-body mannequins can be used together with multidisciplinary teamwork training to emphasize communication and teamwork. Virtual reality and robotic trainers are high-fidelity task trainers that more realistically resemble clinical scenarios to improve skills and technique. The use of cadavers, a fundamental part of the general medical school curriculum, allows the learner to hone surgical skills and

E. Higgins (✉)
Department of Obstetrics and Gynecology, Cleveland Clinic, Cleveland, OH, USA

T. C. Auguste
Department of Obstetrics and Gynecology, MedStar Washington Hospital Center, Washington, DC, USA
e-mail: Tamika.c.auguste@medstar.net

acquire a better understanding of human anatomy. Finally, standardized patients provide learners with the opportunity to interact with a live person to role-play specific scenarios ranging from obtaining a history to delivering bad news.

> **Key Learning Points**
> This chapter will demonstrate the wide range of simulation modalities that exist for medical education and training, allowing instructors to teach virtually any skill or competency. The specific simulator used will depend on the goal to be achieved and can be selected based on available resources at an institution.

Body

Background

While initially used in aviation and military training, simulation-based training has quickly become a key training modality in most medical disciplines [2]. Removing live patients to focus on clinical skills allows the learner to make mistakes in a risk-free environment. Simulation has been identified as a useful tool to help prevent medical errors and improve patient safety. Simulation also allows for repetition as a teaching skill, permitting the learner to develop motor skills and muscle memory necessary for many common tasks while protecting real patients from the risk of novice learners. Additionally, it can be used as an assessment tool, aiding observers in the evaluation of learners of various skill levels [3].

Simulation and Medical Training

Simulation-based training has been shown to be effective at various levels of medical training [3]. For medical students who otherwise would have their first patient encounters on the wards, simulation allows honing of technical skills and interpersonal communication prior to an in situ clinical interaction. Simulation creates a safe learning environment in which errors are not life-threatening and controlled clinical interactions can be used as a teaching device through the use of reflection and discussion [4]. A standardized teaching environment also allows learners to complete tasks and demonstrate proficiency in a reproducible clinical setting that does not vary based on individual patient characteristics. Medical students exposed to simulation training prior to the start of their clinical Ob/Gyn clerkship have demonstrated better technical skills, higher scores on cumulative examinations, and increased levels of confidence compared to students who received traditional lecture-based instruction [5–7]. This confidence translates into increased participation on the clinical side, with simulation-trained students demonstrating more active involvement in real-life clinical encounters [8]. Specifically, high-fidelity models have been shown to improve students' understanding of the pathophysiology of labor and of intrapartum procedures, when compared to low-fidelity models [9].

In graduate medical education, work hour restrictions have limited the clinical exposure residents receive, especially for rare but high-risk events. The use of simulation allows residents to acquire the skills and knowledge necessary to manage infrequent clinical scenarios that require quick intervention [10]. Ob/Gyn residents taught with the use of simulation have been found to be better equipped to handle obstetric emergencies including postpartum hemorrhage and shoulder dystocia [3, 11]. The use of box trainers has similarly shown improved surgical performance in the operating room [12]. Simulation can also be used for evaluation of technical skills in consideration of promotion to the next year of training [13]. Additionally, simulation has been utilized for remediation during residency training, and it has been considered for integration into licensure and reentry programs for attending providers [14].

Implementation of a Simulation Program

Several key elements are necessary prior to the implementation of a simulation program. Identifying and securing a facility in which to carry out simulation training is one of the first steps. While task and box trainers take up relatively little space, full-body mannequins and cadavers must have dedicated storage space and skilled maintenance staff. Virtual reality and other high-fidelity models require regular upkeep and system upgrades from time to time. If training is to be carried out in situ, there remains the issue of storage and maintenance of materials.

A dedicated simulation team is also an important consideration in creating a simulation program. Trained and motivated faculty members are a necessity to develop and conduct simulation training sessions properly. Since simulation is a teaching modality that can be applied to a diverse group of learners, it is important to create a robust curriculum that includes modules ranging from novice to expert level. In addition to faculty, a simulation center benefits from trained staff that are knowledgeable about assembling modules, conducting simulation programs, leading debriefs, and maintaining equipment. A regularly scheduled program (i.e., monthly sessions) and protected time, both for faculty and learners, are also helpful to provide adequate exposure to and opportunity to use the available devices.

Cost remains a significant barrier to widespread implementation of simulation training in undergraduate and graduate medical education. Equipment can be purchased from any of a number of large simulation companies. Low-fidelity models have the benefit of being affordable, requiring little or no maintenance, and being simple to understand and use. High-fidelity models, on the other hand, such as full-body mannequins that can respond to interventions such as medication administration, are often prohibitively expensive and require high-level familiarity with the device to properly execute its functions [2].

Research on the effectiveness of simulation in improving patient safety may be limited by quantity of quality studies, but several of those in the literature undeniably support the use of simulation to improve patient safety. Draycott et al. showed that neonatal outcomes improved following simulation-based training for shoulder dystocia. They were able to show a positive effect of simulation-based training on patient safety through a 51% reduction in the 5-min Apgar <7

[15]. Phipps et al. reviewed an 18-month period after simulation-based team training and saw improvements in patient outcomes, teamwork, and communication, in addition to enhanced perceptions in patient safety [16]. Another example of quality research comes from Pratt et al., who did a Joint Commission study that prospectively collected perinatal morbidity and mortality data from three hospitals, one of which implemented TeamSTEPPS only, one that implemented TeamSTEPPS with simulation, and one that did not implement a safety program at all. For the hospital that did TeamSTEPPS with simulation, there was a statistically significant and persistent reduction of perinatal morbidity by 37% when comparing pre- and post-intervention data [17].

Simulation Modalities in Ob/Gyn

Various models, ranging from low-cost box trainers to sophisticated virtual reality devices, exist for the simulation of skills in medicine, a wide variety of which can be applied to obstetrics and gynecology.

Task Trainers

Task trainers represent the most basic of simulation modalities yet can reliably teach specific procedural tasks to both new providers and those wanting to improve upon existing skills. Commonly used task trainers in Ob/Gyn include the use of a hemi-pelvis for teaching delivery techniques such as vacuum and forceps application, beef tongue or chicken breast for practicing cervical conization procedures, and papayas for simulating manual vacuum aspiration procedures. While often simplistic in their construction, these training devices are inexpensive and intuitive, and many of the supplies can be purchased at easily accessible stores such as grocery stores and craft stores.

Box Trainers

Box trainers approximate the surgical field as a low-fidelity model and provide a setting in which laparoscopic skills can be practiced and enhanced. From simple skills such as peg transfer to more complex techniques like intracorporeal knot tying, learners can gain a number of important skills and additionally benefit from repetition of action. Such trainers allow for the use of real laparoscopic instruments, which helps to replicate the clinical environment with haptic feedback and depth perception. Like task trainers, box trainers can often be created at home using inexpensive items including a box, light bulb, webcam, and home PC or laptop.

Box trainers provide the benefit of being small and portable, allowing learners to practice at home or in the hospital at their own convenience. Performance on box trainers, however, is limited by external evaluation by qualified staff members, and individual scoring is thus vulnerable to inter- and intra-observer differences [18]. Additionally, box trainers tend to have lower anatomic and haptic fidelity than other modalities.

Virtual Reality Trainers

Virtual reality (VR) trainers incorporate both a physical handpiece and a computer-based program to mimic surgical procedures. Utilizing sophisticated software, VR trainers register all movements and are able to provide precise and objective results, aiding evaluation of a trainee's performance. This feedback allows trainees to monitor their performance and focus on self-improvement. VR trainers emphasize hand-eye coordination, manual dexterity, and economy of motion while providing familiarity with instruments and surgical sequence of events [2].

VR can be used to teach basic surgical skills, including laparoscopic suturing and knot tying, and to simulate full clinical scenarios when employed with an anatomically correct mannequin. Haptic feedback can be incorporated into the handpiece but has not been widely utilized to date [19]. Several iterations of VR trainers exist, which each generation incorporating different levels of sophistication. First-generation VR simulators involve the manipulation of abstract objects in space for the development of physical skills, while second-generation trainers incorporate anatomic structures, thereby making the simulation more clinically relevant. Third-generation VR trainers combine advanced software programs with an anatomic mannequin to

create a more realistic model that approximates a surgical setting. Finally, fourth-generation VR trainers combine didactic instruction with hands-on skills practice to create an all-encompassing model to improve surgical competence, including both physical skills and decision-making [2]. These include the commercially available models LapSimGyn® (Surgical Science Sweden, Göteborg, Sweden), SimSurgery® (Simsurgery, Oslo, Norway), and Simbionix® (Simbionix-Baker, Cleveland, OH, USA). Hybrid models incorporate box trainers with VR technology to enhance the training environment with real instruments and physical materials, such as ProMIS® simulator (Haptica, Boston, MA, USA).

VR trainers have demonstrated performance differences between intermediate and expert surgeons, lending construct validity to these models [20]. The same study showed improvement of learners' skills, leading to shortened procedure time. A randomized controlled study by Larsen et al. also demonstrated shorter time to achieve competency when trainees used VR combined with traditional clinical training, compared to traditional training alone [21]. Additionally, a Cochrane review suggested that VR training leads to shorter operating time, fewer errors, and better economy of motion in novice laparoscopic surgeons [22]. Studies have not, however, demonstrated a specific benefit to VR trainers, as learners have been noted to perform at a similar level on the less expensive box trainers with regard to task completion times and number of errors made. Further research remains to be done to determine the predictive validity of these systems.

A limitation to VR devices remains with regard to cost, as such devices are extremely expensive (in excess of $100,000). Additionally, such models require maintenance and periodic upgrades, both of which incur additional expenses.

Robotic Simulators

As robotic laparoscopic surgery becomes more common, there is a need for specific simulation training in this modality. Robotic equipment differs from traditional laparoscopy in that it provides a three-dimensional view and surgeons utilize a console at which one can sit while operating [23]. Robotic instruments provide greater range of motion compared to laparoscopic instruments and eliminate the fulcrum effect, in which surgeons move in directions opposite to that of the instrument. Robotic surgery eliminates haptic feedback, however, which represents a significant disadvantage for those familiar with traditional methods. Additionally, achieving master-level skills in robotics requires a significant investment of time in training [24]. Some of the robotic system manufacturers do provide a simulator of sorts for training purposes. This is often an additional pack that can be placed on the actual robotic system that allows for simulated practice. The cost of such add-ons to the robotic system represents an additional barrier, as the baseline da Vinci Surgical System® (Intuitive Surgical, Sunnyvale, CA, USA) costs over $1 million.

Mannequin Trainers

Full-body mannequins can be employed in Ob/Gyn simulation training. Specifically, they can be used to simulate obstetric emergencies before, during, and after delivery, including such as a maternal code, postpartum hemorrhage, and eclampsia. The system includes vital sign and external fetal monitoring systems. Other mannequin-based systems can be used to simulation gynecologic clinical scenarios, such as intraoperative hemorrhage. These high-tech devices exist in wireless forms, can be programmed for a particular clinical scenario, and are fully responsive to interventions [2]. Mannequin trainers have the benefit of more closely approximating the natural clinical setting compared to less sophisticated modules. Such mannequin-based devices can be cost prohibitive, however, with expenses exceeding $100,000, and require a dedicated storage location, given their large size. Portable devices are becoming increasingly common, which allows for more widespread access to training drills using these mannequins.

Part-task trainers (PTTs) represent a mannequin-based simulation device that replicates an anatomic structure to practice a specific procedural skill, such as cervical cerclage or labor cervical examination [25]. These devices have the advantage of lower cost and smaller size compared to full-body mannequins. PTTs vary in their fidelity, depending on the materials used in their construction.

Cadaveric Trainers

Cadavers, a mainstay of medical education since the sixteenth century, have been deemed the gold standard of surgical training prior to clinical encounters. Cadaveric training is similarly used in Ob/Gyn for ex vivo procedural skill practice, including lymph node dissection and repair of pelvic floor disorders. These models have the benefit of exact representations of human anatomy but are limited by cost, availability, degradation, and the possibility of disease transmission [2]. There are also limitations to the storage and usage of human tissue in some simulation labs, thus creating another barrier. The physical space that stores and utilized human cadavers must be to a certain standard regarding handling of human tissue.

Standardized Patients

Standardized patients (SPs) are trained individuals who portray a patient to teach and evaluate clinical skills in a simulated environment. Commonly used in medical schools nationwide and a prominent part of the United States Medical Licensing Exam (USMLE), SPs help trainees to perfect their bedside manner and exam technique through feedback from an impartial observer [2]. Interactions with SPs can also be used to explore difficult topics and practice counseling techniques for less common clinical scenarios. These encounters can also be videotaped and later reviewed by a larger group in a debriefing session.

The use of SPs is advantageous in the authentic nature of interacting with a live human while protecting real patients. Additionally, SPs are able to simulate a diverse array of clinical scenarios, lending wide applicability of this simulation modality [2]. SPs can provide immediate feedback and are highly standardized, allowing for reduced bias in evaluation. Limitations to the use of SPs include cost (both for training and employment of SPs in an evaluative scenario) and restricted fidelity with regard to specific physical conditions.

Teamwork Training

In previous decades, efforts to improve patient outcomes typically focused on the individual provider level. However, many studies have demonstrated that complications and sentinel events most commonly result from communication failures [1, 15]. The Institute of Medicine's report *To Err is Human* recommended the use of simulation to promote a culture of patient safety and reduce errors [26]. In addition to promoting an individual's skill development, teamwork training has been demonstrated to improve communication between members of the healthcare team and improve overall team performance. Multidisciplinary team-based training, involving inter- and intraprofessional teamwork, can be carried out in a variety of settings to identify lapses in knowledge and training and determine best practices for specific units [27]. Implementation of such trainings on perinatal units, with or without simulation training, has been shown to decrease perinatal morbidity [17]. While most programs to date have focused on obstetrics, there also exists a need for teamwork training in a gynecologic surgery setting.

Summary

Simulation in Ob/Gyn is an exciting field with an active focus on developing new approaches to medical education and training. With a wide range of teaching modalities available, the opportunities for small group, multidisciplinary, and in situ simulation sessions are quickly expanding. While establishing curriculum and purchasing equipment can be a daunting prospect, simulation has repeatedly been shown to be beneficial at all levels of training while simultaneously promoting patient safety through improved communication and teamwork.

References

1. Daniels K, Auguste T. Moving forward in patient safety: multidisciplinary team training. Semin Perinatol. 2013;37(3):146–50.
2. Levine A, De Maria S Jr, Schwartz A, Sim A. *The comprehensive textbook of healthcare simulation.* New York: Springer; 2014. Print.
3. Deering S, Auguste T, Lockrow E. Obstetric simulation for medical student, resident, and fellow education. Semin Perinatol. 2013;37(3):143–5.
4. Macedonia CR, Gherman RB, Satin AJ. Simulation laboratories for training in obstetrics and gynecology. Obstet Gynecol. 2003;102:388–92.
5. Deering SH, Hodor J, Wylen M, Poggi S, Nielsen P, Satin AJ. Additional training with an obstetric simulator improves medical student comfort with basic procedures. Simul Healthc. 2006;1(1):32–4.
6. Jude DC, Gilbert GG, Magrane D. Simulation training in the obstetrics and gynecology clerkship. Am J Obstet Gynecol. 2006;195(5):1489–92. Epub 2006 Jul 17.
7. Nitsche JF, Shumard KM, Fino NF, Denney JM, Quinn KH, Bailey JC, Jijon R, Huang C, Kesty K, Whitecar PW, Grandis AS, Brost BC. Effectiveness of labor cervical examination simulation in medical student education. Obstet Gynecol. 2015;126(Suppl 4):13S–20S.
8. Dayal AK, Fisher N, Magrane D, Goffman D, Bernstein PS, Katz NT. Simulation training improves medical students' learning experiences when performing real vaginal deliveries. Simul Healthc. 2009;4(3):155–9.
9. Scholz C, Mann C, Kopp V, Kost B, Kainer F, Fischer MR. High-fidelity simulation increases obstetric self-assurance and skills in undergraduate medical students. J Perinat Med. 2012;40(6):607–13.
10. Fisher N, Bernstein PS, Satin A, Pardanani S, Heo H, Merkatz IR, Goffman D. Resident training for eclampsia and magnesium toxicity management: simulation or traditional lecture? Am J Obstet Gynecol. 2010;203(4):379.e1–5. https://doi.org/10.1016/j.ajog.2010.06.010. Epub 2010 Aug 5.
11. Deering S, Poggi S, Macedonia C, Gherman R, Satin AJ. Improving resident competency in the management of shoulder dystocia with simulation training. Obstet Gynecol. 2004;103:1224–8.
12. Kiely DJ, Stephanson K, Ross S. Assessing image quality of low-cost laparoscopic box trainers: options for residents training at home. Simul Healthc. 2011;6(5):292–8.
13. Winkel AF, Gillespie C, Uquillas K, Zabar S, Szyld D. Assessment of developmental progress using an objective structured clinical examination-simulation hybrid examination for obstetrics and gynecology residents. J Surg Educ. 2016;73(2):230–7.
14. Chang E. The role of simulation training in obstetrics: a healthcare training strategy dedicated to per-

formance improvement. Curr Opin Obstet Gynecol. 2013;25(6):482–6.

15. Draycott TJ, Crofts JF, Ash JP, et al. Improving neonatal outcome through practical shoulder dystocia training. Obstet Gynecol. 2008;112:14–20.

16. Phipps MG, Lindquist DG, McConaughey E, et al. Outcomes from a labor and delivery team training program with simulation component. Am J Obstet Gynecol. 2012;206(1):3–9.

17. Pratt S, Mann S, Salisbury M, et al. Impact of CRM-based team training in obstetric outcomes and clinician patient safety attitudes. Jt Comm J Qual Patient Saf. 2007;33:720–5.

18. Newmark J, Dandolu V, Milner R, Grewal H, Harbison S, Hernandez E. Correlating virtual reality and box trainer tasks in the assessment of laparoscopic surgical skills. Am J Obstet Gynecol. 2007;197(5):546.e1–4.

19. Botden SM, Torab F, Buzink SN, Jakimowicz JJ. The importance of haptic feedback in laparoscopic suturing training and the additive value of virtual reality simulation. Surg Endosc. 2008;22(5):1214–22. Epub 2007 Oct 18.

20. Burden C, Oestergaard J, Larsen CR. Integration of laparoscopic virtual-reality simulation into gynaecology training. BJOG. 2011;118(Suppl 3):5–10.

21. Larsen CR, Soerensen JL, Grantcharov TP, Dalsgaard T, Schouenborg L, Ottosen C, et al. Effect of virtual reality training on laparoscopic surgery: randomised controlled trial. BMJ. 2009;338:61802.

22. Gurusamy KS, Aggarwal R, Palanivelu L, Davidson BR. Virtual reality training for surgical trainees in laparoscopic surgery. Cochrane Database Syst Rev. 2009;1:CD006575.

23. Ballantyne GH, Moll F. The da Vinci telerobotic surgical system: the virtual operative field and the telepresence surgery. Surg Clin N Am. 2003;83(6):1293–304.

24. Schreuder HW, Wolswijk R, Zweemer RP, Schijven MP, Verheijen RH. Training and learning robotic surgery, time for a more structured approach: a systematic review. BJOG. 2012;119(2):137–49. https://doi.org/10.1111/j.1471-0528.2011.03139.x. Epub 2011 Oct 10.

25. Nitsche JF, Brost BC. A cervical cerclage task trainer for maternal-fetal medicine fellows and obstetrics/gynecology residents. Simul Healthc. 2012;7(5):321–5.

26. Kohn LT, Corrigan JM, Donaldson MS, editors. To err is human: building a safer health system. Washington, DC: Institute of Medicine (US) Committee on Quality of Health Care in America/ National Academies Press (US); 2000.

27. Eppich W, Howard V, Vozenilek J, Curran I. Simulation-based team training in healthcare. Simul Healthc. 2011;6(Suppl):S14–9.

Part III

Simulation of Obstetrics

Fundamental Obstetric Procedures

12

Komal Bajaj and Michael Meguerdichian

Introduction

Pregnant women receive care from a myriad of health professionals, especially during the intrapartum and postpartum periods. Fundamental clinical obstetrics skills such as cervical exams, vaginal deliveries, and episiotomy repair may be difficult to acquire for several reasons. First, they necessarily involve an intimate examination. Second, the fast pace of labor and delivery can limit the time that students and new providers have to spend learning these skills, and work hour restrictions may further compound these time constraints. Within the United States, obstetrics and gynecology residents have seen an 18.6%

decrease in the number of vaginal births performed during residency from 320 in 2002 to 273 in 2012 [1]. This is speculated to be attributable to changing patient populations, a changing medicolegal climate, and updates in evidence-based practices. Male healthcare trainees may have further limited opportunity to practice core obstetric skills due to patient preference for female providers [2]. Simulation has been effectively integrated into the majority of medical, nursing, and midwifery training programs to teach basic obstetric procedures and address these potential barriers to gaining experience [3, 4]. In fact, a 2011 survey by the Association of American Medical Colleges revealed that 60% of obstetrics-gynecology clerkships in training hospitals utilize simulation to teach undergraduate medical education [5]. Simulation is also a core component of nursing training in obstetrics and has been shown to improve perceptions of learning and self-efficacy [6].

Furthermore, simulation for basic obstetric procedures has been deployed in a variety of healthcare settings ranging from rural, resource-limited environments to tertiary care centers [7]. With simulation, educators can focus learners on both the technical and communication skills required for these procedures [8]. This chapter highlights the application of simulation to augment training for cervical exams, assessment of fetal position, spontaneous vaginal delivery, and perineal laceration repair.

K. Bajaj (✉)
NYC Health + Hospitals Simulation Center, Bronx, NY, USA

Albert Einstein College of Medicine, Bronx, NY, USA
e-mail: komal.bajaj@nychhc.org

M. Meguerdichian
NYC Health + Hospitals Simulation Center, Bronx, NY, USA

Harlem Hospital Center, Emergency Department/ H+H Simulation Center, New York, NY, USA
e-mail: michael.meguerdichian@nychhc.org

© Springer International Publishing AG, part of Springer Nature 2019
S. Deering et al. (eds.), *Comprehensive Healthcare Simulation: Obstetrics and Gynecology*,
Comprehensive Healthcare Simulation, https://doi.org/10.1007/978-3-319-98995-2_12

Key Learning Points
- A wide array of obstetric procedures can be trained for with currently available task trainer simulators.
- There are many low-cost options that are available to create simulators to train many obstetric procedures.
- Sometimes simulation training for obstetric procedures can include a hybrid simulation where both communication and technical skills are assessed.

Cervical Exams

Digital cervical exams are a critical skill in the management of patients on the labor and delivery unit. A cervical exam includes assessment of cervical dilation (measured in centimeters), cervical effacement, and fetal station [9]. When the presenting part is a fetal head, the position of the vertex can be determined by palpating the fetal sutures and fontanelles. Determination of the position of the fetal vertex is a mandatory component of planning for operative delivery as misapplication can result in significant injury to the fetus. Furthermore, knowledge of position of the fetal vertex can guide counseling during labor. For example, a persistent occiput posterior position complicates 4.7% of pregnancies and is associated with a longer labor and increased risk of cesarean birth [10].

In the traditional training paradigm for cervical examinations, both the trainee and a supervising provider examine a patient in order to assess the trainee's skill and provide feedback. This paradigm exposes women to additional cervical examinations which can be uncomfortable and can potentially increase the risk of infection during labor if the membranes are ruptured. With the advances in simulation education and technology, the cervical exam can now effectively be coached without exposing the patients to undue stress. Several different approaches to digital labor cervical exam simulation training have been described in the literature.

After a 30-minute standardized course on cervical examination, Arias et al. randomized fifth-year medical students to perform 0, 10, or 30 examinations using a shoebox-shaped simulator with silicon external genitalia prior to examinations in the clinical environment (Health Edco) [11]. Cervical exam accuracy was ascertained by comparing student examination of a patient with his/her clinical supervisor's exam, and there was a significant improvement in the accuracy scores between the control group and the groups that performed at least ten simulated procedures.

Nitsche et al. also sought to assess the effectiveness of cervical exam simulation during the medical student obstetrics and gynecology clerkship [12]. Medical students were assigned to receive a series of simulation-based training in either cervical examination or vaginal delivery. For the cervical examination simulation, both a self-produced simulator made from polyvinyl chloride pipe and silicon rubber models made by Human Analog Applications were utilized [12, 13]. During their final assessments, all students were assessed on their cervical exam skills by completing ten cervical examinations on standardized task trainers where dilation was predetermined. The students who underwent cervical examination simulation training were significantly more accurate in assessing dilation and effacement when compared to students who received vaginal delivery simulation training. The majority of students were able to achieve competence after an average of 76 repetitions, and the investigators estimated that in order to get all trainees to competence, a training program would require at least 100 repetitions of the cervical exam on the simulator.

In an effort to develop a low-cost task trainer utilizing commonly available household items, Shea and Rivera crafted a simulator using citrus fruit and tube socks [14]. The technical report describes circles of various sizes cut into the fruit rind representing the dilating "cervix" and placement of the fruit in the tube sock as a "vagina." The model aimed to train prelicensure nursing students to ascertain cervical dilation and effacement. Another inexpensive task trainer which has the added feature of simulating a fetal vertex has been using models created from a softball and clay [15].

Implementation Considerations

Simulation-based cervical examination training draws heavily on the use of task trainers. Prior to acquiring a commercially available part-task trainer or producing one locally, one must carefully consider the needs of the learner group and the learning objectives. It is usually advisable to design a simulation program where participants can perform multiple repetitions on a range of clinical circumstances – from a closed, uneffaced cervix to one where the fetal vertex is at +2 station. In assessing the fetal station and the position of the vertex, it is important to select a trainer that incorporates the fetal head and can address these exam components. Also, remember that the simulation component can be augmented by additional educational strategies, including a didactic and/or cervical examination within the clinical unit.

Manual Assessment of Fetal Position

Determining fetal position is an essential part of antepartum and intrapartum counseling. While ultrasound is often applied to confirm fetal position, this modality may not always be readily available and requires additional technical expertise. The Leopold maneuvers are a systematic set of four maneuvers aimed at determining fetal position and estimating fetal weight through palpation of the fetus through the maternal abdomen.

Diez-Goni et al. sought to perform a learning curve-cumulative summation (LC-CUSUM) test regarding the ability of students to correctly carry out Leopold maneuvers by combining simulation-based training and clinical experience [16]. Medical students were trained to carry out 50 Leopold maneuvers on different fetal positions using a thoracic abdominal maternity model (Maternity Model G4000, Medical Simulator), and a LC-CUSUM was plotted for each student. Sixty percent of students achieved proficiency, with between 13 and 37 attempts required to attain this level. Two months later, the students performed the Leopold maneuvers on five pregnant women, and all students had at least a 60% success rate when carrying out the maneuvers on

pregnant patients. The authors determined that because of the differences observed between students in the number of attempts needed for achieving proficiency in Leopold maneuvers, students learning curves can be different and may need to be individualized.

Deering et al. assessed the use of simulators to train third-year medical students on basic obstetrical procedural skills, including Leopold maneuvers, during their obstetric clerkship. One group received training on a computerized anthropomorphic robotic birthing simulator (NOELLE, Gaumard Scientific) at the beginning of the rotation, and the other group received standard didactics without simulation. At the end of rotation evaluations, the team found that simulation-trained students were significantly more comfortable with basic procedures including Leopold maneuvers than the didactic-only group [17].

Implementation Considerations

As mentioned previously, there are multiple simulator options that can be used for this training. After an explanation and demonstration of how to perform Leopold maneuvers, the simulation-based component should allow for multiple repetitions of the procedure spanning a variety of fetal positions with feedback after each attempt. As this is not an invasive procedure, performing this on actual patients on labor and delivery after training is an excellent way to both practice and demonstrate transfer of skills.

Spontaneous Vaginal Delivery

A spontaneous vaginal delivery is an emotional event that requires a well-choreographed sequence of steps. The procedure begins with the positioning of the patient, the protection of the perineum to avoid lacerations as the head crowns, the delivery itself, and the third stage of labor which is the delivery of the placenta. Each of these steps can be the subject of a simulated opportunity to provide coaching and feedback. Furthermore, a simulated vaginal birth scenario can provide an opportunity to debrief and focus on the critical teamwork and communication skills needed. It also provides a chance to practice the nuances of more complex deliveries such as those complicated by prematurity, precipitous birth, or even a shoulder dystocia.

Along with technical skills and team training, simulated vaginal birth can be considered as a tool to maintain skills of providers who rarely perform the procedure. Reese et al. surveyed active duty Army family physicians regarding their comfort level in performing procedures prior to and after deployment. Family physicians deployed to support combat operations felt less comfortable with critical clinical skills including vaginal deliveries after returning back to their regular hospitals, highlighting an opportunity for refresher training for health professionals who desire to return to their obstetric practices [18]. Similarly, to train emergency department staff on the teamwork and skills associated with rarely encountered obstetric procedures such as vaginal delivery, Cooper et al. developed a simulation-based curriculum using PROMPT (Limbs N' Things) task trainers [19].

Simulation training embedded into medical student OB/GYN clerkships has also demonstrated increased student confidence and/or involvement in actual births [17, 20–22]. For example, Dayal et al. randomized 33 students to receive either standard didactics or simulation-based training utilizing a Noelle birthing simulator [20]. All students were then assessed on 11 critical skills using a competency-based assessment tool (see Table 12.1) both 1 week and

Table 12.1 Students clinical skills assessment (for simulated vaginal deliveries) [20]

Critical action	Action performed	
	Yes	No
Controls fetal head		
Supports perineum		
Checks for nuchal cord		
Delivers anterior shoulder		
Delivers posterior shoulder		
Delivers abdomen and legs		
Clamps and cuts cord		
Delivers placenta		
Performs fundal massage		
Placental inspection		
Inspection of the perineum		

5 weeks into their clerkship. Clerkship logs demonstrated that simulation-trained students participated in more deliveries than control students (9.8 versus 6.2) and reported increased confidence in their skills. The overall delivery performance score was also significantly higher in the simulation group when compared with controls at week 1 and week 5.

Physician assistant programs also include preclinical and clinical instruction in pediatrics and women's health. Donkers et al. sought to determine whether a simulation experience would increase physician assistant students' comfort level in caring for obstetric patients [15]. Each student participated in a series of simulations, including a normal vaginal delivery and blind cervical dilation assessment using the softball and clay model previously discussed. Students were asked to rate their comfort level before and after the simulation and provide information regarding their obstetrics clinical experience level. Comfort levels were significantly increased post session and were not affected by experience level.

Easter et al. designed a simulation-based curriculum for OB/GYN residents focusing on twin vaginal delivery, a procedure which is declining in frequency. Using a Noelle maternal birthing simulator (Gaumard), the delivery of the second twin was complicated by bradycardia, prompting the residents to consider mode of delivery. The trainees were surveyed pre- and post-simulation regarding knowledge, experience, attitudes, and comfort with twin vaginal birth. The debriefing centered around expedited-delivery decision-making. Knowledge of twin delivery improved after simulation, and more residents reported they would strongly counsel a patient to attempt vaginal birth (33.3–50%) [23].

Implementation Considerations for Teaching Vaginal Delivery

Simulation for vaginal delivery can be done with a focus on technical skills, such as hand placement and maneuvers, or in a more comprehensive manner combining both technical and communication/teamwork skills. The simulator you will need is determined by how you choose to approach the training. Some suggestions with regard to curriculum focus and simulators are outlined in Table 12.2 (Fig. 12.1).

After determining the learning objectives and choosing a simulator, you will need to design the simulation station to address these. If you are attempting to provide more structured feedback, then creating an evaluation form (as seen in Table 12.1) may also be helpful.

Perineal Repair

Third- and fourth-degree perineal lacerations complicate 0.1–15% of births and are associated with instrumental delivery and episiotomy [25, 26]. Third-degree lacerations (where the anal sphincter is torn) and fourth-degree lacerations (involving the sphincter as well as rectal mucosa)

Table 12.2 Outline of curriculum focus and simulators

Curriculum focus	Considerations
Management of the patient positioning	If this skill is a desirable component of a simulation program, part-task trainers with lower extremities or a full-body simulator will be required
Communication with patient	For curricula that include elements of patient counseling or coaching during labor, a hybrid simulation is required, where a part-task trainer and standardized/simulated patient can be combined to allow for practice of technical and communication skills simultaneously [24] (see Fig. 12.1)
Ability to standardize delivery parameters (vital signs/delivery mechanics)	A full-body, high-technology simulator will allow for a pre-programmed, highly reproducible labor and delivery experience
Portability of simulator	If the use of the simulator is to be utilized in multiple center-based sites and/or in situ environments, consider portability and ease of operability. A full-body mannequin will likely have additional technical and storage requirements compared to a part-task trainer

can have long-term sequelae including anal incontinence and sexual dysfunction [27, 28]. A survey of practicing obstetricians in Canada revealed a wide range of experience and approach to the repair of obstetric anal sphincter injuries, highlighting the need for additional training in this area [28].

Several part-task trainers used to simulate obstetric anal sphincter injury have been shown to be effective teaching tools. For example, after experiencing a workshop that included a lecture, instructional video, and practice on a task trainer, OB/GYN residents completed a written exam and objective structured assessment of technical skills (OSATS). Six months later, the same residents, along with another group that had not completed the workshop, took the same posttests. Residents who had participated in the simulation workshop demonstrated higher written examination and OSATS scores and maintained their skills for 6 months [29].

With regard to actual models, a beef tongue model has been applied in several studies demonstrating improved learner confidence [30]. When comparing the beef tongue model to a "sponge perineum" model constructed from a two-layer car washing sponge, both models proved to be effective tools at increasing residents' knowledge and confidence related to obstetric laceration repair [31].

Recently, Illston et al. reported a modification to enhance the realism of the previously described beef tongue model, substituting beef tripe for anal mucosa and chicken leg muscles for the anal sphincter [32].

Implementation Considerations

Task trainers are the mainstay of simulation-based perineal laceration repair training and can be seamlessly integrated into a mixed-modality training program. Commercial models constructed from a variety of synthetic materials are also available. Trainers made from locally sourced items are low cost and therefore afford a lower participant-to-model ratio. Furthermore, the beef model may allow for a more realistic sur-

Fig. 12.1 Hybrid birthing simulator

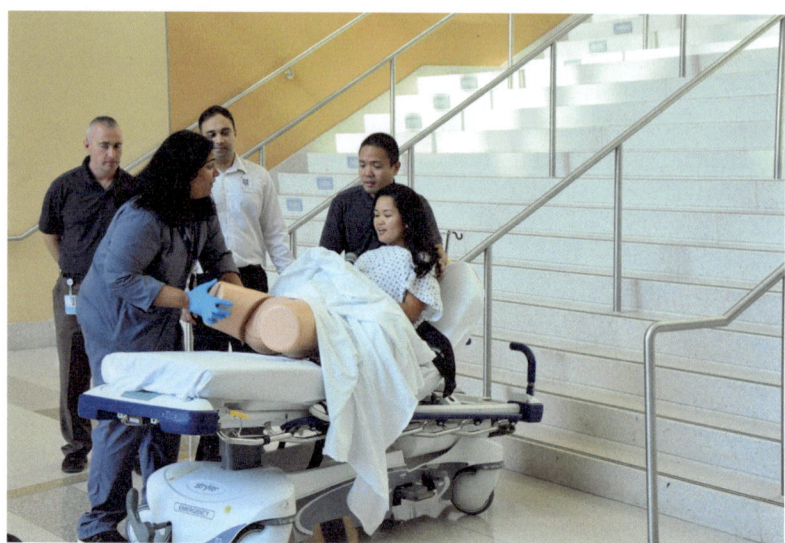

gical experience as it is crafted from mammalian tissue. The fact that it is a biologically based model, however, means that it does not have the longevity of a synthetic model. While greater in cost than the locally sourced models described, commercial models made of materials such as silicon have the advantage of long-term storage/ use, reproducibility, and multiple uses per trainer.

In terms of structuring the simulation training experience, Winkel et al. proposed a framework for assessment of OB/GYN resident technical skills during an observed structured clinical examination (OSCE) involving a hybrid simulation where the resident ascertained history from a standardized patient and performed vaginal laceration repair on a pelvic model [33]. Respect for tissue, time and motion required for each step of the procedure, instrument handling, and knowledge of instruments were measured as key components of vaginal laceration repair.

Additionally, there are well-written examples of this type of simulation training available online. One helpful collection is the ACOG Simulation Toolkit which can be found at https://www.acog.org/About-ACOG/ACOG-Departments/Simulations-Consortium/Simulations-Consortium-Tool-Kit. This toolkit includes instructions on how to create/use simulators for teaching basic surgical skills as well as obstetric and gynecologic procedures for vaginal laceration repair, tubal ligation, and even cesarean section, though it does require you to be a member of ACOG to access the materials. Resources can also be found simply by searching YouTube, and as an example, there is an in-depth explanation of the beef tongue model found at the following link: https://www.youtube.com/watch?v=pJ0GG635M1Q.

Summary

Simulation-based training can be effectively applied to basic obstetric procedures such as cervical exams, Leopold maneuvers, vaginal delivery, and perineal repair to enhance learner confidence and support knowledge acquisition. Many of the simulators are inexpensive, and there are examples of curriculum readily available, making training for these common but important skills within the reach of any institution.

References

1. Gupta N, Dragovic K, Trester R, Blankstein J. The changing scenario of obstetrics and gynecology residency training. J Grad Med Educ. 2015;7:401. https://doi.org/10.4300/JGME-D-14-00730.1.

2. Higham J, Steer PJ. Gender gap in undergraduate experience and performance in obstetrics and gynaecology: analysis of clinical experience logs. Br Med J. 2004;328(7432):142–3. https://doi.org/10.1136/bmj.328.7432.142.

3. Cooper S, Cant R, Porter J, et al. Simulation based learning in midwifery education: a systematic review. Women Birth. 2012;25(2):64–78. https://doi.org/10.1016/j.wombi.2011.03.004.

4. Deering S, Auguste T, Lockrow E. Obstetric simulation for medical student, resident, and fellow education. Semin Perinatol. 2013;37:143. https://doi.org/10.1053/j.semperi.2013.02.003.

5. Medical Simulation in Medical Education: Results of an AAMC Survey. 2011. https://www.aamc.org/download/259760/data/medicalsimulationinmedical-educationanaamcsurvey.pdf. Accessed 5 Apr 2017.

6. Pinar G, Knight CC, Gaioso VP, et al. International Archives of Nursing and Health Care. The effects of high fidelity simulation on nursing students' perceptions and self-efficacy of obstetric skills. Int Libr Cit Int Arch Nurs Heal Care Pinar al Int Arch Nurs Heal Care. 2015;1(12). https://www.researchgate.net/profile/Gul_Pinar2/publication/303951328_International_Archives_of_Nursing_and_Health_Care_The_Effects_of_High_Fidelity_Simulation_on_Nursing_Students'_Perceptions_and_Self-Efficacy_of_Obstetric_Skills/links/5760023b08ae97c1231434de.pdf. Accessed 5 Apr 2017.

7. Fritz J, Walker DM, Cohen S, Angeles G, Lamadrid-Figueroa H. Can a simulation-based training program impact the use of evidence based routine practices at birth? Results of a hospital-based cluster randomized trial in Mexico. https://doi.org/10.1371/journal.pone.0172623.

8. Kumar A, Gilmour C, Nestel D, Aldridge R, MCLelland G, Wallace E. Can we teach core clinical obstetrics and gynaecology skills using low fidelity simulation in an interprofessional setting? Aust N Z J Obstet Gynaecol. 2014;54(6):589–92. https://doi.org/10.1111/AJO.12252.

9. Cunningham FG. Williams obstetrics. New York: McGraw-Hill Education; 2008.

10. Gardberg M, Tuppurainen M. Persistent occiput posterior presentation – a clinical problem. Acta Obstet Gynecol Scand. 1994;73(1):45–47. http://www.ncbi.nlm.nih.gov/pubmed/8304024. Accessed 4 Apr 2017.

11. Arias T, Tran A, Breaud J, Fournier JP, Bongain A, Delotte J. A prospective study into the benefits of simulation training in teaching obstetric vaginal examination. Int J Gynecol Obstet. 133:380. https://doi.org/10.1016/j.ijgo.2015.08.028.

12. Nitsche JF, Shumard KM, Fino NF, et al. Effectiveness of labor cervical examination simulation in medical student education. Obstet Gynecol. 2015;126(4 Supplement):13S–20S. https://doi.org/10.1097/AOG.0000000000001027.

13. Huhn KA, Brost BC. Accuracy of simulated cervical dilation and effacement measurements among practitioners. Am J Obstet Gynecol. 2004;191(5):1797–9. https://doi.org/10.1016/j.ajog.2004.07.062.

14. Shea KL, Rovera EJ. Vaginal examination simulation using citrus fruit to simulate cervical dilation and effacement. Cureus. 2015;7(9):e314. https://doi.org/10.7759/cureus.314.

15. Donkers K, Delong D. High-fidelity simulation use in preparation of physician assistant students for neonatal and obstetric care. https://doi.org/10.1097/JPA.0000000000000070.

16. Diez-Goni N, Guillen S, Rodriguez-Diez MC, Pineda L, Alcazar JL. Use of the learning curve-cumulative summation test for Leopold maneuvers assessment in a simulator: a pilot study. Simul Healthc. 2015;10(5):277–82. https://doi.org/10.1097/SIH.0000000000000109.

17. Deering SH, Hodor JG, Wylen M, Poggi S, Nielsen PE, Satin AJ. Additional training with an obstetric simulator improves medical student comfort with basic procedures. Simul Healthc J Soc Simul Healthc. 2006;1(1):32–4. http://www.ncbi.nlm.nih.gov/pubmed/19088571

18. Reese TR, Deering SH, Kavanagh LB, Maurer DM. Perceived clinical skill degradation of Army family physicians after deployment. Fam Med. 2015;47(5):343–348. http://www.ncbi.nlm.nih.gov/pubmed/25905875. Accessed 5 Apr 2017.

19. Cooper M, Papanagnou D, Meguerdichian M, Bajaj K. Emergency obstetrics for the emergency medicine provider. MedEdPORTAL Publ. 2016;12. https://doi.org/10.15766/mep_2374-8265.10481.

20. Dayal AK, Fisher N, Magrane D, Goffman D, Bernstein PS, Katz NT. Simulation training improves medical students' learning experiences when performing real vaginal deliveries. Simul Healthc. 2009;4(3):155–9. https://doi.org/10.1097/SIH.0b013e3181b3e4ab.

21. Reynolds A, Ayres-de-Campos D, Bastos L, van Meurs W, Bernardes J. Impact of labor and delivery simulation classes in undergraduate medical learning. Med Educ Online. 2008;13:14. https://doi.org/10.3885/meo.2008.Res00285.

22. Holmström SW, Downes K, Mayer JC, Learman LA. Simulation training in an obstetric clerkship: a randomized controlled trial. Obstet Gynecol. 2011;118(3):649–54. https://doi.org/10.1097/AOG.0b013e31822ad988.

23. Easter SR, Gardner R, Barrett J, Robinson JN, Carusi D. Simulation to improve trainee knowledge and comfort about twin vaginal birth. Obstet Gynecol. 2016;128(4):34S–9S. https://doi.org/10.1097/AOG.0000000000001598.

24. Ion STEDIT, Downing D, Hargreaves O, et al. Healthcare simulation. 2016;(June):1–50. www.ssih.org/dictionary.

25. Blondel B, Alexander S, Bjarnadóttir RI, et al. Variations in rates of severe perineal tears and episiotomies in 20 European countries: a study based on routine national data in Euro-Peristat Project. Acta Obstet Gynecol Scand. 2016;95(7):746–54. https://doi.org/10.1111/aogs.12894.

26. Hirayama F, Koyanagi A, Mori R, Zhang J, Souza JP, Gülmezoglu AM. Prevalence and risk factors for third- and fourth-degree perineal lacerations during vaginal delivery: a multi-country study. BJOG Int J Obstet Gynaecol. 2012;119(3):340–7. https://doi.org/10.1111/j.1471-0528.2011.03210.x.

27. Ampt AJ, Ford JB. Ascertaining severe perineal trauma and associated risk factors by comparing birth data with multiple sources. Public Health Res Pract. 2015;2525(44). https://doi.org/10.17061/phrp2541544.

28. Best C, Drutz HP, Alarab M. OBSTETRICS obstetric anal sphincter injuries: a survey of clinical practice among Canadian obstetricians. J Obstet Gynaecol Can. 2012;34(8):747–54. https://doi.org/10.1016/S1701-2163(16)35338-5.

29. Martinez A, Cassling C, Keller J. Objective structured assessment of technical skills to teach and study retention of fourth-degree laceration repair skills. J Grad Med Educ. 2015;7(1):32–5. https://doi.org/10.4300/JGME-D-14-00233.1.

30. Patel M, LaSala C, Tulikangas P, O'Sullivan DM, Steinberg AC. Use of a beef tongue model and instructional video for teaching residents fourth-degree laceration repair. Int Urogynecol J. 2010;21(3):353–8. https://doi.org/10.1007/s00192-009-1042-3.

31. Dancz CE, Sun V, Moon HB, Chen JH, Özel B. Comparison of 2 simulation models for teaching obstetric anal sphincter repair. Simul Healthc J Soc Simul Healthc. 2014;9(5):325–30. https://doi.org/10.1097/SIH.0000000000000043.

32. Illston JD, Ballard AC, Ellington DR, Richter HE. Modified beef tongue model for fourth-degree laceration repair simulation. Obstet Gynecol. 2017;129(3):491–6. https://doi.org/10.1097/AOG.0000000000001908.

33. Winkel AF, Lerner V, Zabar SR, Szyld D. A simple framework for assessing technical skills in a resident Observed Structured Clinical Examination (OSCE): vaginal laceration repair. J Surg Educ. 2012;70:10–4. https://doi.org/10.1016/j.jsurg.2012.08.005.

Practical Approaches to Simulating Obstetric Emergencies

13

Kimberly S. Harney and Colleen A. Lee

Introduction

This chapter will discuss the various steps involved in developing obstetric emergency scenarios as well as how to establish appropriate learning objectives, including cognitive, technical, and behavioral goals for training. It will also summarize the evidence supporting simulation's effectiveness in preparing teams to deal with these emergencies. Developing a structured debriefing based on the learning objectives will be reviewed and is covered extensively in the chapter entitled "Essentials of Debriefing and Feedback." Information will also be presented about the various types of models and equipment with respect to features, advantages, and disadvantages of each. The chapter will conclude with a description of sample scenarios, including learning objectives, helpful hints, and advanced modifications for each of the obstetric emergencies mentioned above.

> **Key Learning Points**
>
> - OB emergencies are time-sensitive, low-frequency, high-consequence events.
> - Communication errors play a role in 70% of sentinel events on L&D, making teamwork a key focus of simulation and debriefing.
> - Technical skills are best taught in task training sessions when you have early learners.
> - Simulation equipment does not have to involve expensive, high-fidelity models.
> - Creating an environment that is similar to your unit or training on your unit allows the identification of facilities and systems issues that may impede care during emergencies.
> - Establishing a safe zone of confidentiality for the simulation is important, and acknowledging that your participants are highly intelligent professionals who care deeply about patient safety and have come together to practice, improve, and find ways to optimize outcomes from the beginning will help to do this.
> - There are multiple ways to simulate each emergency, and scenarios can be customized to meet the needs of learners with available resources.

K. S. Harney (✉)
Stanford University School of Medicine, Department of Obstetrics & Gynecology, Stanford, CA, USA
e-mail: kharney@stanford.edu

C. A. Lee
Department of Quality and Patient Safety, New York Presbyterian/Weill Cornell Medical Center, New York, NY, USA

© Springer International Publishing AG, part of Springer Nature 2019
S. Deering et al. (eds.), *Comprehensive Healthcare Simulation: Obstetrics and Gynecology*,
Comprehensive Healthcare Simulation, https://doi.org/10.1007/978-3-319-98995-2_13

Evidence for Effectiveness and Training

Evidence for the effectiveness of simulation in training teams to respond to obstetric emergencies is becoming more robust. In fact, the most recent ACOG Practice Bulletin on shoulder dystocia states "Simulation exercises and shoulder dystocia protocols are recommended to improve team communication and maneuver use because this may reduce the incidence of brachial plexus palsy associated with shoulder dystocia." Obstetric simulation is an effective tool for this emergency because shoulder dystocia is unpredictable and a high-acuity/low-frequency event. Studies have shown that simulation results in improved communication, use of obstetric maneuvers, and documentation of events [2–15]. Specifically, Draycott and Crofts were able to demonstrate a reduction in fetal injury after widespread use of their shoulder dystocia simulation in a group of National Health Service hospitals. This represented the first time an evidence-based study showed the effectiveness of simulation in improving clinical outcomes in obstetrics [3]. A follow-up study evaluating 12 years of simulation training by the same team demonstrated a 100% reduction in permanent brachial plexus injuries in 562 dystocias where 34% involved a posterior arm delivery [7].

Eclampsia drills have been run in the UK as in situ simulations since the early 2000s. When studied, Thompson et al. showed that simulation was effective in the rapid activation of an emergency team after one call and resulted in the development and dissemination of an evidence-based protocol for eclampsia and strategically placed "eclampsia boxes" which also came out of this [16]. Data from both the USA and the UK have shown that although death rates from eclampsia have improved over the years, the predominant risk remains cerebral hemorrhage from hypertension [17, 18]. Because of this, simulation studies have focused on the value of checklists for accomplishing timely administration of antihypertensive therapy. One multi-institutional study demonstrated that for eclampsia, there were trends toward higher completion of checklist items noted for blood pressure and airway management [19]. The concept is that training and socialization of a checklist can be done via simulation with the hope that clinical teams will begin to incorporate the tool into actual practice during emergencies [20].

Much has also been written on the preparation for and simulation of postpartum hemorrhage, including it being recommended in the most recent ACOG Postpartum Hemorrhage Practice Bulletin, and the effectiveness of simulation in correcting system errors and implementing patient safety bundles has also been well-established [21–27].

Vaginal breech delivery simulations rely heavily on technical learning objectives. Jordan et al. have published their OSAT (Objective Structured Assessment Tool) for vaginal breech delivery, which they developed using a modified Delphi process and validated in simulation comparing a group of 20 novices with 20 experts [28].

In their 2016 study of over 6,000 forceps deliveries pre- and post-simulation training, Gossett et al. identified a 22% reduction in severe lacerations for actual patients, which when corrected for a priori risk factors became a 30% reduction for the simulation training group [29].

Clinical emergencies requiring prompt movement for emergent cesarean have also been simulated and studied. In 2013, Lipman et al. evaluated OB teams and found they required nearly 10 min to move from the labor room to the OR and make the incision for a simulated uterine rupture. Through the use of simulation, they were able to identify and correct institution-specific barriers responsible for the delay [30]. Diagnosis to delivery intervals were shown to improve urgent cesarean delivery secondary to cord prolapse when comparing actual patient cases pre-and post-introduction of annual simulations for this complication. A number of measures of neonatal well-being also improved, and there was a trend to greater use of spinal anesthesia, implying that teams were more likely to consider taking time to assess the fetal heart rate after arrival in the OR [31].

Scenario Development

Learning Objectives

The primary types of learning objectives for team training simulations are technical, cognitive, and behavioral. Debriefing will flow from the learning objectives, so it is important to write them with the scenario sequence in mind. Although it may be preferable to teach certain technical skills in a separate task training session, it is important to incorporate these tasks into the scenario as realistically as possible, as the act of performing technically challenging procedures may impact a provider's ability to communicate effectively in the moment. This is also a valuable area to focus on during debriefing. Cognitive learning objectives may be very clear for homogenous groups, such as OB residents; however, when including various disciplines in your participant teams, the cognitive objectives may need to be tailored specifically for each group. Interdisciplinary learning is a highly valuable aspect of simulation, and it is enhanced by participants sharing their thought processes during debriefing. Behavioral objectives focus on teamwork and should be specific to the scenario. If the organization has adopted a particular team training curriculum, such as TeamSTEPPS or crisis resource management, it will be helpful to frame objectives utilizing the language specific to that program. In the absence of a formal team training curriculum, team skills may still be practiced in simulation by incorporating the use of emergency checklists or algorithms, identifying roles, and calling for assistance or any number of communication strategies such as directed or closed-loop communication. In writing learning objectives, it is most effective to start with an active verb for each sentence (see Table 13.1).

Debriefing

The debriefing session following the scenario is often the most important part of the simulation experience for participants. This is where they can reflect and process the events of the emergency. It is often helpful to start out by asking one of the first participants to describe what they encountered as the emergency began, what the challenges were, what kind of help they needed, and whether they received appropriate assistance. If there were lapses in technique, shortcomings in timeliness of the response, or communication failures, the participants will often note their own deficits.

In order to facilitate a good debriefing, it is also critical to create an atmosphere that allows participants to openly discuss issues. One goal is to have them reveal what they were thinking but may not have verbalized. Try and avoid having senior faculty interrupt debriefing conversations to interject with corrections, as this can interfere with the learning process and inhibit participation by the learners. Factual information may be provided at the end, if needed; and participants may also share the key learning points that they have gleaned from the experience. Try to focus the conversation on the learning objectives, but allow some free flow as well.

In debriefing obstetric emergencies, it is important to recognize that some participants may have had a traumatic experience with a similar event. If they spontaneously share this with the group, try to keep the discussion focused while showing support for the emotional challenges associated with professional experiences. If participants have questions about technique, having the task trainers available to practice on once debriefing is concluded is also helpful.

Table 13.1 Learning objectives

Type of objective	Examples of words	Example objective
Cognitive	Identify or recognize	The learner will recognize severe hypertension requiring intervention during the simulation
Technical	Demonstrate	The learner will be able to demonstrate proper technique for posterior arm delivery
Behavioral	Utilize	The learner will utilize patient friendly language during the emergency

Choosing a Simulator for Your Scenario

Full-Body Mannequin

Full-body mannequins may be high fidelity with software-controlled vital signs, automatic pulses, breath sounds, voice, uterine blood flow, and seizure mechanisms. Many programs, however, utilize a less expensive full-body mannequin where external vital signs are controlled remotely and displayed on a separate screen or tablet. Other enhancements include replacement of the abdominal wall to allow surgery or insertion of a uterus that allows intracavity exploration, bimanual massage, and placement of tamponade devices in a hemorrhage simulation. Full-body mannequins usually have a bleeding uterus component that may have advantages (inflation to simulate increased tone) and disadvantages (no access for intrauterine massage or a cavity that is hollow such that an intrauterine hand is surrounded by air). Many of the available models have automatic birthing mechanisms, but these do have some limitations as sometimes the mechanism will stall or the pace of the programmed delivery is out of sync with the actions of the care team. If the mechanism stalls or the timing is not right, the fetus can always be pushed out mechanically by a confederate faculty member. The patient voice can be done with a remote microphone or the scenario can be created so that a confederate family member helps with answering patient questions. Overall, a full-body mannequin is good for scenarios such as postpartum hemorrhage, eclampsia, umbilical cord prolapse, maternal cardiac arrest, or other emergencies which may require airway management, compressions, or general anesthesia.

Hybrid Model: Pelvis and Standardized Patient

For some scenarios, a hybrid model has advantages. A hybrid model generally includes a pelvic model that is either fixed to the bed or worn by a standardized patient. When the confederate is wearing a patient gown draped over the top of the pelvis, the effect is fairly realistic, though they will often need to remain in an upright position, particularly in scenarios such as shoulder dystocia, vaginal breech, or failed operative vaginal delivery where they may need to hold the fetus to keep it from delivering. The standardized patient is able to act faint, express pain, and even demonstrate a seizure. In addition, the hybrid patient allows participants the opportunity to interact with a real person, which has the added value of practicing and being able to discuss communication learning objectives.

Some models designed for shoulder dystocia (e.g., PROMPT and PROMPT Flex – Limbs & Things, Bristol, UK) can be purchased with a strain gauge embedded within the fetus to evaluate force used to accomplish delivery. Although these models are marketed for shoulder dystocia, breech delivery, or operative vaginal delivery, there are some disadvantages for teaching these advanced maneuvers as there is much open space between the fetus and pelvic wall. There are more anatomically correct models which are composed of a soft, compliant material (Sophie's Mum & Lucy's Mum from MODEL-med, Australia) that are better for task training purposes as the fetus fits tightly within the pelvis and creates the pressure expected when the posterior arm is delivered, forceps are placed, or an arm is swept out for a breech. (It is important to note that these models must be used with water-based lubricant and not ultrasound gel.)

There are also simple, easily portable models which may be loaded in a backpack and taken to any location to run drills. One such model is the MamaNatalie pelvis (Laerdal Medical). This simulator works well for postpartum hemorrhage and has an excellent contained system with 1.5 L of simulated blood. Additionally, a simple hemipelvis with a soft cloth abdominal wall can also be used with a neoprene uterus which allows intrauterine and intraabdominal procedures. These same features may also be created in a full-body mannequin with a cloth abdominal perineal overlay (see ACOG Simulations Group Toolkit available at https://www.acog.org/About-ACOG/ACOG-Departments/Simulations-Consortium/Simulations-Consortium-Tool-Kit).

When no vaginal procedures will be done, having a standardized patient wear a pregnant belly, like the MamaNatalie, under a skin-colored shirt and monitor belts and a gown works well for eclampsia or other medical complications as the patient can have oxygen, pulse oximetry monitor, and blood pressure cuff applied to create higher fidelity. However, injections, cardiac compressions, and airway management techniques cannot be practiced on a live patient, and this should be reviewed during orientation to the scenario.

Room Orientation

Before bringing participants into the room, it may be helpful to run through a "room ready" checklist to ensure that all equipment is present and functional. Important things to point out relate to how the participants will interact with the model and whether "simulated equipment" has been provided in lieu of obtaining supplies from their usual source. Be sure to cover whether this "patient" can have certain procedures such as a Foley catheter placed, cervical exam, vaginal delivery, forceps or vacuum delivery, cesarean section, intubation, defibrillation, IM injections in particular sites, and IVs placed. Demonstrate the patient's carotid or femoral pulses if active; and if simulated blood is being used, demonstrate how it will appear, where it will collect and warn about wearing gloves as it can stain. Discuss whether IV bags and med syringes are fluid filled or not, and demonstrate how to utilize them in the scenario. Show where medications, IV catheters, and other equipment may be obtained; and make it clear where and how vital signs will be displayed. Also, demonstrate the patient voice if appropriate. Introduce confederates and their roles to ensure that participants know exactly what to expect from them (i.e., whether or not the confederate is able to offer assistance or if they are just there to operate the simulator, etc.). If the scenario includes multidisciplinary teams, assign roles to the individuals, and have each participant say their name/role. If possible, have name tags available, especially for personnel who may not always work together.

Finally, inform the team that patient information will be provided to the initial responders utilizing the unit's typical handoff format. Request that participants suspend disbelief as much as possible in order to promote an optimal learning environment. This should include using personal protective equipment.

Obstetric Emergency Simulation Scenarios

Shoulder Dystocia

Shoulder dystocia is one of the easiest simulations to set up as it requires minimal equipment and a full scenario generally runs no more than 5 min for each participant. It can also be done as simple task training initially, with discussion and clarification, followed by performance of the whole sequence of maneuvers and practice of each one until the provider is confident with them. When running a full scenario, it is valuable to set up in a delivery room, using a hybrid patient in the labor bed, RN participants, and even a pediatric team that receives a depressed infant at their resuscitation bed. Having an anesthesia team member involved also allows for a discussion of the logistics for the Zavanelli maneuver, even if it is not considered as a core part of the emergency response.

Shoulder Dystocia: Room/Model Setup, Orientation, and Scenario Hints

A full-body mannequin can be used, but the ability to communicate with a hybrid patient adds substantial value in exploring teamwork learning objectives. In either case the fetus will need to be held back from delivering. Some of the higher-fidelity simulators have an internal mechanism that will do this and release when the operator allows it through the software. Otherwise, the fetus is held by the standardized patient. It is important for the operator to practice this as it can be more difficult than expected since some participants will pull with sudden vigorous force and the lubricant required for the simulator may make the fetus slippery and hard to hold onto. If the Zavanelli maneuver is an option in the scenario, it may be valuable to have the team take the time to move the patient the full distance to the OR from the labor room during the simulation. This can provide some realism to the gravity of this choice as it is not an instantaneous solution, and the fetal oxygenation may be compromised during the time it takes to prepare the patient for surgery.

Orientation to this scenario should include an opportunity for the participants to see and handle the baby to know how the joints work. Orientation to the room should include explanation of confederates who are playing family members and access to props to allow them to time the procedure (fetal monitor strip with paper rolling, digital clock, smartphone, or tablet timer). If there is no fetal monitor associated with the particular model in use, the smartphone/tablet metronome app (see Box 13.1) can simulate a terminal bradycardia when the head is crowning to establish a realistic sense of urgency as the scenario starts. (*Make sure to remind participants not to cut the

---

Box 13.1 Demonstrating Fetal Heart Rate (FHR) During Simulation

Many high-tech mannequins have a FHR program imbedded, some of which can be manipulated in real time. There are, however, some low-tech options for communicating the FHR during simulations. Some of these include the following:

Paper FHR Strips and Metronome

A predrawn paper strip can be inserted into the standard fetal monitoring equipment. If there are repetitive decelerations which are all similar, it is not actually necessary to make the strip move. Using a metronome App on a tablet or smartphone can create the auditory output for the sequence of decelerations, especially if coordinated with the patient's contractions. This works very well for repetitive deep variables, especially for busy scenarios when the team does not have time to come over and

look at the monitor. You may have to explain in the room orientation that the paper does not move and they should listen to the auditory signal and metronome numerical read out.

If there is a progression in the decelerations which is predictable (deterioration to bradycardia regardless of team's interventions), the predrawn paper strip can also be put in motion but paused strategically when the scenario is playing out more slowly than usual. This will be less precise, but if the participants tune into the metronome and become reliant on its large numerical display of the FHR, you can use this to override information from the paper monitor, which you can remove visually. It is important not to create conflicting information as this impairs the realism of the scenario.

Tapping on the FHR Monitor

Another low-tech approach is to take the US disc of the FHR monitor, place a small amount of gel on it, and tap on the surface at the rate you need. When you bring the volume up, this can be effective in simulating the sound of an external monitor. The simulation team member doing this will need to practice a bit and will benefit from having additional gel and a towel nearby. Realize that this technique will tie up one simulation team member completely, but it can be easily changed to follow the scenario.

Switching from External to Internal Monitors

If you offer the option to place a scalp electrode in the scenario (not all fetal head models allow this), then you can start with "tapping" and switch to the metronome to provide a distinct change in the tone that the whole room can appreciate. In order to demonstrate the change visually, it may help to switch from blank paper picking up the tapping signal to a predrawn FHR strip which shows a clear continuous tracing. Alternatively you can switch to an electronic program on a nearby screen, if available.

model, but to verbalize if they would perform an episiotomy.) Some institutions use an alternative instrument for scissors (such as a Kelly clamp labeled as scissors) to provide an additional safeguard to avoid damage to the simulator.

Advanced Modifications

Strain Gauge/Force Monitoring

Some of the most commonly used models for shoulder dystocia are the PROMPT and PROMPT Flex (Limbs & Things, Bristol, UK). The latter provides a Bluetooth-operated strain gauge embedded within the fetus. The axial traction force applied during the delivery is displayed in newtons (the force required to move 1 kg 1 m in 1 s) as a continuous color column starting out as green in the low range, climbing to orange then red at 100 N when in meter mode. This gives continuous visual feedback to the OB provider of the actual force applied as they progress through maneuvers. It can be utilized during task training sessions or the scenario if desired. Another feature of the PROMPT Flex is the "drill mode" which gives the ability to measure traction force at specific points in the scenario by marking the tracing with a particular maneuver. The ability to visualize how much "force" they apply during the scenario can be eye-opening for providers.

Advanced Models for Shoulder Dystocia Task Training

One of the most realistic models with for teaching internal maneuvers is Sophie's Mum (MODEL-med, Australia). Because there is almost no extra space in the pelvis, this model allows the learner to appreciate how difficult it can be to accomplish rotational maneuvers or to manipulate the posterior arm. It does have the disadvantage of a higher cost, and the joints of the fetus do not always move through a normal range of motion. Because the shoulder girdle is not broad and the anterior shoulder is visible upon head delivery, a metal rod can be screwed into the base of the spine in the buttocks to pull back on and create a turtle sign. Despite these problems, it is an extremely realistic model for task training for shoulder dystocia and other difficult delivery scenarios such as breech vaginal delivery.

Eclampsia

Responding to a simulated eclamptic seizure offers a valuable experience to OB providers and helps organize the multidisciplinary team in their response to this emergency. The patient scenario does not need to be complex in order to be effective. Additionally, this scenario is also a good opportunity to review and practice urgent treatment of severe hypertension.

Eclampsia: Room/Model Setup, Orientation, and Scenario Hints

In the absence of a high-fidelity model, any full-body mannequin can be laid on a foam bed with an embedded mechanical box which generates jerking movements under her torso (SimSeize, SimAction, Bozeman, MT). The on/off switch can be placed at a distance from the model. You may demonstrate the seizure in the room orientation when it is a known scenario, or a simulation team member playing a nurse can comment "Is she having a seizure?" if the case is presented as an unknown (Fig. 13.1). It can help to have a patient voice so that the mannequin is very talkative at first and then complains of a bad headache and stops talking just before the seizure box is activated.

A standardized patient can also be a good option as she can portray the full-body tonic-clonic seizures. If you do use a real person in this simulation, make sure to orient the team that they will not actually be placing IV lines or any other invasive procedures.

In general, we recommend starting the scenario with only 1–2 providers in the room when the seizure starts. This makes the team call for help and makes them communicate the situation when additional help arrives. Also, having providers have to leave the room to get supplies and medications will not only make the scenario more realistic but also give them the opportunity to practice communication techniques such as "checkbacks." Because the "patient" will not be talking during the seizure, having a family member for the team to explain interventions to is helpful.

Many units have an acute hypertension or eclampsia box. If you are running the simulation on the actual hospital ward, then make the team

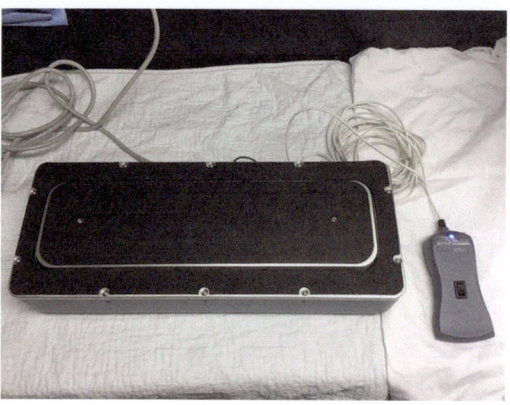

Fig. 13.1 SimSeize (SimAction, Bozeman, MT)

bring in the actual box. If you are in another location, such as a simulation center, then you can replicate it with a tackle box which has the same visual markings and information inside and out. If this is not something typically utilized by the staff, then you can bring a container with magnesium sulfate for IV and IM routes, labetalol, hydralazine, nifedipine, and calcium gluconate and have a simulation team member supervise administration to ensure that a realistic amount of time is taken to actually procure the desired medication.

Because eclampsia can be associated with severe range hypertension, there is also an opportunity to provide cues or demonstrate blood pressure readings in that range within the scenario which should alert teams to acutely address this with IV medication.

Fetal monitoring, particularly portrayal of the classic 5–6 min prolonged deceleration, can also add value to this simulation. It reminds the team that uterine tachysystole is part of the physiologic response to acute hypoxia and provides a realistic distraction for advanced teams in the midst of their effort to stabilize the mother. One of the most important learning objectives and powerful take-aways from this scenario is that participants must resist the urge to rush to emergent cesarean in this context.

Postpartum Hemorrhage

One key item to keep in mind when developing a postpartum hemorrhage (PPH) scenario is that while atony is the cause in 80% of hemorrhages,

there are other possible causes, such as retained products, lacerations, DIC, and uterine inversion. Although rare, these other causes of PPH can be highly consequential if not recognized. Fortunately, the first steps in treating PPH, a vigorous uterine exploration and internal massage, are both diagnostic and therapeutic and therefore should be emphasized during simulation. Since taking care of a patient requires a team, running the simulation with a multidisciplinary team is encouraged. With regard to picking a scenario endpoint, it depends on the learning objectives. If your goal is basic recognition and treatment, then you can use a uterine atony scenario that improves after basic evaluation, uterine exploration and massage, and the administration of two uterotonics. If you want to push the team to the point of operative intervention, then you can continue to have the patient decompensate with initial treatment until they are in need of transfusion [21].

Postpartum Hemorrhage: Room/Model Setup, Orientation, and Scenario Hints

Some high-fidelity mannequins have blood flow tubing exiting into a uterine cavity, but most do not have the anatomy to allow intrauterine massage. While this is a disadvantage, it can be mitigated by briefing participants before the simulation about the limitation and making the scenario that the primary OB cannot take their arm out of the vaginal canal due to the need for continuous intrauterine massage. The ACOG simulations group website shows an alternative neoprene uterus that can be placed in any full-body mannequin or pelvis (https://www.acog.org/About-ACOG/ACOG-Departments/Simulations-Consortium/Simulations-Consortium-Tool-Kit). It requires some limited construction utilizing surgical suture but allows intrauterine massage and provides the haptic feel of persistent atony.

If the simulator has the ability to demonstrate bleeding automatically, then these systems can be used for the scenario. However, if your simulator does not have this feature, or you wish to have more control over the flow and volume of hemorrhage, there are other options you can use. You may place the simulated blood in a well-sealed container that can be hung on an IV pole, some bags are available commercially from simulation companies (Gaumard Scientific, Miami FL), and others can be found in the hospital (dialysis bags). The bag can be covered with an opaque surface that makes it look like a plain IV bag, and you should choose a gauge of tubing that allows maximum flow of 500 mL per minute if possible. Flow can be modulated by one of the simulation staff with any surgical clamp on the tubing. It also helps to plan a signal for flow rate (faster, slower, and stop) for the simulation team. Depending on the clinical scenario you have written, loading around 2000 mL of blood in one or two containers is adequate, although it is important to do a trial run. Where the blood comes out will depend on the mannequin. While blood flow from the vagina creates realism, having blood flow directly into the collection drape limits the cleanup issues, and it requires that someone other than the OB doing massage will have to look at the amount of blood accumulating. This reinforces the concept that cumulative quantitative blood loss assessment is a key feature in the successful management of PPH. You may tape the tubing alongside the model's torso, but avoid placing it under the weight of her pelvis as that may inhibit flow. If you have it enter the under buttocks collection drape from the side, tape it securely so it ends in the midline. A small absorbent cloth may also be placed over the tip at the end for more realistic staining as opposed to allowing the blood to stream out in a line. Additionally, as a backup, having some smaller capped bottles of simulated blood held aside for adding to the perineum is helpful in case technical difficulties arise during the case. An alternative to simulated blood is to use a long swath of red utility nylon fabric soaked in warm water to represent blood flow. This can fill the pelvis and be subtly pulled out by a simulation team member who is standing by as a confederate RN. Practice how quickly to withdraw it based on how long the scenario is expected to run with continued bleeding. Depending on whether the material is colorfast, it may stain, and participants should be made aware of this possibility. Similarly, blood transfusions are best done dry to limit the hazards of spilling on clinical surfaces. Images of the real transfusion units can be taped to the surface of appropriate size IV bags so that team members can look up and see that blood products are being transfused. The process of checking in blood is labor intensive, so it may be helpful to provide all the typical paperwork with each unit in order to simulate this workflow.

It is also possible to have bleeding from atony continue to the point where the team should place an intrauterine balloon for tamponade. This can be done with or without an actual uterus in the mannequin, as the kinetic learning experience of placing it and filling it with fluid can be valuable either way, though it is much more realistic if there is a physical uterine cavity inside. This part of the simulation can also be enhanced by making sure they place a vaginal packing after the balloon is placed and even having a simulation team member subtly pull outward to dislodge the balloon from the uterus if they fail to do this in order to demonstrate a failure of the tamponade balloon.

Advanced Options

Surgical Intervention: If a B-Lynch, O'Leary, or other operative procedures are part of the learning objectives, a surgical abdominal wall can be placed on any model. An example is available on the ACOG simulations website under Abdominal Wall and Perineum (https://www.acog.org/About-ACOG/ACOG-Departments/Simulations-Consortium/Simulations-Consortium-Tool-Kit). If utilizing both a labor room and an OR, one option is to start the scenario with a hybrid model and then have a full-body mannequin (with the surgical abdominal wall in place) in the OR for a surgical procedure when the patient is "transferred" there.

Individual Skill Task Training: The neoprene uterine model shown on the ACOG website can be placed in a simple pelvis and used to demonstrate how to do bimanual massage, safely use a Banjo curette (with or without retained POC), inspect for cervical lacerations, reposition an inverted uterus, and place the Bakri balloon. Technique for placement of a B-Lynch suture or O'Leary uterine artery ligation can be taught with or without the pelvis or abdominal wall. These are all good task training sessions to have before the scenario or for junior providers, especially if laparotomy is the expected endpoint of the scenario.

Uterine Inversion: There is a separate neo-prene model which can be used to teach and reinforce the management of a uterine inversion, instructions for which are also on the ACOG simulations website. The uterus is fixed in place in the pelvis of any model but requires a confederate to push outward from the abdomen with a mechanism which maintains the uterine inversion until appropriate treatment is given. The scenario can have the inversion resolve at any stage of treatment, or it can escalate to the point that the patient requires general anesthesia. Once the uterus is replaced, it is atonic, and heavy bleeding continues, requiring active intrauterine massage until adequate uterotonics are given.

Vaginal Breech Delivery

Although the mechanics are nearly the same, the two scenarios of assisted vaginal breech delivery and second twin breech extraction are very different clinical entities. Current practice guidelines have steered away from the former and encouraged more training for providers in the latter. Nevertheless, all obstetricians need to be able to assist a singleton breech, as vaginal deliveries may be precipitous, even when a cesarean was planned. Although it is rare to need to place Piper forceps, simulation offers an excellent opportunity to become familiar with this technique.

Vaginal Breech Delivery: Room/Model Setup, Orientation, and Scenario Hints

Task training is critical to the process of building competency for breech extractions, and ensuring that all obstetrical participants have been trained on models before they are asked to participate in a scenario is helpful. In case technical issues arise during the scenario, try to incorporate time for the participants to practice with the model afterward in order to solidify these learning objectives. It can also be very helpful to have posters or a binder of the images for breech maneuvers from classic texts to refer to during either the task training or afterward. This allows the observers to connect what they are seeing in real time with the two-dimensional images they have seen.

Assisted breech delivery for a precipitous singleton breech is easy to teach on most any model with an articulating delivery baby. However, similar to the discussion about using simulators for shoulder dystocia maneuvers, many of the current commercial models have significantly more room for maneuvers than real patients. As mentioned before, the Sophie's Mum (MODEL-med, Australia) has a fetus that fits much more snuggly into the pelvis and is more realistic for the delivery. (Of note, caution should be applied when attempting a frank breech delivery with this model as it is sometimes difficult to perform a typical Pinard maneuver due to a rotation of her hip joint which can lock the knee joints in an unnatural position. If she continues to descend with the legs straight, they will suddenly and forcibly extend from the hip causing possible trauma to the model's perineum, which is best avoided.)

In contrast to hybrid models or a simple birthing pelvis simulator, using a full-body mannequin may help engage the team in some of the common prep for a breech vaginal delivery in the operating room such as setting up stirrups and can involve the anesthesia team in conversation as they stand by for possible conversion to cesarean section.

Advanced Options

Breech Extraction of the Second Twin

There are currently no commercial models which allow extraction of Twin B from an intact fluid-filled amniotic sac, though some homemade models are in use.

Operative Vaginal Delivery (OVD)

Operative vaginal delivery (OVD) simulations can be purely task training sessions, or they can involve a scenario with an indication for operative delivery (i.e., maternal exhaustion, fetal bradycardia). Given the decline in the rate of operative vaginal deliveries, practicing with simulation is critical in order to teach both indications as well as hands-on technique. Simulation can also be valuable to simulate a failed operative vaginal delivery.

Operative Vaginal Delivery: Room/Model Setup, Orientation, and Scenario Hints

One of the most important prerequisite skills, determining vertex position, is not typically taught on a formal basis. Simulated models can be used to help with this education. Trainees should learn to think of LOA as "posterior fontanelle at 1–2 o'clock," ROA as "posterior fontanelle at 10–11 o'clock," etc. as they visualize how they will both apply the instruments and provide traction in the correct vector. Examining and inspecting the models is helpful to solidify this skill. Before beginning the teaching session with any of the models below, test the provider with several of the commonly misidentified positions such as LOT, ROP, etc. Performing ultrasound for vertex position can be taught as well, and while this is not yet a part of simulation products, a simple set of ultrasound images on paper or a computer screen can be used to convey all of the typical positions.

Vacuum

Though many people think of vacuum application as requiring less certain knowledge of the exact vertex position, if position is not determined accurately, incorrect placement and traction in the wrong direction may occur. Vacuum delivery has been taught with a variety of simulators, and it is important to see if the type your institution has will hold suction on the simulated baby. Often, this will require application of a small amount of lubricant to keep a good seal.

Forceps

Forceps can be placed on any pelvic model if the fetal head has landmarks, but most pelvises have too much empty space surrounding the head. The Lucy's Mum (Paradigm Medical Systems, Portland, OR) pelvis has realistic haptics, with no empty space; however, resistance of the pelvic floor is minimal. This can be mitigated by pulling back on the fetal head to slow the pace of the delivery. A graded approach may work well where interns are introduced to the types of forceps and shown how they travel into place along the fetal head outside of a pelvis. They can then try an application without the resistance of pelvic floor tissues

on a simple pelvic model or full-body mannequin. They may also benefit from looking into the pelvis as they perform the procedure. The perineal attenuation and risk of 3rd- and 4th-degree lacerations are clearly demonstrated on these models in the final stages of forceps delivery. The timing for when to take the forceps off can be simulated nicely, and a modified Ritgen maneuver can be simulated as well. After mastery of appropriate techniques, providers can advance to applying them on a higher-fidelity model (such as Lucy's Mum or Sophie's Mum) with a variety of vertex positions.

Failed operative delivery, with or without fetal bradycardia, is a helpful scenario for determining the team's ability to both recognize when to stop the operative delivery attempt and the process required to quickly convert to a cesarean section. If a full-body mannequin is used, a confederate must be present alongside the bed to reach in through the top of the abdominal wall and hold the baby back, prohibiting delivery. A hybrid model can be used so that the realism of coaching a patient to push and the need to quickly explain the failure are presented to the obstetrical provider.

Emergency Cesarean Section

Various scenarios which lead to emergent cesarean section can be simulated including umbilical cord prolapse, uterine rupture, failed operative vaginal delivery, or a simple fetal bradycardia. For fetal bradycardia, use of a high-tech mannequin's electronic FHR program or the metronome App on a smartphone (see Box 13.1) should be sufficient to produce the desired sense of urgency.

Emergency Cesarean Section: Room/Model Setup, Orientation, and Scenario Hints

There are several simple models for an abdominal wall which can be placed on a full-body mannequin or pelvis for a cesarean section (https://www.acog.org/About-ACOG/ACOG-Departments/Simulations-Consortium/Simulations-Consortium-Tool-Kit). Additionally, many of the higher fidelity models now have abdominal covers that can be used to make the necessary abdominal incision, though most do not have a uterus inside. There is a very realistic, but expensive, simulator called C-Celia (Operative Experience) that allows for the provider to perform a complete cesarean section and even simulates operative complications.

Advanced Options

The complication of an impacted fetal head is becoming more common with changing guidelines in diagnosing active phase arrest and allowing for longer second stages. Manning et al. published a literature review of 11 international studies on the "pull versus push" technique for delivery in these cases. The "pull techniques" have been shown to significantly reduce the incidence of lower uterine segment and cervicovaginal lacerations, blood loss, and operating times [1]. Given the literature about these techniques, even experienced obstetricians can benefit from practicing with these techniques before needing to perform them in the time-sensitive situation of impacted fetal head. There is even a model which has been created to apply graded pressure of the head into the pelvic cavity using a tightening mechanism to simulate this situation (Desperate Debra, Adam,Rouilly, UK). The PROMPT Flex (Limbs & Things, UK) pelvis also has a modification for the impacted head which works reasonably well to signify that the problem is an impacted head, and then, with its soft flexible abdominal wall inserted and incised, it can be used to practice the two "pull techniques," reverse breech extraction, or the "shoulders first" delivery method, also known as the Patwardhan maneuver. These techniques can be simulated on any model with a cesarean abdominal wall that is flexible and well-lubricated and an articulated baby model that will flex at the waist.

Summary

There is a recognized need for OB/GYN providers to train learners and multidisciplinary teams to optimally manage obstetric emergencies, especially given that many are time-sensitive, low-frequency, high-consequence events.

References

1. Manning JB, Tolcher MC, Chandraharan E, Rose C. Delivery of an impacted fetal head at cesarean: literature review and proposed management algorithm. Obstet Gynecol Surv. 2015;70(11):719–24.
2. Deering S, Poggi S, Macedonia C, Gherman R, Satin AJ. Improving resident competency in the management of shoulder dystocia with simulation training. Obstet Gynecol. 2004;103(6):1224–8.
3. Draycott TJ, Crofts JF, Ash JP, Wilson LV, Yard E, Sibanda T, Whitelaw A. Improving neonatal outcome through practical shoulder dystocia training. Obstet Gynecol. 2008;112(1):14–20.
4. Seminars in Perinatology. 2009;33:76–81. Crofts JF, Fox R, Ellis D, Winter C, Hinshaw K, Draycott TJ. Observations from 450 shoulder dystocia simulations: lessons for skills training. Obstet Gynecol. 2008;112:906912.
5. Grobman WA, Miller D, Burke C, Hornbogen A, Tam K, Costello R. Outcomes associated with introduction of a shoulder dystocia protocol. Am J Obstet Gynecol. 2011;205(6):513–7.
6. Inglis SR, Feier N, Chetiyaar JB, et al. Effects of shoulder dystocia training on the incidence of brachial plexus injury. Am J Obstet Gynecol. 2011;204(322):e1–6.
7. Crofts JF, Lenguerrand E, Bentham GL, Tawfik S, Claireaux HA, Odd D, et al. Prevention of brachial plexus injury- 12 years of shoulder dystocia training: an interrupted time-series study. BJOG. 2016;123(1):111–8.
8. Goffman D, Heo H, Pardanani S, Merkatz IR, Bernstein PS. Improving shoulder dystocia management for resident and attendings using simulation. Am J Obstet Gynecol. 2008;122:1284–7.
9. Hoffman MK, Bailit JL, Branch DW, Burkman RT, VanVeldhusien P, Lu L, et al. A comparison of obstetric maneuvers for the acute management of shoulder dystocia. Consortium on safe labor. Obstet Gynecol. 2011;117:1272–8.
10. Poggi SH, Spong CY, Allen RH. Prioritizing posterior arm delivery during severe shoulder dystocia. Obstet Gynecol. 2003;101:1068–72.
11. Grimm MJ, Costello RE, Gonik B. Effect of clinician-applied maneuvers on brachial plexus stretch during a shoulder dystocia event: investigation using a computer simulation model. Am J Obstet Gynecol. 2010;203:339.e1–5.
12. Deering SH, Weeks L, Benedetti T. Evaluation of force applied during deliveries complicated by shoulder dystocia using simulation. Am J Obstet Gynecol. 2011;204:234. e1–5.
13. Leung TY, Stuart O, Suen SS, Sahota DS, Lau TK, Lao TT. Comparison of perinatal outcomes of shoulder dystocia alleviated by different type and sequence of manoeuvres: a retrospective review. BJOG. 2011;118:985–90.
14. Crofts JF, Bartlett C, Ellis D, Hunt LP, Fox R, Draycott TJ. Management of shoulder dystocia: skill reten-

tion 6 and 12 months after training. Obstet Gynecol. 2007;110:1069–74.

15. Daniels K, Arafeh J, Clark A, Waller S, Druzin M, Chueh J. Prospective randomized trial of simulation versus didactic teaching for obstetrical emergencies. Simul Healthc. 2010;5(1):40–5.

16. Thompson S, Neal S, Clark V. Clinical risk management in obstetrics: eclampsia drills. BMJ. 2004;328(7434):269–71.

17. Knight M, UKOSS. Eclampsia in the United Kingdom 2005. BJOG. 2007;114(9):1072–8.

18. Main EK, McCain CL, Morton CH, Holtby S, Lawton CS. Pregnancy-related mortality in California: causes, characteristics and improvement opportunities. Obstet Gynecol. 2015;125(4):938–47.

19. Bajaj K, Rivera-Chiauzzi EY, Lee C, Shepard C, Bernstein PS, Moore-Murray T. Am J Obstet Gynecol. 2016;33(12):1182–90. https://doi.org/10.1055/s-0036-1586118. Epub 2016 Jul 25, Validating obstetric emergency checklists using simulation: a randomized controlled trial.

20. Hilton G, Daniels K, Carvahlo B. Simulation study assessing healthcare provider's knowledge of preeclampsia and eclampsia in a tertiary referral center. Simul Healthc. 2016;11(1):25–31.

21. Bingham D, Melson K, Main E. CMQCC obstetric hemorrhage hospital level implementation guide. The California Maternal Quality Care Collaborative (CMQCC). Palo Alto: Stanford University; 2010.

22. Shields LE, Wiesner S, Fulton J, Pelletreau B. Comprehensive maternal hemorrhage protocols reduce the use of blood products and improve patient safety. Am J Obstet Gynecol. 2015;212:272–80.

23. Einerson BD, Miller ES, Grobman WA. Does a postpartum hemorrhage patient safety program result in sustained changes in management and outcomes? Am J Obstet Gynecol. 2015;212:140–4.e1.

24. Main EK, Goffman D, Scavone BM, Low LK, Bingham D, Fontaine PL, et al. National Partnership for maternal safety: consensus bundle on obstetric hemorrhage. Obstet Gynecol. 2015;126:155–62.

25. Hilton G, Daniels K, Goldhaber-Fiebert SN, Lipman S, Carvalho B, Butwick A. Checklists and multidisciplinary team performance during simulated obstetric hemorrhage. Int J Obstet Anesth. 2016;25:9–16.

26. Clark EA, Fisher J, Arafeh J, Druzin ML. Team Training/Simulation. Clin Obstet Gynecol. 2010;53(1):265–77. Lippincott Williams and Wilkins.

27. Skupski DW, Brady D, Lowenwirt IP, Sample J, Lin SN. Improvement in outcomes of major obstetric hemorrhage through systematic change. Obstet Gynecol. 2017;130(4):770–7.

28. Jordan A, Antomarchi J, Bongain A, Tran A, Delotte J. Development and validation of an objective structured assessment of technical skill tool for the practice of breech presentation delivery. Arch Gynecol Obstet. 2016;294(2):327–32.

29. Gossett DR, Gilchrist-Scott D, Wayne DB, Gerber SE. Simulation training for forceps-assisted vaginal delivery and rates of maternal perineal trauma. Obstet Gynecol. 2016;128(3):429–35.

30. Lipman SS, Carvalho B, Cohen SE, Druzin ML, Daniels K. Response times for emergency cesarean delivery: use of simulation drills to assess and improve obstetric team performance. J Perinatol. 2013;33(4):259–63.

31. Siassakos D, Hasafa Z, Sibanda T, Fox R, Donald F, Winter C, Draycott T. Retrospective study of diagnosis-delivery interval with umbilical cord prolapse: the effect of team training. BJOG. 2009;116(8):1089–96.

Obstetric Critical Care

14

Jean-Ju Sheen, Colleen A. Lee, and Dena Goffman

Introduction

In the United States, increasing rates of maternal morbidity and mortality over the last two decades have prompted calls to action to reverse this disturbing trend [1]. In 1900, the maternal mortality ratio in the United States was 850/100,000 live births; by 1986, this ratio had fallen to 7.4/100,000 live births [2]. For a variety of complex and likely interrelated reasons, the maternal mortality ratio recently has doubled to 14.5/100,000, rising as high as 37.7/100,000 in African American women [2]. Maternal morbidity is even more prevalent than maternal death, affecting many thousands of women each year [3, 4]. In 2013, D'Alton et al. explored potential contributors to the rise in maternal morbidity and mortality as well as potential interventions to improve maternal outcomes [5]. Assisted reproductive technology has allowed women to delay childbearing to more advanced ages [5], resulting in a greater number of pregnancies complicated by one or more diseases associated with older women, such as cardiovascular disease, cancer, type 2 diabetes, and hypertension. The combination of the obesity epidemic, the increasing rates of chronic diseases affecting pregnancy [6], a steadily rising cesarean delivery rate with resultant complications such as abnormal placentation [7, 8], and medical advances allowing women with rare and serious medical or genetic diseases to conceive [5] contributes to the climbing rates of maternal morbidity and mortality.

Despite the growing number of critically ill obstetrical patients, the opportunities to care for them remain limited, particularly in single hospital settings. With the population of obstetrical patients shifting toward women with significant comorbidities, the American Board of Obstetrics and Gynecology (ABOG) sponsored a meeting in 2012 with the American Congress of Obstetricians and Gynecologists (ACOG), the Society for Maternal-Fetal Medicine (SMFM), and the Eunice Kennedy Shriver National Institute of Child Health and Human Development (NICHD) to provide recommendations for each of three objectives established at the meeting: (1) to enhance education and training in maternal care, (2) to improve medical management of pregnant women around the country, and (3) to address critical research gaps in maternal medicine [5]. To address the first two objectives, the group endorsed medical simulation over more

J.-J. Sheen (✉)
Department of Obstetrics and Gynecology,
New York Presbyterian/Columbia University Irving
Medical Center, New York, NY, USA
e-mail: dg2018@cumc.columbia.edu

C. A. Lee
Department of Quality and Patient Safety,
New York Presbyterian/Weill Cornell Medical Center,
New York, NY, USA

D. Goffman
Department of Obstetrics and Gynecology,
Columbia University Irving Medical Center,
New York, NY, USA

© Springer International Publishing AG, part of Springer Nature 2019
S. Deering et al. (eds.), *Comprehensive Healthcare Simulation: Obstetrics and Gynecology*,
Comprehensive Healthcare Simulation, https://doi.org/10.1007/978-3-319-98995-2_14

traditional teaching methods [5]. Simulation offers an alternative learning opportunity in a safe environment where multidisciplinary team members can improve their skills caring for critically ill patients with rare complications.

Key Learning Points
- Rising rates of maternal morbidity and mortality have prompted action to enhance education and training for maternal care, and to improve medical management for pregnant women.
- Medical simulation education has been used effectively in a variety of other high-risk specialties including anesthesiology, neonatology, and critical care.
- Several studies in obstetric simulation have demonstrated improvement in both management and outcomes for neonatal emergencies.
- Maternal cardiac arrest simulation studies have shown improvement in management and provide a logical starting point for development of further maternal critical care simulation scenarios.

Background

Medical simulation education has been used effectively in many medical specialties, such as anesthesiology, neonatology, and critical care. The Neonatal Resuscitation Program (NRP), required for all neonatal providers, has been restructured to present most content in the form of simulation scenarios [9]. Anesthesiology, a pioneer of medical simulation education, has long required simulation for its maintenance of certification process [10]. Additionally, a newly published study in the journal of the Neurocritical Care Society showed significant improvement in critical care fellows' medical knowledge and confidence after completion of a simulation course involving three different neurological disease states [11].

In the fast-paced field of obstetrics, with numerous high-stakes, low-frequency, rapidly evolving emergencies requiring astute clinical judgment and expert technical skill to optimize outcomes, simulation has proven to be an invaluable learning tool. Although evidence of obstetrical simulation improving clinical practice or reducing adverse events is limited to date [5], several studies have shown promising results. In 2008, after requiring all staff to attend an annual one-day course involving emergency drills and fetal heart rate tracing interpretation, Draycott et al. from the United Kingdom showed a significant decrease in birth injury rates, despite similar rates of shoulder dystocia [12]. This same group used an interrupted time-series study to demonstrate improvements in both medical management and clinical outcomes – specifically, a reduction in the incidence of brachial plexus injuries – after the introduction of an obstetric emergency training program for management of shoulder dystocia [13]. In the United States, Inglis et al. demonstrated a similar decrease in the frequency of brachial plexus injuries over nine years during which a simulated shoulder dystocia protocol was initiated at their institution [14].

Another complex obstetric emergency scenario amenable to simulation is umbilical cord prolapse. One retrospective cohort study noted a statistically significant reduction in the median diagnosis-to-delivery interval (DDI) after introduction of multidisciplinary simulation training [15]. With such promising data and increasingly robust obstetrical simulation programs, a logical next step would be the incorporation of obstetric critical care scenarios into standardized simulation curricula. This chapter will discuss the use of medical simulation training for teaching critical care obstetrics.

Evidence

The incidence of intensive care unit (ICU) admissions for obstetric patients is 2–4/1,000 deliveries in developed countries and 2–13.5/1,000 deliveries in developing countries [16]. Critically ill obstetric patients pose unique challenges to multidisciplinary care teams, which may include obstetricians, anesthesiologists, and intensivists, among others [17]. Obstetric patients tend to be younger and healthier than the typical nonpregnant ICU patient and may be able to tolerate a variety of physiologic insults initially. However, once their physiologic reserve is exhausted, decompensation may be swift, and care teams must be prepared to work cohesively to provide prompt appropriate treatment.

Obstetric ICU admissions are associated with both obstetric causes (hemorrhage, hypertensive disease, and puerperal sepsis) and nonobstetric causes (maternal cardiac disease, trauma, anesthetic complications, cerebrovascular disorders, and illicit drug use), all of which may be exacerbated by existing medical comorbidities [18]. While some technical procedures performed on pregnant patients are unchanged and adaptable from those performed on nonpregnant patients, the anatomic and physiologic changes of pregnancy may pose unique challenges for critical procedures such as intubation and cardiopulmonary resuscitation. In the anesthesia literature, one review found that maternal mortality during cesarean deliveries was 2.3/100,000 patients undergoing general anesthesia, but 1/90 if failed intubation occurred [19]. Additionally, the overall number of pregnant patients requiring critical care procedures is fewer than in nonpregnant patients, resulting in less practical clinical experience. For example, while endotracheal intubation requires 30–74 cases to reach a 90% success rate [20, 21], anesthesiologists perform fewer intubations for obstetric patients during their training, as general anesthesia is only used in 8% of all cesarean deliveries, most being emergency cases [22]. Because critically ill patients in the ICU require a cohesive, efficient, and well-trained interprofessional team for optimal patient care, simulation-based education has been important in improving both teamwork and communication skills, in addition to elevating technical skills and care quality during medical crises [23]. A 2013 meta-analysis of 182 studies using simulation technology for resuscitation training involving over 16,000 participants concluded that simulation-based training improved knowledge, skill, patient outcomes, and learner satisfaction, when compared with no intervention [24]. Recognition of the challenges the obstetric patient poses in critical care medicine has resulted in the creation of a subset of pregnancy-specific team-based simulations by subspecialists involved in the care of these critically ill patients, but this literature remains sparse.

Maternal cardiac arrest is the primary obstetrical critical care simulation scenario that has demonstrated improved learner performance. Maternal cardiac arrest is a rare and catastrophic occurrence with survival rates below those of nonpregnant adults (as low as 6.9%) [25, 26]. Timely initiation and continuation of high-quality chest compressions are critical to resuscitation success [27]. Fisher et al. demonstrated that after implementation of a maternal arrest simulation program, maternal-fetal medicine staff demonstrated statistically significant improvement in the timely initiation of cardiopulmonary resuscitation in follow-up simulations [28]. Another prospective study by Adams et al. demonstrated improved obstetrics/gynecology resident knowledge, confidence, and competence in the management of a simulated third trimester cardiac arrest after implementation of a simulation-based curriculum including maternal cardiac arrest [29].

How to Implement

The experience gained from maternal cardiac arrest simulation studies provides a springboard for modeling other critical care obstetric simulations. Simulation programs are able to be tailored depending on the needs of the individuals or institutions involved. In critical care obstetrics, multiple disciplines with varying levels of learners may be involved, from trainees to nurses to therapists to subspecialists. Conversely, the simulated scenario may focus on learners from a single discipline, whose primary responsibility is stabilization of the simulated patient until the critical care team arrives. The goal for the participants may be to provide tiered care depending on the case complexity and timing of their introduction into the scenario.

The scenario and simulators chosen should reflect specific learning objectives and teaching points. The teaching focus may be technical, such as central line placement, intubation and chest compressions, with an emphasis on the modifications for the anatomic and physiologic changes of pregnancy. Alternatively, the focus may be to improve clinician communications and teamwork. Scenarios to achieve these goals may range from a single complex medical condition such as diabetic ketoacidosis, to a multistage progression of disease such as pyelonephritis evolving to septic shock.

Simulators used can range from low or moderate fidelity for procedures isolated to a particular organ or organ system, to higher fidelity commercial models, allowing for sophisticated real-time presentation of vital signs and physiologic state changes. For multidisciplinary critical care obstetric simulations, high-fidelity simulators or human actors are ideal for demonstrating complex medical situations involving multiple organ systems with issues needing to be addressed simultaneously. High-fidelity simulators not only allow for real-time response rates to critical vital signs and physiologic state changes but also encourage more realistic patient interactions, potentially reinforcing communication skills, since less effort is required to achieve the suspension of disbelief necessary for successful simulation exercises.

The location where simulations may be performed ranges from being in situ, which has the advantage of helping uncover both systems and team interaction issues, to being in a simulation center, which may allow for more complex scenarios and high-fidelity simulations. Designing clear objectives and recognizing the level of learners involved are important first steps to designing and implementing a successful obstetrics critical care curriculum. If individual institutions do not have the means to support and sustain their own simulation curriculum, hospitals may want to consider collaborating and pooling resources.

Examples

Because developing obstetric critical care curricula may be overwhelming given the depth and breadth of possible clinical scenarios, institutions may ben-

efit from collaboration with others. Additionally, they may build on information obtained from work that already has been done in this area by other centers. For example, Banner University Medical Center in Arizona, in collaboration with the Society for Maternal-Fetal Medicine (SMFM), hosts an annual three-day Critical Care in Obstetrics Course. This program focuses on essential learning in critical care obstetrics, is open to all disciplines (including high-risk obstetrical nurses, emergency medicine physicians, MFM attendings and fellows, obstetric hospitalists, physicians, residents, and medical students), and employs multiple educational methods such as interactive didactics, virtual reality experiences, case-based group learning, and hands-on simulation drills led by expert faculty. Scenarios range from postpartum hemorrhage and the morbidly adherent placenta to diabetic ketoacidosis and respiratory distress syndrome (Table 14.1). Course objectives include understanding pregnancy physiology, recognizing the risks for maternal complications posed by critical illness in pregnancies, and reinforcing knowledge about the care and treatment for multiple critical care conditions in pregnancy. Simulation courses such as this provide an invaluable framework for developing one's own critical care curriculum or

Table 14.1 Brief description of two simulation scenarios presented at the Critical Care in Obstetrics course (Banner University Medical Center in Arizona, in collaboration with the Society for Maternal-Fetal Medicine)

	Megasim 1: DKA » sepsis/intubation » cardiac arrest	Megasim 2: thyroid storm » preeclampsia/ eclampsia » abruption/PPH
State 1	Initial presentation and diagnosis/initial management of diabetic ketoacidosis	Initial presentation and diagnosis/initial management of thyroid storm
State 2	Diagnosis of sepsis requiring additional treatment, intubation, invasive monitoring, and medication for hypotension	Diagnosis of severe preeclampsia and then treatment of an eclamptic seizure
State 3	Maternal cardiac arrest	Placental abruption with precipitous vaginal delivery and postpartum hemorrhage

for creating collaborations with other local institutions. Data from and feedback on this work over time will help formally define the utility of medical simulations in obstetrical critical care education.

A national focus on building obstetric critical care simulation opportunities has the potential to address two of the three objectives set out by ABOG, ACOG, SMFM, and NICHD in 2012. This type of education provides a mechanism to train a cadre of skilled and confident clinicians who can then continue to teach others, both through ongoing formal educational efforts and at the bedside while providing optimal care to complex and critically ill maternal patients. Participants will also develop the skill set and obtain tools to facilitate the creation of local simulation opportunities to help develop obstetric critical care competencies in future trainees and current multidisciplinary teams.

Summary

Although maternal morbidity and mortality rates are on the rise, in part due to advancing maternal age and increasing medical comorbidities, opportunities to care for critically ill obstetric patients at individual institutions remain few. Medical simulation education already has been used effectively in a multitude of specialties. While utility in obstetrics requires further research, the use of simulation for multidisciplinary management of maternal cardiac arrest has been studied extensively, revealing improved learner performance. Critical care simulation training in obstetrics may result in improved medical knowledge, technical skill, and multidisciplinary teamwork, with the ultimate hope of decreasing maternal morbidity and mortality rates.

References

1. Main EK, Menard MK. Maternal mortality: time for national action. Obstet Gynecol. 2013;122(4):735–6.
2. Centers for Disease Control and Prevention (CDC). Healthier mothers and babies. MMWR Morb Mortal Wkly Rep. 1999;48:849–58.
3. Callaghan WM, Mackay AP, Berg CJ. Identification of severe maternal morbidity during delivery hospitalizations, United States 2001–2003. Am J Obstet Gynecol. 2008;199(133):e1–8.
4. Danel I, Berg C, Johnson CH, Atrash H. Magnitude of maternal morbidity during labor and delivery: United States 1993–1997. Am J Public Health. 2003;93:631–4.
5. D'Alton ME, Bonanno CA, Berkowitz RL, et al. Putting the "M" back in maternal-fetal medicine. Am J Obstet Gynecol. 2013;208(6):442–8.
6. Berg CJ, Mackay AP, Qin C, Callaghan WM. Overview of maternal morbidity during hospitalization for labor and delivery in the United States: 1993–1997 and 2001–2005. Obstet Gynecol. 2009;113:1075–81.
7. Solheim KM, Esakoff TF, Little SE, et al. The effect of cesarean delivery rates on the future incidence of placenta prevue, placenta accreta, and maternal mortality. J Matern Fetal Neonatal Med. 2011;24:1341–6.
8. Blanchette H. The rising cesarean delivery rate in America: what are the consequences? Obstet Gynecol. 2011;118:687–90.
9. American Academy of Pediatrics (AAP). Neonatal resuscitation program. http://www2.aap.org/nrp/7thedinfo.html. Accessed 24 Feb 2017.
10. American Society of Anesthesiologists (ASA). Maintenance of certification. http://www.asahq.org/education/moca. Accessed 24 Feb 2017.
11. Bracksick SA, Kashani K, Hocker S. Neurology education for critical care fellows using high-fidelity simulation. Neurocrit Care. 2017;26:96–102.
12. Draycott TJ, Crofts JF, Ash JP, Wilson LV, Yard E, Sibanda T, Whitelaw A. Improving neonatal outcome through practical shoulder dystocia training. Obstet Gynecol. 2008;112(1):14–20.
13. Crofts JF, et al. Prevention of brachial plexus injury—12 years of shoulder dystocia training: an interrupted time-series study. BJOG Int J Obstet Gynaecol. 2016;123(1):111–8.
14. Inglis SR, et al. Effects of shoulder dystocia training on the incidence of brachial plexus injury. Am J Obstet Gynecol. 2011;204(4):322–e1.
15. Siassakos D, et al. Retrospective cohort study of diagnosis-delivery interval with umbilical cord prolapse: the effect of team training. BJOG. 2009;116(8):1089–96.
16. Pollock W, Rose L, Dennis CL. Pregnant and postpartum admissions to the intensive care unit: a systematic review. Intensive Care Med. 2010;36:1465–74.
17. Bajwa SK, Bajwa SJ, Kaur J, Singh K, Kaur J. Is intensive care the only answer for high risk pregnancies in developing nations? J Emerg Trauma Shock. 2010;3:331–6.
18. Bajwa SJ, Kaur J. Critical care challenges in obstetrics: an acute need for dedicated and coordinated teamwork. Anesth Essays Res. 2014;8(3):267–9.
19. Kinsella SM, Winton AL, Mushambi MC, et al. Failed tracheal intubation during obstetric general anaesthesia: a literature review. Int J Obstet Anesth. 2015;24:356–74.
20. Toda J, Toda AA, Arakawa J. Learning curve for paramedic endotracheal intubation and complications. Int J Emerg Med. 2013;6:38.

21. Je S, Cho Y, Choi HJ, et al. An application of the learning curve-cumulative summation test to evaluate training for endotracheal intubation in emergency medicine. Emerg Med J. 2013;emermed-2013-202470.

22. Winter J. Hospital episode statistics analysis, health and social care information centre. NHS Maternity Statistics-England, 2012–3.

23. Brunette V, Thibodeau-Jarry N. Simulation as a tool to ensure competency and quality of care in the cardiac critical care unit. Can J Cardiol. 2017;33:119–27.

24. Mundell WC, Kennedy CC, Szostek JH, Cook DA. Simulation technology for resuscitation training: a systematic review and meta-analysis. Resuscitation. 2013;84:1174–83.

25. Department of Health, Welsh Office, Scottish Office Department of Health, Department of Health and Social Services, Northern Ireland. Why mothers die: report on confidential enquiries into maternal deaths in the United Kingdom 2000–2002. London: The Stationery Office; 2004.

26. Dijkman A, Huisman CM, Smit M, et al. Cardiac arrest in pregnancy: increasing use of perimortem cesarean section due to emergency skills training? BJOG. 2010;117:282–7.

27. Jeejeebhoy FM, Zelop CM, Lipman S, et al. AHA scientific statement: cardiac arrest in pregnancy, a scientific statement from the American Heart Association. Circulation. 2015;132:1747–73.

28. Fisher N, Eisen LA, Bayya JV, et al. Improved performance of maternal-fetal medicine staff after maternal cardiac arrest simulation-based training. Am J Obstet Gynecol. 2011;205:239.e1–5.

29. Adams J, Cepeda Brito JR, Baker L, et al. Management of maternal cardiac arrest in the third trimester of pregnancy: a simulation-based pilot study. Crit Care Res Pract. 2016;2016:5283765.

Obstetric Ultrasound-Guided Invasive Procedure Simulation

Joshua F. Nitsche and Brian C. Brost

Introduction

Adequately training obstetrics and gynecology (OB/GYN) residents and maternal-fetal medicine (MFM) fellows in ultrasound-guided invasive procedures has become quite challenging due to a steady decline in clinical training opportunities. The decline has become particularly marked since the introduction of cell-free DNA (cfDNA) testing. This technology allows for a noninvasive and highly sensitive evaluation for an increasing number of aneuploidies and microduplication/microdeletion disorders. As such, many more women are choosing this form of initial genetic screening, rather than the gold standard of determining a karyotype from an amniocentesis or chorionic villus sampling (CVS) specimen. Studies suggest that proficiency is obtained after one has performed between 50 and 100 amniocenteses [1–3], 100 CVS procedures [4], and 60 PUBS procedures [5]. Currently in many fellowships, there are insufficient numbers of procedures being performed to insure all graduating fellows are able to perform these procedures independently.

A robust simulation curriculum can help to make up for this deficit. Utilizing task trainers with incremental structured training offers several advantages over the traditional approach of using only real-life procedures to train residents and fellows. First, it allows trainees to practice the skills and sequence of steps required to complete the procedure in a safe environment where errors cannot cause patient harm. As the steps of the procedure and dealing with common issues become familiar, there is a significant decrease in the trainee's (and therefore patients) anxiety when novices perform their initial real-life procedures. In addition, the knowledge and skill obtained during simulation will allow the trainee to better appreciate the challenges of their initial procedures and learn more from each clinical experience. The safe environment provided by simulation also allows instructors to more easily and objectively provide timely feedback and to assess a trainee's ability. These can be done either as summative or formative assessments, but in either event, allow the instructor to better measure a trainee's readiness to perform these procedures on real patients. Knowing that a trainee possesses the requisite knowledge and skills will likely lead to faculty being more agreeable to having the trainee actively participate in or perform procedures for which they are ultimately responsible.

Unfortunately, there has been little study of how to best utilize simulation as an adjunct to

J. F. Nitsche (✉) · B. C. Brost
Wake Forest School of Medicine, Department of Obstetrics and Gynecology, Division of Maternal-Fetal Medicine, Winston-Salem, NC, USA
e-mail: jnitsche@wakehealth.edu

© Springer International Publishing AG, part of Springer Nature 2019   157
S. Deering et al. (eds.), *Comprehensive Healthcare Simulation: Obstetrics and Gynecology*,
Comprehensive Healthcare Simulation, https://doi.org/10.1007/978-3-319-98995-2_15

resident or fellowship training. The optimal amount of simulation, the most effective simulators, and the most efficient curriculum structure have not been determined. This lack of evidence leaves us with common sense, expert opinion, and the understanding of adult learning theory to guide the important decisions that must be made when fashioning a simulation curriculum. Here we provide a summary of the available simulators and our approach for training fellows in obstetric ultrasound-guided invasive procedures.

Key Learning Points
- With the decrease in real-life ultrasound-guided invasive procedure training opportunities, the use of simulation is necessary to insure that trainees continue to obtain competence in these procedures during residency and fellowship.
- There is significant overlap in the guidance skills needed to perform obstetric ultrasound-guided procedures. These similarities can be exploited by having trainees practice the core guidance skills common to all invasive procedures.
- Practicing these core guidance skills will help trainees be better prepared for their initial simulated and real-life invasive procedures.
- Procedure-specific task trainers for nearly all obstetric ultrasound-guided invasive procedures are available and should be used to augment training after the core guidance skills have been mastered.
- A structured curriculum with ample opportunity for deliberative practice is an essential part of training for ultrasound-guided invasive procedures.
- Clearly defined performance milestones should be used to make certain that trainees have sufficient technical skill prior to performing their first real-life procedures.

Background: Common Skills and Unique Aspects

Historically, each invasive procedure has been taught independently of the other ultrasound-guided needle procedures. Amniocentesis has traditionally been the first procedure taught to senior OB/GYN residents or junior MFM fellows. It is not until that skill has been mastered that trainees—typically MFM fellows—would be taught how to perform a chorionic villus sampling (CVS). Next come more advanced procedures such as percutaneous umbilical blood sampling (PUBS) and in utero stenting. This stepwise approach to training leaves little time to teach the more complex procedures during the course of the 3 years of fellowship.

In reality there is significant overlap in the overall approach and psychomotor skills used in these procedures. Key elements to optimize and make these invasive tasks as easy as possible include the following: planning your approach, selection of the instrument insertion site, localization of the needle, and guiding it to the target without losing ultrasound visualization of the needle during the procedure. What is done after the needle or a device reaches the desired space or target is what distinguishes these procedures. Thus, performing one procedure such as an amniocentesis will actually improve one's skill with transabdominal CVS. Although there are clearly differences in how to perform amniocentesis and transabdominal CVS, it is intuitive that someone who has mastered amniocentesis should be able to readily master transabdominal CVS as well with additional focused procedure-specific instruction and practice. The same logic applies when considering very rare procedures such as percutaneous umbilical blood sampling (PUBS) and in utero stenting. However, it should be noted that transcervical CVS guidance skills are unique and have very little overlap with other obstetric invasive procedures and will require more procedure-specific simulation as a result.

With the rapidly diminishing volume of real-life procedures, many fellows will have difficulty obtaining clinical privileges for these procedures considering their training logs are typically judged as if skill with one ultrasound-guided invasive procedure has no relevance to any other. If the trend in clinical training opportunities continues, 1 day applying this concept of "cross competency" may be the only way many providers will be able to obtain clinical privileges for these procedures.

The idea of cross competency is echoed by the American Institute of Ultrasound in Medicine (AIUM) in their Practice Statement on the Performance of Selected Ultrasound-Guided Invasive procedures [6]. They outline a set of core guidance skills that all providers performing these procedures, regardless of specialty, should master. Specific recommendations include provider proficiency with both the in-plane guidance approach—where the needle path and ultrasound beam are within the same plane—and out-of-plane guidance approach, where the needle path crosses the ultrasound beam at a single point. They also outline a variety of needle visualization optimization techniques that can be used during in-plane needle guidance. These techniques include *probe translation*, moving the probe toward the needle along the plane of the

needle path so as to center the needle in the ultrasound screen; *rotation*, turning the probe so that the ultrasound beam aligns with the plane of the needle path; and the *heel-toe oblique standoff technique*, pushing or rocking the transducer toward the needle tip so that the long axis of the ultrasound beam and needle path are closer to perpendicular. This focus on a set of core skills common to all ultrasound-guided procedures is a shift from the recommendations of many professional specialty and subspecialty organizations that most often treat specific procedures as a separate entity from all others. The common skills and unique aspects of the various obstetric ultrasound-guided invasive procedures are outlined in Table 15.1.

Evidence

Numerous studies have demonstrated improvements in trainee performance in both cognitive and procedural tasks with the use of simulation [7]. Thus far, the majority of the study of simulation effectiveness has been in the fields of surgery

Table 15.1 Common skills and unique aspects of obstetric ultrasound-guided invasive procedures

Procedure	Common skills	Unique aspects
Amniocentesis	In-plane guidance Probe translation Probe rotation Probe heel-toe standoff	Acute angle of entry into the uterus Avoidance of the placenta Attaching and removing syringe Fluid aspiration
Transabdominal chorionic villus sampling	In-plane guidance Probe translation Probe rotation Probe heel-toe standoff	Obtuse angle of entry into the uterus Targeting of the placenta Possible use of coaxial needles Solid material (villi) aspiration
Transcervical chorionic villus sampling		Transabdominal guidance of transcervical device Inability to self-guide Targeting of the placenta Attaching and removing syringe
In utero stenting	In-plane guidance Probe translation Probe rotation Probe heel-toe standoff	Insertion into the fetus Stent deployment steps
Percutaneous umbilical blood sampling	In-plane guidance Probe translation Probe rotation Probe heel-toe standoff	Insertion into the umbilical vein Attaching and removing syringe Blood aspiration Use of transfusion setup Prolonged procedure

[8], anesthesiology [9], and emergency medicine [10]. In the field of OB/GYN, simulation has been used in training for cognitive tasks such as the management of shoulder dystocia [11–15], eclamptic seizure [16], and obstetric hemorrhage [16] and in procedural training for abdominal surgery [17–19], endoscopic surgery [18–22], hysteroscopic surgery [23], and the LEEP procedure [24].

Unfortunately, there has been only one empirical study of the effectiveness of simulation in the training of ultrasound-guided invasive procedures [25]. Trainees were required to successfully aspirate simulated blood from an umbilical cord segment 20 times/day for a 15-day period. Simulation-trained learners had a higher success rate and shorter procedure duration compared with learners that did not receive the simulation training. Although there has been minimal investigation of the effectiveness of simulation training for obstetric ultrasound-guided invasive procedures, there have been several studies examining the number of procedures that need to be performed in order to obtain competence. These studies suggest that between 50 and 100 amniocenteses [1–3], 100 CVS procedures [4], and 60 PUBS procedures are required to decrease fetal loss rates and to acquire competence [5].

In the United States, relevant stakeholder organizations, such as the American Board of OB/GYN, the American Institute of Ultrasound in Medicine, and American Council of Graduate Medical Education, among others, have not designated specific minimum procedure numbers needed to acquire and maintain competency in ultrasound-guided invasive procedures. In the United Kingdom, the Royal College of Obstetrics and Gynecology has set clear guidelines and recommends that a minimum of 30 invasive procedures (amniocentesis and CVS combined) be performed to initially obtain competence and the same amount per year to maintain competence [26]. Although the exact number of procedures needed for competence is a subject of legitimate debate, it is clear that in many programs there are insufficient numbers of real-life procedures to ensure that their trainees graduate with the skill needed to perform these procedures independently.

Many program directors have turned to simulation as a way to improve the training in these increasingly rare procedures. Below we describe our approach to the use of simulation in the training of ultrasound-guided invasive procedures.

How to Implement

Needle Guidance Basics

Even before starting to teach fellows these core guidance skills outlined by the AIUM, we start with what we refer to as needle guidance basics. We have trainees perform a series of short exercises to illustrate (1) how needle placement in relation to the probe affects where the needle appears on the ultrasound screen, (2) how their hand movements affect the location of the needle on the screen, and (3) the pros and cons of holding the probe parallel or perpendicular to their shoulders. Fellows first place the needle into the task trainer directly adjacent to one end of the probe illustrating that this will result in the needle rapidly appearing near the upper corner of the screen. As the needle is moved further away from the probe, the fellows see how the needle then appears further down the side of the screen and has to be inserted further prior to visualizing it on the ultrasound screen. The fellow performs these tasks placing the needle both next to the end of the probe with the orientation mark and the end opposite the orientation mark. This allows them to see what it is like to guide a needle when the needle appears on the same side of the screen as their dominant hand and when this relationship is flipped. They are also instructed to move their needle hand within the ultrasound plane to demonstrate how this causes the needle tip to move on the screen and perpendicular to the ultrasound plane to demonstrate how this causes the needle to appear and disappear from the screen. Finally, all of these short tasks just described are performed with the probe held parallel and perpendicular to their shoulders to illustrate how this variable affects needle guidance.

Oftentimes a fellow's exposure to one or more of these needle/probe orientations may be lacking if their faculty only use a subset of the possible combinations. We encourage our fellows to try out all of the possible combinations of appearance of the needle on the screen (mirror image vs. flipped) and relationship of the probe to the fellows' shoulders (parallel vs. perpendicular). By practicing these variations, they gain a broad set of guidance skills allowing them to use the optimal approach based on the anatomy of the patient for the specific procedure at hand. In addition, they will be familiar with the individual approaches used by different faculty members. In fact our faculty members use the task trainer to practice the orientations they are less familiar with, so they can better instruct the fellows. We have even practiced needle guidance with our left hands to better teach our left-handed fellows

Core Guidance Skills

Traditionally, fellows did not receive specific instruction on the core guidance skills outlined by the AIUM but rather obtained them gradually through performing individual procedures either in real-life or in a simulated environment. We have devised a task trainer and targeting curriculum that allows providers to practice these individual core guidance skills in isolation from a specific procedure [27]. This has several advantages over procedure-specific practice. First, it removes many aspects of procedures that may interfere with the trainees' acquisition of guidance skills. For example, the presence of the fetus and loops of umbilical cord encountered during a real-life or simulated amniocentesis can increase the cognitive load of an already nervous trainee such that they lose focus on guiding the needle. Second, the level of difficulty can be easily increased to suit learners with intermediate and advanced levels of skill. In addition, while procedure-specific training will still be required, deliberately practicing the core guidance skills in isolation has the advantage of simultaneously preparing novice trainees for nearly all of the ultrasound-guided invasive procedures they will eventually be called upon to perform.

Amniocentesis

Amniocentesis, for fetal lung maturity testing or genetic evaluation for aneuploidy, is the most common ultrasound-guided needle procedure performed in obstetrics. While historically both OB/GYN residents and MFM fellows received training in this procedure, it is no longer a required skill for graduation from OB/GYN residency. While it may be necessary for a small number of general OB/GYNs to perform amniocentesis, particularly those practicing in remote locations, it is now almost exclusively performed by maternal-fetal medicine providers. The use of amniocentesis simulators is an important adjunct to learning the procedure before performance by novice learners in a clinical setting.

Commercially produced simulators (CAE, Montreal; SynDaver, Tampa, FL), "homemade" gelatin-based simulator, and "homemade" fetal pig-based simulator [28] have been available for some time (Fig. 15.1). The purchase of commercially available task trainers does not necessarily confer an increased degree of realism or "high fidelity." Preassembled commercial models often suffer from a "one size fits all" approach to their construction. The model purchased contains a single fetus, in a set position, with an immutable configuration of fluid pockets. This limits the models use for trainees as they soon memorize its limited number of configurations or utilize the same puncture mark on the skin which diminishes interest and engagement in the simulation. In addition, static models also do not provide the needed escalation of variability and difficulty of the clinical setting required for a truly effective training model. We prefer the "homemade" fetal pig model that has been previously described [28] as it allows for the adjustment of factors such as fetal size and position, maternal body habitus, and amniotic fluid depth and pocket volume.

We typically begin with a straightforward procedure where fellows must access a generous fluid pocket with a fetal pig of similar size to an 18-week human fetus. After these easier simulations have been mastered, the amniotic fluid volume can be decreased, the fetal position or size

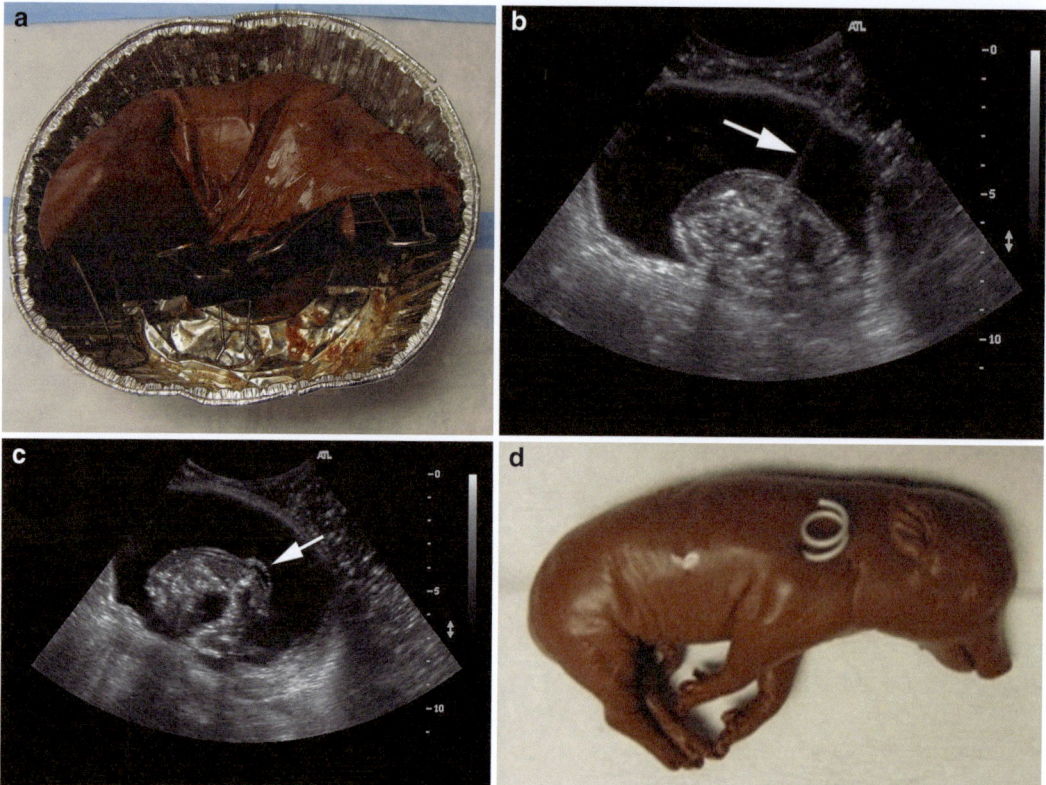

Fig. 15.1 Amniocentesis and in utero stent task trainer. (**a**) Photograph of an assembled task trainer with a fetal pig placed inside of a water-filled segment of gravid pig uterus. (**b**) An ultrasound image depicting trocar place-ment for an in utero stent procedure within the assembled task trainer. (**c**) An ultrasound image depicting in utero stent after deployment. (**d**) Photograph showing thoracic shunt location after simulated stent placement

changed, increasingly challenging pockets of fluid targeted, and the amount of simulated adipose tissue increased to create more difficult simulations. The model can also be modified to simulate anhydramnios, and the fellow may perform a transabdominal amnioinfusion. This versatility extends the model's usefulness further into training as the many different possible configurations prevent memorization by the trainees and maintains their interest for greater number of training sessions.

We introduce our fellows to the amniocentesis simulator after they have practiced and become comfortable with the core guidance skills discussed above. This allows the fellows to come to the simulation with the ability to plan an approach, find their needle, and guide it to the desired target before adding the distractions of the procedure specific to amniocentesis. For example, fellows should take the time to set up the needles and other needed equipment to make them conveniently within reach, just as they would during an actual procedure on a patient. They can assess the anatomic relationship between the placenta, fetus, and umbilical cord that guide selection of an appropriate pocket of fluid. After insertion of the needle into the pocket, the focus then shifts to the more procedure-specific tasks of attaching a syringe to the needle, aspirating amniotic fluid, and detaching the needle all without allowing the needle to migrate out of the fluid pocket selected. Through direct observation or use of a checklist, faculty can then determine the trainee is "ultrasound guided needle ready" and has the necessary skill and confidence to work in a clinical setting with an actual patient.

Chorionic Villus Sampling

Like amniocentesis, the number of CVS procedures is steadily decreasing due to the introduction of cfDNA screening. It is increasingly difficult for fellows in small to medium volume programs to graduate with sufficient experience to perform CVS independently. If the current downward trend in procedure numbers continues, at some point only the highest-volume academic centers will be able to train fellows to perform CVS. This can be avoided if simulation training is more widely adopted and the performance of simulated procedures is counted along with real-life procedures when providers apply for clinical privileges.

Although no commercially produced CVS simulators are available, we and others have developed "homemade models" [29, 30]. We began using a novel bovine heart and fetal porcine-based model [29] (Fig. 15.2) but have abandoned it due to the substantial amount of work needed to first create and then set up this model and trainee/faculty reluctance to use animal tissue. Instead we now use a silicone pastry bag as the simulated uterus. Although it does not accurately reproduce the thickness of a first trimester uterus, compared to the pig heart model, the pastry bag requires no time to create, is easier to set up, and provides superior ultrasound images of the simulated placenta. We then insert a piece of tofu inside the bag to serve as a simu-

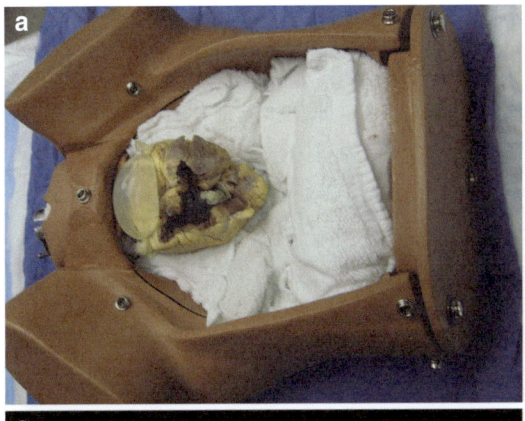
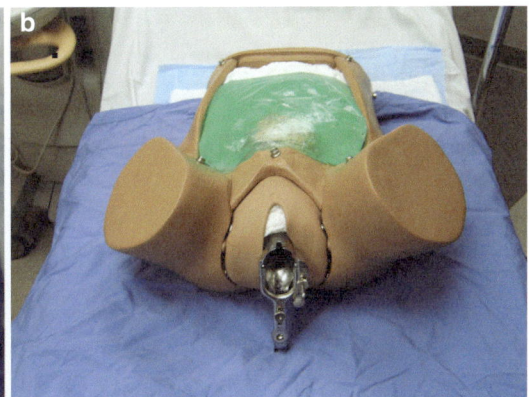
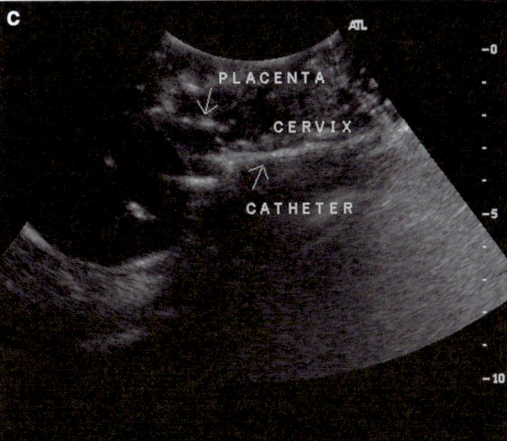

Fig. 15.2 Chorionic villus sampling task trainer. (**a**) Photograph of the task trainer with ultrasound gel-filled Ziploc bag removed to demonstrate configuration of the heart within the pelvis model. (**b**) Photograph of the fully assembled task trainer for performing transcervical CVS. (**c**) Ultrasound image depicting sampling catheter passing through the simulated cervix into the placenta

lated placenta [30] and next place a water-filled condom inside the pastry bag which pressures the tofu up against the inside of the pastry bag. A Ziploc freezer bag filled with ultrasound gel is then placed on top of the assembled task trainer and serves as the skin and adipose tissue.

Transabdominal CVS can be performed by introducing a needle or coaxial needle set into the gel bag, through the pastry bag, and into the simulated placenta. Transcervical CVS can be performed by cutting a circular hole in one end of the plastic container and passing the small end of the pastry bag through the hole. A CVS catheter is then introduced through the small end of the bag, or simulated cervix, between the condom and pastry bag, and into the placenta. The pastry bag can be rotated to simulate a variety of anatomic positions, i.e., anterior, posterior, left, right, etc., and distances from the cervical os. As we do with amniocentesis, we typically start training with the placenta in a favorable position, anterolateral and away from the cervix for transabdominal and a posterior previa for transcervical. The difficulty of the simulated transabdominal and transcervical CVS can then be altered by moving the position of the simulated placenta within the pastry bag.

There is significant overlap in the skill set required to perform amniocentesis and transabdominal CVS. We find that trainees and established providers comfortable performing amniocentesis have little difficulty performing a simulated transabdominal CVS on our models when trained about site selection and selecting the appropriate needle path. The main difference between the two procedures is the approach angle of the needle with regard to the uterine wall and placenta. In amniocentesis, the placenta is avoided when possible, and the needle is introduced as close to 90 degrees to the uterine wall as possible. However, when performing a transabdominal CVS, the placenta is the target, and the needle must often be introduced into the placenta at an obtuse angle to the uterine wall. This subtle difference can quickly be mastered by established amniocentesis providers with expert faculty instruction. Similarly, we find more novice providers who have extensively practiced their

core guidance skills but have not performed many real-life procedures grasp the difference in needle approach between amniocentesis and CVS rather quickly.

Transcervical CVS is unique among obstetric ultrasound guidance procedures as it is the only one not performed transabdominally. There are several notable differences between transcervical and transabdominal procedures. For example, one cannot self-guide the procedures as holding a transabdominal ultrasound probe while simultaneously guiding a catheter through the cervix is impractical if not impossible. Furthermore, while it is easy to line up the target and needle in the same ultrasound plane during a transabdominal procedure, this is not always possible in a transcervical procedure due to a non-straight cervical canal or a placenta that lies laterally to the cervix. As a result the guidance skills used in other procedures do not transfer very well for transcervical CVS. Given the uniqueness of the guidance skills needed for transcervical CVS, it is often necessary for fellows to spend proportionally more time to master this procedure.

Percutaneous Umbilical Blood Sampling

Percutaneous umbilical blood sampling (PUBS) is a rare procedure utilized mainly to assess for anemia, thrombocytopenia, and the need for fetal intrauterine transfusion. As a result, training in PUBS during Maternal-Fetal Medicine fellowship training is limited in many portions of the United States [31]. In fact, many fellows will not have performed enough procedures to reach an acceptable level of competence prior to graduation except through the use of simulation.

By the time a fellow has reached the point in their training when they may be called upon to participate in or perform a PUBS procedure, they will likely have already received considerable experience in ultrasound-guided needle procedures through simulated and real-life amniocentesis and CVS. However, there are pieces of equipment and several motor tasks specific to PUBS that are not a part of the other ultrasound-guided needle procedures. Unlike the other invasive procedures discussed thus far, which tend to be brief, even in experienced hands it is not uncommon for a PUBS and intrauterine transfusion to take an hour or more to complete while awaiting analysis of the blood and preparation and infusion of blood products. Fellows will not be accustomed to having to hold a needle steady for such a prolonged period of time. It is important to provide fellows with an opportunity to familiarize themselves with the needed equipment and practice steadying a needle for extended periods of time.

Fortunately there are several options for simulating a PUBS including using a delivered placenta and/or umbilical cord or a commercially available task trainer [25, 32–34]. As is the case with all phantom-based simulators, the commercially available task trainers have a limited number of configurations. However, models made from recently delivered placentas and umbilical cords allow for much greater flexibility in terms of anatomic arrangements and degree of procedural difficulty. All the placental models allow the manipulation of the placental umbilical cord insertion site and cord orientation.

Prior to performing the needle guidance portion of the procedure, the fellows should lay out all of the needed equipment and practice assembling and dissembling the transfusion apparatus. Mock donor blood can even be injected through the tubing while the fellow manipulates the stopcocks or other parts of the transfusion setup. It may also be beneficial to have one fellow manage the transfusion apparatus and transfuse the blood, while another fellow or faculty member inserts the needle into the cord and steadies the needle. Once this has been mastered, simulation of a PUBS and intrauterine transfusion can be created starting with a favorable anatomic relationship of the placenta and cord allowing learners to begin practicing with a technically easy and lower stress procedure. Once these easier procedures have been mastered, the model can be altered to simulate procedures that require awkward angles of vascular access due to unfavorable placenta and cord locations. In all of these cases, the fellow should transfuse a sizeable volume of simulated blood so they can experience how difficult it can be to keep the needle tip within the cord throughout the procedure.

Prior to actual clinical procedures, we have the most junior fellow in attendance perform the initial ultrasound and choose their needle insertion site, with successively senior fellows doing the same. This approach allows all fellows to participate in a critical portion of the PUBS procedures—planning the needle insertion and target orientation site.

In Utero Stenting

Although not an FDA-approved device, in utero stents have been granted a compassionate care exemption for treatment of bladder outlet obstruction and type I CPAMs with a dominant cyst. The conditions are rare (1 in 4000–5000 births) such that even the most experienced providers will seldom perform more than 10 procedures throughout their careers. With that statistic in mind, it is not reasonable to expect a provider to perform 25 or more of these procedures (which is the case for CVS and amniocentesis) prior to being granted clinical privileges leading many to advocate that these procedures only be performed in specialized, "higher-volume" centers. Others contend that a provider with extensive experience in amniocentesis and CVS has the requisite skills to perform an in utero stenting procedure to guide the trocar to its target. Although this seems a plausible assumption, it does not naturally follow that they would be sufficiently familiar with the steps necessary to deploy the stent once the trocar has been appropriately placed or how to handle the more complex clinical situations and possible complications.

Simulation can be a valuable tool in the training or reviewing the steps for stent deployment for both experienced and novice providers. Unfortunately, there are no commercially available simulators available for this procedure. However, we have described a homemade fetal pig-based simulator for in utero stenting [35] (Fig. 15.1). Although the latter model provides a higher-fidelity representation of the uterine and fetal anatomy, it has many of the same problems with construction and setup we encountered with our bovine heart CVS model. Once again we opted for a more convenient model with lower fidelity but greater utility that allows trainees to focus on the steps of stent deployment without and then with ultrasound guidance. In our new approach, we use two pint-sized Ziploc freezer bags filled with ultrasound gel. Once the upper surface of one of the bags is covered with ultrasound gel, the second bag is placed on top allowing one to deploy the shaft of the stent across the interface of the two bags with a single coil in each bag. While this does not reproduce the guidance of the trocar into the relevant fetal body cavity, it does allow the stent to be deployed. Deployment is first performed under direct visualization of the trocar and stent within the bags. Once the provider is comfortable with the movements enabling stent deployment, the procedure can be performed under ultrasound guidance. This model allows the provider to practice multiple deployments in quick succession as the stent can easily be retrieved by gasping the straight segment of the stent as it crosses the interface between the two bags. This availability of repetitive practice is particularly valuable for novice trainees learning this skill for the first time. Experienced providers can practice the procedure prior to an actual procedure as their deployment skill can deteriorate over the many months and even years that pass between the need for these procedures.

Putting It All Together

Utilization of the above models can allow beginning and intermediate learners to gain the requisite skills to be ready to perform an amniocentesis or chorionic villus sampling procedure in an actual clinical setting. Any areas needing improvement noted on actual clinical procedures can be readily taught and practiced immediately afterward using the task trainers set to the maternal condition and oriented to the fetal position or placental location. Any anxiety with a problem during an actual procedure can be reduced for both the faculty and the trainee by focused post-procedural practice.

The amount of instructional time each fellowship devotes to ultrasound-guided procedure training will likely determine which of the above simulators are used in fellow training and how much time will be devoted to each. As amniocentesis is the only ultrasound-guided invasive procedure in which fellows must demonstrate competency to perform prior to graduation, it is essential to devote a significant amount of time to training to this procedure. For the remainder of the procedures discussed above, i.e., CVS, in utero stenting, and PUBS, fellows must only demonstrate an understanding of their indications, contraindications, risk, and principles but need not demonstrate competency in performing them prior to graduation. Many programs may still wish to devote considerable amount of time to training in one or more of these additional procedures.

Examples

Our approach has been to devote a significant amount of time to training in the core ultrasound guidance skills. When this is complete, we focus on both amniocentesis and CVS and to a lesser extent to in utero stenting and PUBS. For these very rare procedures, we tend to practice more after one of them has been scheduled. In these rarer cases, we practice extensively in the few days prior to the procedure with our senior fellows who have already demonstrated sufficient needle guidance skill and if possible arrange the simulator in such a way that mimics the relevant maternal, fetal, and placental anatomy specific to the patient.

At our institution we have six ultrasound-guided invasive procedure simulation sessions each year. An outline of our curricular topics is provided in Table 15.2. We devote much of the first session to explaining how the relationship of the needle to the probe affects where the needle appears and how hand movements alter the needles position on the ultrasound screen (see section "Needle Guidance Basics" above). During this first session we also demonstrate targeting tasks (see section "Core Guidance Skills" above) and have the fellows perform them. Their completion time and number of targeting errors are recorded to establish their baseline level of ultra-

Table 15.2 Ultrasound-guided invasive procedure simulation curriculum

Session	Simulation
1	Needle guidance basics and core basic guidance skills
2	Amniocentesis
3	Intermediate core guidance skills
4	Chorionic villus sampling
5	Advanced core guidance skills
6	In utero stenting and PUBS

sound guidance skill. We then alternate procedure-specific simulation sessions with core guidance skill sessions for the remainder of the curriculum. During the procedure-specific session, we introduce the unique aspects of each procedure, such as syringe attachment, aspiration of fluid (amniocentesis) or villi (CVS), attachment of transfusion apparatus (PUBS), or the steps of stent deployment (in utero stenting). In addition, at the end of the procedure-specific sessions, we perform a baseline assessment using a checklist of critical procedural steps. We compare an individual fellow's checklist scores and targeting task performance each year and attempt to identify specific areas of improvement that should be focused upon in the coming year. We often employ our senior fellow as instructors during these sessions as we find this helps solidify the knowledge and procedural skills they will need after graduation.

Conclusions

The number of real-life obstetric ultrasound-guided invasive procedures has decreased to the point that it is no longer possible to sufficiently train residents and fellows to perform these procedures without the use of simulation. While participation in real-life procedures will always be necessary, utilization of a robust simulation educational curriculum with appropriate task trainers has become a critical adjunct to real-life training in ultrasound-guided invasive procedures. To be truly effective the curriculum should be clearly structured and provide ample time for deliberative practice. In addition, performance milestones should be clearly defined to make sure a trainee grasps the central concepts and has a considerable amount of technical skill prior to performing a procedure on an actual patient.

In this chapter we have provided the theoretic framework needed to construct such a curriculum and described our approach to invasive procedure training. However, we do not wish for our approach to be rigidly applied to other training programs, as we acknowledge that each program will have its own set of challenges to overcome regarding baseline skill level of their trainees, available instructor time, and funds for simulation equipment, among others. Rather, we recommend that each program structure their training regimen based on the educational needs of their trainees and the educational resources they have available. However, we feel that it is more efficient to "cross train" between procedures by focusing on the core skills of planning the approach, localization of the needle, and guiding it to the intended target. Once these skills have been mastered, procedure-specific training is also needed to obtain proficiency in the steps that are required once needle reaches its intended destination.

References

1. Leschot NJ, Verjaal M, Treffers PE. Risks of midtrimester amniocentesis; assessment in 3000 pregnancies. Br J Obstet Gynaecol. 1985;92:804–7.
2. Verjaal M, Leschot NJ, Treffers PE. Risk of amniocentesis and laboratory findings in a series of 1500 prenatal diagnoses. Prenat Diagn. 1981;1:173–81.
3. Nizard J, Duyme M, Ville Y. Teaching ultrasound-guided invasive procedures in fetal medicine: learning curves with and without an electronic guidance system. Ultrasound Obstet Gynecol. 2002;19:274–7.
4. Wijnberger LD, van der Schouw YT, Christiaens GC. Learning in medicine: chorionic villus sampling. Prenat Diagn. 2000;20:241–6.
5. Tongprasert F, Srisupundit K, Luewan S, Phadungkiatwattana P, Pranpanus S, Tongsong T. Midpregnancy cordocentesis training of maternal-fetal medicine fellows. Ultrasound Obstet Gynecol. 2010;36:65–8.
6. AIUM practice parameter for the performance of selected ultrasound-guided procedures. http://www.aium.org/resources/guidelines/usGuidedProcedures.pdf. Cited 7 Mar 2017.
7. Cook DA, Hatala R, Brydges R, Zendejas B, Szostek JH, Wang AT, et al. Technology-enhanced simulation for health professions education: a systematic review and meta-analysis. JAMA. 2011;306:978–88.

8. Cooke DT, Jamshidi R, Guitron J, Karamichalis J. The virtual surgeon: using medical simulation to train the modern surgical resident. Bull Am Coll Surg. 2008;93:26–31.

9. Ross AJ, Kodate N, Anderson JE, Thomas L, Jaye P. Review of simulation studies in anaesthesia journals, 2001–2010: mapping and content analysis. Br J Anaesth. 2012;109:99–109.

10. McLaughlin S, Fitch MT, Goyal DG, Hayden E, Kauh CY, Laack TA, et al. Simulation in graduate medical education 2008: a review for emergency medicine. Acad Emerg Med. 2008;15:1117–29.

11. Crofts JF, Bartlett C, Ellis D, Fox R, Draycott TJ. Documentation of simulated shoulder dystocia: accurate and complete? BJOG. 2008;115:1303–8.

12. Crofts JF, Fox R, Ellis D, Winter C, Hinshaw K, Draycott TJ. Observations from 450 shoulder dystocia simulations: lessons for skills training. Obstet Gynecol. 2008;112:906–12.

13. Draycott TJ, Crofts JF, Ash JP, Wilson LV, Yard E, Sibanda T, et al. Improving neonatal outcome through practical shoulder dystocia training. Obstet Gynecol. 2008;112:14–20.

14. Goffman D, Heo H, Chazotte C, Merkatz IR, Bernstein PS. Using simulation training to improve shoulder dystocia documentation. Obstet Gynecol. 2008;112:1284–7.

15. Goffman D, Heo H, Pardanani S, Merkatz IR, Bernstein PS. Improving shoulder dystocia management among resident and attending physicians using simulations. Am J Obstet Gynecol. 2008;199:294 e1–5.

16. Daniels K, Parness AJ. Development and use of mechanical devices for simulation of seizure and hemorrhage in obstetrical team training. Simul Healthc. 2008;3:42–6.

17. Hong A, Mullin PM, Al-Marayati L, Peyre SE, Muderspach L, Macdonald H, et al. A low-fidelity total abdominal hysterectomy teaching model for obstetrics and gynecology residents. Simul Healthc. 2012;7:123–6.

18. Lentz GM, Mandel LS, Goff BA. A six-year study of surgical teaching and skills evaluation for obstetric/gynecologic residents in porcine and inanimate surgical models. Am J Obstet Gynecol. 2005;193:2056–61.

19. Lentz GM, Mandel LS, Lee D, Gardella C, Melville J, Goff BA. Testing surgical skills of obstetric and gynecologic residents in a bench laboratory setting: validity and reliability. Am J Obstet Gynecol. 2001;184:1462–8; discussion 1468–70.

20. Goff BA, VanBlaricom A, Mandel L, Chinn M, Nielsen P. Comparison of objective, structured assessment of technical skills with a virtual reality hysteroscopy trainer and standard latex hysteroscopy model. J Reprod Med. 2007;52:407–12.

21. Gurusamy K, Aggarwal R, Palanivelu L, Davidson BR. Systematic review of randomized controlled trials on the effectiveness of virtual reality training for laparoscopic surgery. Br J Surg. 2008;95:1088–97.

22. Gurusamy KS, Aggarwal R, Palanivelu L, Davidson BR. Virtual reality training for surgical trainees in laparoscopic surgery. Cochrane Database Syst Rev. 2009;8:CD006575.

23. Savran MM, Sorensen SM, Konge L, Tolsgaard MG, Bjerrum F. Training and assessment of hysteroscopic skills: a systematic review. J Surg Educ. 2016;73:906–18.

24. Hefler L, Grimm C, Kueronya V, Tempfer C, Reinthaller A, Polterauer S. A novel training model for the loop electrosurgical excision procedure: an innovative replica helped workshop participants improve their LEEP. Am J Obstet Gynecol. 2012;206:535 e1–4.

25. Tongprasert F, Wanapirak C, Sirichotiyakul S, Piyamongkol W, Tongsong T. Training in cordocentesis: the first 50 case experience with and without a cordocentesis training model. Prenat Diagn. 2010;30:467–70.

26. Amniocentesis and Chorionic Villus Sampling. Royal College of Obstetricians and Gynaecologists. https://www.rcog.org.uk/globalassets/documents/guidelines/gtg_8.pdf. Accessed 9 Sep 2018.

27. Nitsche JF, Shumard KM, Brost BC. Development and assessment of a novel task trainer and targeting tasks for ultrasound-guided invasive procedures. Acad Radiol. 24(6):700–8.

28. Zubair I, Marcotte MP, Weinstein L, Brost BC. A novel amniocentesis model for learning stereotactic skills. Am J Obstet Gynecol. 2006;194:846–8.

29. McWeeney DT, Schwendemann WD, Nitsche JF, Rose CH, Davies NP, Watson WJ, et al. Transabdominal and transcervical chorionic villus sampling models to teach maternal-fetal medicine fellows. Am J Perinatol. 2012;29:497–502.

30. Wax JR, Cartin A, Pinette MG. The birds and the beans: a low-fidelity simulator for chorionic villus sampling skill acquisition. J Ultrasound Med. 2012;31:1271–5.

31. Grace D, Thornburg LL, Grey A, Ozcan T, Pressman EK. Training for percutaneous umbilical blood sampling during Maternal Fetal Medicine fellowship in the United States. Prenat Diagn. 2009;29:790–3.

32. Mcweeney D, Nitsche J, White W, Rose C, Davies N, Watson W, et al. Periumbilical blood sampling and intravascular transfusion model to teach maternal-fetal medicine fellows. Am J Obstet Gynecol. 2009;201:380.

33. Timor-Tritsch IE, Yeh MN. In vitro training model for diagnostic and therapeutic fetal intravascular needle puncture. Am J Obstet Gynecol. 1987;157:858–9.

34. Angel JL, O'Brien WF, Michelson JA, Knuppel RA, Morales WJ. Instructional model for percutaneous fetal umbilical blood sampling. Obstet Gynecol. 1989;73:669–71.

35. Nitsche JF, McWeeney DT, Schwendemann WD, Rose CH, Davies NP, Watson W, et al. In-utero stenting: development of a low-cost high-fidelity task trainer. Ultrasound Obstet Gynecol. 2009;34:720–3.

Part IV

Simulation of Gynecology

Basic Gynecologic Encounters and Procedures

16

Mary K. Collins, Meleen Chuang, Shad Deering, and Tamika C. Auguste

Introduction

The annual "well-woman" visit is important for recognizing general health risk factors, promoting prevention practices and identifying gynecological problems. It should include screening, evaluation, and counseling. The intimate nature of women's health issues often presented during a gynecological visit makes it an important priority that a patient's comfort be optimized [2].

The clinician's ability to provide a nonjudgmental, non-threatening experience can enable the patient to feel at ease and facilitate a positive as well as purposeful encounter. A skilled clinician who is proficient with history taking and performing a physical exam can help to alleviate patient anxiety and improve the patient's overall experience [3]. The use of simulation in this area enables these skills to be practiced prior to an encounter with a real patient, and we will review how simulation can be used for gynecological history taking as well as to address aspects of the physical exam and common gynecologic procedures.

> **Key Learning Points**
> - As gynecologic procedures can involve intimate examinations, simulation is a useful method to improve provider familiarity and competency before seeing actual patients.
> - Both task trainers as well as standardized patients can be used depending on the learning objectives.

M. K. Collins (✉)
Walter Reed National Military Medical Center, Bethesda, MD, USA

M. Chuang
Albert Einstein College of Medicine/Montefiore Medical Center, Bronx, NY, USA

S. Deering
Department of Obstetrics and Gynecology, Uniformed Services University of the Health Sciences, Bethesda, MD, USA

T. C. Auguste
Department of Obstetrics and Gynecology, MedStar Washington Hospital Center, Washington, DC, USA

Learning Techniques

Individuals who take part in the gynecologic visit include medical students, nurses, resident physicians, physician assistants, attending physicians, midwives, and nurse practitioners. Just as there are a wide variety of providers that need to learn how to perform the exams, there are a numerous methods used to teach these learners how to perform gynecologic procedures. Discussions as well as demonstrations are often used. Because gynecologic exams can be uncomfortable for the patient, it is often difficult to teach via a hands-on learning approach. A paradox exists in that patients prefer exams to be performed by experienced and well-practiced providers, yet understandably patients prefer not to be practiced on [4]. Because of this, simulation is well-suited to enable the provider to learn exam techniques with task trainers which allow for the opportunity to practice the technical steps with supervision and feedback.

Another simulation teaching method that allows learners to practice skills and be evaluated on their ability to perform tasks before actual patients is the use of standardized patients. This is when a trained individual portray the role of a patient for learners to practice their skills. This process was pioneered by the University of Southern California in the 1960s and is now used in the majority of medical schools in the United States [5]. A thorough discussion about the use of standardized patients for gynecologic examinations can be found in Chap. 11 of this book.

A 2016 survey conducted with respondents from 95 US allopathic medical school obstetrics and gynecology clerkship directors found that only 40% of respondents rated their school's pelvic examination training as excellent and only 18% rated breast examination training as excellent. This study also found that pelvic and breast examinations are most commonly taught during obstetrics and gynecology clerkships. Therefore suggesting that it is an area that could focus improved integration with simulations [6].

History Taking

The importance of obtaining a medical history is vital in patient encounters, as it establishes why the patient presented and leads to potential plans of care. The interviewer should begin by introducing themselves and state their role in the patient's care. Next the interviewer establishes names and relationship of the patient and any other individuals present. The patient's agenda/reason for visit should be elicited. Optimally this part of the encounter should be in a relaxed, private setting with the patient dressed. The questions should be open-ended, and the clinician should allow the patient to describe her concerns without interruption. Body language, such as maintaining eye contact and smiling, is an essential non-verbal cue that interviewers should be aware of. Enhancing the conversation through practice with standardized patients can help the learner to be better prepared and make the patient feel more at ease disclosing and when partaking in physical examinations.

Breast Examination

Gynecologists and all women healthcare provider routinely discuss breast health, awareness, screening guidelines, risk factors, and review recommendations. The breast examination is usually included in the routine annual well-women physical examination.

A 2013 meta-analysis for simulation training found that eight studies of breast simulation training showed moderate to large positive results for both skills and outcomes (i.e., successful ability to detect breast abnormalities), though these results were not consistent across all of the studies. Breast models that had technological advancements (i.e., inflatable masses, pulsating lumps, and pressure sensors) were found to be superior at training students as compared to static silicone breast models [4]. Additionally a 2014 study reported that not only were simulation methods like standardized patients and models able to improve student's abilities to perform patient histories and physical exams and detect breast cancers but also in their ability to communicate bad news to patients effectively. Specifically, students taught with the aid of standardized patients were more accurate, thorough, and professional at performing breast examinations [7].

There are a variety of task trainers for breast exams that are commercially available. Listed below are some examples that can be used:

- The Breast Examination Model (3B Scientific Atlanta, GA) is a female breast trainer that can be used to teach detection of breast nodules and cysts. It allows in either the sitting or prone position.

- The Advanced Breast Exam Simulator (Anatomy Warehouse.Com, Skokie, IL) allows for general breast examinations. The tissue density varies within the simulated breast, and there is the option of inserting masses of different sizes and densities.
- The Standard Breast Examination Trainer (Limbs and Things, Savannah, GA) provides the ability for a trainer to actually wear the simulator. It can also be worn by the trainee so they can learn how to perform/teach self-breast examination. There are interchangeable inserts that allow for different masses to be palpated as well (Fig. 16.1).

Pelvic Examination

The pelvic examination can be a very challenging examination to execute because of associated patient discomfort, anxiety, and embarrassment. The American College of Physicians reported that 35 percent of surveyed women experience fear, anxiety, discomfort, and/or pain during their pelvic examination [8]. Women who experienced pain with their pelvic examination were found to be less likely to return for their visit than those

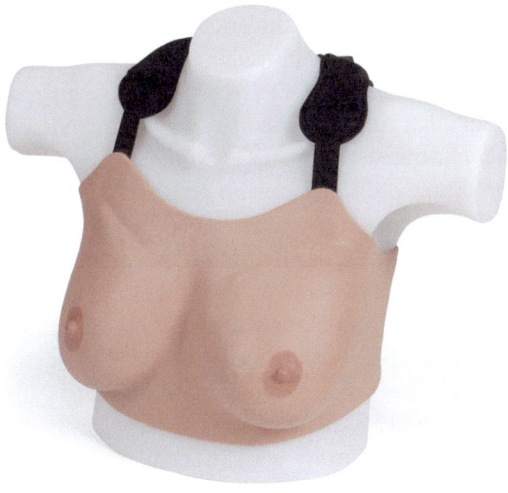

Fig. 16.1 Standard Breast Examination Trainer. Reproduced with permission of Limbs and Things, Inc.

who did not have a negative experience [9]. Another study sought to address suggestions to improve the examination process from patients that had negative experience. Explaining each step of the examination in advance, providing information about the reproductive organs, warming the instruments, increased gentleness, and maintaining eye contact have been suggested by the patients as ways to improve the overall experience of the basic GYN examination [10]. All of these areas can be addressed with simulation training.

The pelvic examination is conducted to screen for pathology, with the examination made of three elements: inspection of the external genitalia; speculum examination of the vagina and cervix; and bimanual examination of the adnexa, uterus, ovaries, and bladder and sometimes a rectovaginal examination.

Teaching the pelvic examination portion of the basic GYN exam can start with an overview of the necessary materials. Reviewing the various swabs, Pap smear collection devices, bacterial wound culture, viral culture container, review of various specula (pediatric, nulliparous, multiparous speculum), and urine culture collection are some of the many various useful materials that a learner may not have seen before. Becoming familiar with these materials, recognizing what they look like, and indications and uses of collecting samples may be very helpful for the learner and lead to a more efficient and streamlined exam.

Having the opportunity to be instructed by a standardized patient on proper techniques for performing pelvic examinations is ideal as the anatomy is real and the feedback is immediate. Standardized patients are often utilized as both instructors and patients for these sessions. The standardized patient is able to talk the learner through proper bedside manner and work though a pelvic examination and bimanual examination usually with an instructor present to further provide brief lecture to the students prior to the examination. Often, the standardized patient provides the learner with feedback and helpful critiques to allow for improvement in clinical skills as both the content expert and patient.

A hemi-pelvis simulator can also be used for most aspects of the pelvic examination. Some of the tasks that can be trained include placement of a speculum, cytology sampling, obtaining vaginal and cervical cultures, and bimanual examinations.

It is important to ensure the patient is as comfortable as possible during the exam. This can be optimized by describing each step of the exam before doing it, maintaining the patient's modesty, and performing the exam in a gentle and professional manner. It is also important to make clear to the patient that they can stop the exam at any point throughout the process.

Below is an outline for steps of the pelvic exam that can be taught with both standardized patients and task trainers:

Basic Steps for Pelvic Exam

(a) Position patient properly.
(b) Visually examine external genitalia.
(c) Insert speculum.
(d) Inspect the vaginal mucosa and cervix.
(e) Obtain Pap smear or cultures (when indicated).
(f) Bimanual exam:
   (i) Palpate the cervix, uterine fundus, and bilateral adnexa.

Available Simulation Models

There are a variety of task trainers for pelvic exams. Listed below are some examples that can be used:

- The Advanced Pelvic Examination and Gynecological Simulator (Anatomy Warehouse. Com, Skokie, IL.). This simulator can be used for gynecological exam, education, and training. Skills that can be trained include the bimanual exam, speculum exam, and cytology sampling.
- EVA Gynecologic Mannequin (Simulaids, Saugerties, NY). This is a female pelvis that can be used for practicing gynecologic procedures to include abdominal palpation and

speculum insertion. It also allows for palpation of different pelvic masses.
- Life/form Pelvic Examination Simulator, Normal (NASCO, Fort Atkinson, WI). This task trainer contains a normal simulated cervix, uterus, and ovaries. It is designed for digital exam only and is not recommended for speculum examinations.
- Cervical Exam and Pap Smear Test Trainer (3B Scientific, Atlanta, GA). This simulator can be used to train for both external and internal examinations. You can also practice speculum insertion and cytological sampling techniques.
- Clinical Female Pelvic Trainer (CFPT) (Limbs and Things, Savannah, GA). This simulator comes with a standard hemi-pelvis base and includes interchangeable pelvic inserts to simulate different pathologies such as fibroids and cervical polyps.

Colposcopy Simulation

The volume of colposcopies performed has drastically declined after changes in screening and management recommendations. A 2016 study showed a two thirds decline in colposcopy appointments from 2010 to 2015 [11]. But, despite declining procedure volume, adequate training to ensure detection of cervical cancer continues to be important. At present, there are several types of simulations that have been described to assist in training for this examination. An example of a low-cost colposcopy simulator that utilizes kielbasa as the cervix is demonstrated at the ACOG simulation working group's toolkit and can be accessed at: https://www.acog.org/About-ACOG/ACOG-Departments/Simulations-Consortium/Simulations-Consortium-Tool-Kit.

Other types of simulators are commercially available and are able to display cervical cytological dysplasia. One example of this is the Gynecologic Skills Trainer that is made by 3B Scientific (https://www.a3bs.com/gynecologic-skills-trainer-p91-1021592-p91-3b-scientific,p_1453_30133.html). Another is the "Colleen" Cervical Procedure Trainer (Remedy Simulation Group, Perkasie, PA) that can be used for the simulation of cervical procedures including Pap smears, colposcopies, and biopsies. It is actually an insert that fits into existing mannequins and other task trainers. The tissue is realistic enough to allow for use with a speculum.

Endometrial Biopsy Simulation

The endometrial cavity is routinely sampled to evaluate the endometrium for a variety of reasons, most often when a woman has abnormal bleeding. Though some simulators are manufactured to try and mimic this procedure, there are well-documented low-cost models as well. The most widely known is the Papaya Model which has not only been studied, but there are multiple resources available online that describe how to set up and use the model [12]. This includes using a ripe papaya that represents the uterus, and a small hole is made in the stem to represent the cervix. A biopsy is performed by inserting a pipelle into a small hole made in the stem, and the flesh of the papaya mimics endometrial tissue. The papaya can also be placed in a hemipelvis to mimic a uterus in a pelvis that can be accessed by the vaginal canal of the simulator.

Ultrasound Simulators

Ultrasound training is difficult to practice as it can be stressful for trainees and patients, particularly in cases where transvaginal sonography is needed or there is a fetal malformation present. Currently, what has been published with regard to ultrasound training in OB/GYN has found improvements in students' anxiety levels, performance, efficiency, competence, and reconciliation of clinical scenarios [13].

There are a variety of ultrasound simulators, generally divided into their method of image generation. These include:

- Phantom-based: This is where a simulator contains a physical "phantom" that is encased in a shell that the trainee can use a normal ultrasound on. This allows for real-time scanning, but only of the phantom that is contained

in the simulator, and there will not be any movement or blood flow. In order to demonstrate different images/pathology, it is often necessary to either switch out the internal phantom or purchase a separate simulator.

- Interpolative model-based: These simulators presents 2D images generated from 3D volumes that were previously captured in ultrasound examinations. This allows for realistic imagines to be shown, and the probe movements should allow the trainee to obtain different angles through the target being imaged.
- Generative model-based: This type shows 2D imaging that is constructed completely by software. While they continue to improve in quality, these are sometimes critiqued for only having more simplified images [13].

A disadvantage of the interpolative and generative model-based ultrasound simulators is that, as with other virtual reality simulators, they are more expensive and the tactile feedback is not as real as the physical phantom-based ones. What many of the virtual simulators do offer, however, is a more comprehensive case-based and scenario-driven didactic curriculum that can be very helpful for training.

Some of the currently available sonogram simulation training programs offer opportunities to practice skills but also include didactic courses, hands-on training, and knowledge assessments that are integrated in the learning.

Some commercially available simulators in ultrasound include:

- Sonosim (SonoSim, Santa Monica, CA). This product used a simulated ultrasound probe connected to a computer that allows you to practice multiple different examination, including female pelvic ultrasound. It has a full educational curriculum included as well.
- Blue Phantom (CAE Healthcare): This company has a full range of phantom-type ultrasound simulators. They include models for ectopic pregnancy, general gynecologic pathology, and even one with the ability to perform a sonohysterogram.
- ScanTrainer (MedaPhor): This gynecologic ultrasound training platform is focused on the

transvaginal approach and uses actual patient scans as the basis for the images seen. It has a physical ultrasound probe that provides tactile feedback and a full curriculum for gynecologic pathology.

Conclusion

There are many ways to optimize learning for those partaking in gynecological patient care. These opportunities range from the use of simulation, pelvic trainers, standardized patients, and even virtual reality simulators for ultrasound. Providers are able to hone their skills with these and can improve the patient experience, which is especially important in these gynecologic encounters where patients often feel uncomfortable and vulnerable.

References

1. Dennerstein L, Lehert P, Koochaki PE, et al. A symptomatic approach to understanding women's health experiences: a cross-cultural comparison of women aged 20 to 70 years. Menopause. 2007;14(4):688–96.
2. Van Dulmen AM. Communication during gynecological out-patient encounters. J Psychosom Obstet Gynaecol. 1999 Sep;20(3):119–26.
3. Carr SE, Carmody D. Outcomes of teaching medical students core skills for women's health: the pelvic examination educational program. Am J Obstet Gynecol. 2004;190(5):1382.
4. Dilaveri C, Szostek J, Wang A, Cook D. Simulation training for breast and pelvis physical examination: a systematic review and meta-analysis. BJOG. 2013;120:1171–82.
5. Wallace, P. Following the threads of an innovation: the history of standardized patients in medical education. https://web.archive.org/web/20081228115335/http://aspeducators.org/wallace.htm. Accessed 26 Dec 2017. Originally published in Caduceus, A Humanities Journal for Medicine and the Health Sciences, Department of Medical Humanities, Southern Illinois University School of Medicine.1997;13(2):5–28.
6. Dugoff L, et al. Pelvic and breast examination skills curricula in United States medical schools: a survey of obstetrics and gynecology clerkship directors. BMC Med Educ. 2016;16:314.
7. Simpson J. The education utility of simulation in treating history and physical examination skills in diagnosing breast Cancer: a review of the literature. J Breast Cancer. 2014;17(2):107–12.
8. Ubel P, Jepson C, Silver-Isenstadt A. Don't ask, don't tell: a change in medical student attitudes after obstetrics/gynecology clerkships toward seeking consent for pelvic examinations on an anesthetized patient. Am J Obstet Gynecol. 2003;188:575–9.
9. Avery D, McDonald J. The declining number of family physicians practicing obstetrics: rural impact, reasons, recommendations and considerations. Am J Clin Med. 2014;10(2):70–8.
10. Qaseem A, Humphrey LL, Harris R, Starkey M, Denberg TD, Clinical Guidelines Committee of the American College of Physicians. Screening pelvic examination in adult women: a clinical practice guideline from the American College of Physicians. Ann Intern Med. 2014;161(1):67.
11. Landers E, Erickson B, Bae S, Huh W. Trends in colposcopy volume: where do we go from Here? J Low Genit Tract Dis. 2016;20(4):292–5.
12. Steinauer J, Preskill F, Devaskar S, Landy U, Darney P. The papaya workshop: using the papaya to teach intrauterine gynecologic procedures. MedEdPORTAL. 2013;9:9388. https://doi.org/10.15766/mep_2374-8265.9388.
13. Chalouhi G. Ultrasound simulators in obstetrics and gynecology: state of the art. Ultrasound Obstet Gynecol. 2014;43(3):257.

Surgical Simulation in Gynecology

Chetna Arora, Jin Hee Jeannie Kim,
and Arnold Patrick Advincula

Introduction

Our surgical heritage is defined by self-education, apprenticeship, arduous repetition, and, ultimately, autonomy. This pathway of learning is tried-and-true for our experienced surgical role models—those who have written our textbooks, drawn our atlases, and guided our millennial hands in the operating room. These proven methods are neither incorrect nor archaic, but with the ongoing remodeling of our standards of care and increasing lack of confidence in graduating surgical trainees, restructuring our approach to education is crucial. With the integration of duty hours and assimilation of advancements in surgical technology, learning curves are steeper, and hands-on trainee opportunity is narrowed [1, 2].

In addition to the progression of technology and surgery are the changes in the perspective and approach to education of our current learners. We have shifted from lecture-based classrooms and box trainers to interactive peer-to-peer teaching, high-fidelity simulation, and a wider capacity to adjust to an ever-expanding work-life balance [3]. While this may be interpreted with more scrutiny from older generations of educators, this contrast in approach allows and attunes to a wider breadth of successful education. Without acknowledging this difference, we only further disrupt communication and expectations [3, 4].

With the evolution of surgical simulation, our educational practices have spanned from rudimentary box trainers to high-fidelity virtual reality simulators. Basic skill training in standard topics of hand-eye coordination, tissue handling, and instrument handling are still enforced, but the improved functionality allows for a more realistic approach in surgical anatomy, the capacity to complete a wide array of full procedures independently, and provides objective metrics of assessment and instant feedback. With the data reported to the trainee at the completion of the simulation, they can subsequently interpret areas in need of improvement as well as validation of mastery in simulation surgical skillsets.

In gynecologic surgery, all routes of surgery allow for integration and improvement in surgical education via simulation. With the basic principles of surgical education in mind, the use of simulation pushes us beyond the outdated and

C. Arora (✉) · J. H. J. Kim
Columbia University Medical Center/New York-Presbyterian Hospital, Department of Obstetrics and Gynecology, New York, NY, USA
e-mail: ca2773@cumc.columbia.edu

A. P. Advincula
Columbia University Medical Center/New York-Presbyterian Hospital, Department of Obstetrics and Gynecology, New York, NY, USA

Mary & Michael Jaharis Simulation Center, New York, NY, USA

© Springer International Publishing AG, part of Springer Nature 2019
S. Deering et al. (eds.), *Comprehensive Healthcare Simulation: Obstetrics and Gynecology*,
Comprehensive Healthcare Simulation, https://doi.org/10.1007/978-3-319-98995-2_17

dangerous apprenticeship model of "see one, do one, teach one" [5]. In this chapter, we will highlight the current literature and applications of surgical simulation in commonly performed gynecologic procedures.

> **Key Learning Points**
> - Gynecologic surgical techniques can be taught with both low and high-fidelity simulators.
> - Many of the simulation training options include curricula to review relevant anatomy and also provide the opportunity to practice technical skills.
> - Initial training for robotic surgical techniques is largely simulation-based and done on high-fidelity simulators.

Hysteroscopic Surgery

Skill Gap Hysteroscopic surgery allows for direct endoscopic visualization of the uterine cavity for both diagnostic and therapeutic purpose. Via this intrauterine approach, one can readily identify and surgically treat pathologies causing abnormal uterine bleeding, infertility, pelvic pain, and neoplasm. While the majority of these procedures can be completed quickly in an outpatient setting and are traditionally low-risk, operative hysteroscopic experience minimizes the possibility of significant procedure-related complications [5]. It has also been repeatedly evidenced in our literature that there are significant differences in the hands of a novice or inexperienced surgeon versus an expert in hysteroscopic surgery [6, 7]. It is also of noteworthy importance that many residents feel a lack of preparedness in hysteroscopic surgery upon graduation [8–10]. In a recent study, only three-fourths of residents feel prepared with hysteroscopic myomectomy under 3 cm, less than 50% feel competent in global endometrial ablation, and only 20–30% feel competent in advanced skills such as lysis of moderate-severe adhesions or myomas >3 cm [9].

Solution In an effort to bridge this gap, hysteroscopic simulation can be readily integrated into obstetric and gynecologic residency surgical curriculums. Simulation via inanimate models as a low-fidelity model as well as high-fidelity virtual simulators has been described and implemented with positive results.

Inanimate models with box trainers from various sources have been used in dry labs with trainees and confirm that direct simulated procedures measurably improve performance compared to controls and are well-received by the participants (Fig. 17.1). For example, the simplicity in the design and readily implementable hysteroscopy training program as developed by Rackow et al. using trainers developed by the Chamberlain Group © allows for the necessary and characteristic repetition to mastery [11]. Many simulators are available and include trainers focused in skills from endometrial ablation to hysteroscopic resection with energy devices. In the event commercialized simulation products are not available, vegetable and fruit models have been employed with success with the use of

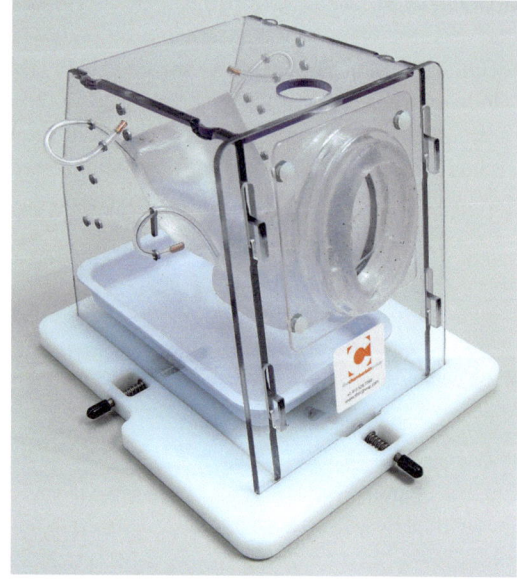

Fig. 17.1 Endometrial ablation trainer from the Chamberlain Group ©. (Used with permission from the Chamberlain Group)

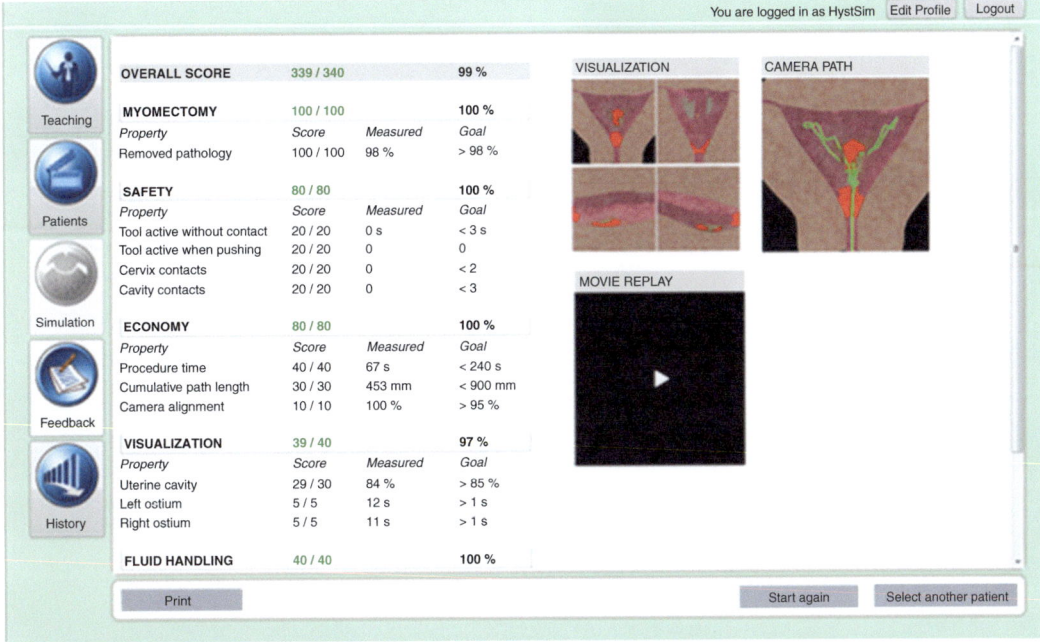

Fig. 17.2 An example of a comprehensive objective feedback report automatically generated upon completion of the task, HYST Mentor 3D Systems™, Littleton, CO. (Used with permission)

hysteroscopic instruments at hand from an institution's operating room [12, 13]. Alternatively, animal models using pig bladders, porcine hearts, and cattle uteri have also been studied in the literature [12, 14].

With the advent of technology, hysteroscopic surgical simulation continues to evolve in the arena of virtual reality (VR). Many proprietors such as 3D systems™ (Cleveland, OH) have developed high-fidelity simulators in which technical skills and theoretical knowledge were demonstrated to have improved after use, as well as positive feedback for realism and training capacity from the trainees [15, 16].

With the purchase of the simulators, complete training curriculums are available that focus on essential surgical skills for varying anatomic pathologies and changeable levels of difficulty. This allows for applicability to not only the novice trainees but also experienced surgeons. Common troubleshooting techniques are simulated such as establishing and maintaining clear views, detecting and coagulating bleeding sources, fluid management and handling, as well

as instrument failure. The trainee can then repeatedly perform these sessions without need for new specimens and at their own pace independently from their starting skill levels.

One important aspect and running theme of high-fidelity VR is the automated return of objective feedback reports (Fig. 17.2). These reports include performance assessments and scoring (as determined by the institution or surgeon) on topics such as economy of motion, visualization, safety, and fluid handling. The whole encounter is also recorded and allows for the learner to immediately watch their performance to modify skills and learn from their mistakes.

In an effort to make the experience as realistic as possible, libraries of modules are available to practice from. Courses from diagnostic hysteroscopy, polyp removal, myomectomy, ablation, resection, and sterilization to morcellation are available (Fig. 17.3).

With the use of simulation in hysteroscopic surgery, whether via box trainers or VR, the training has aided learning and been proven to be well-received.

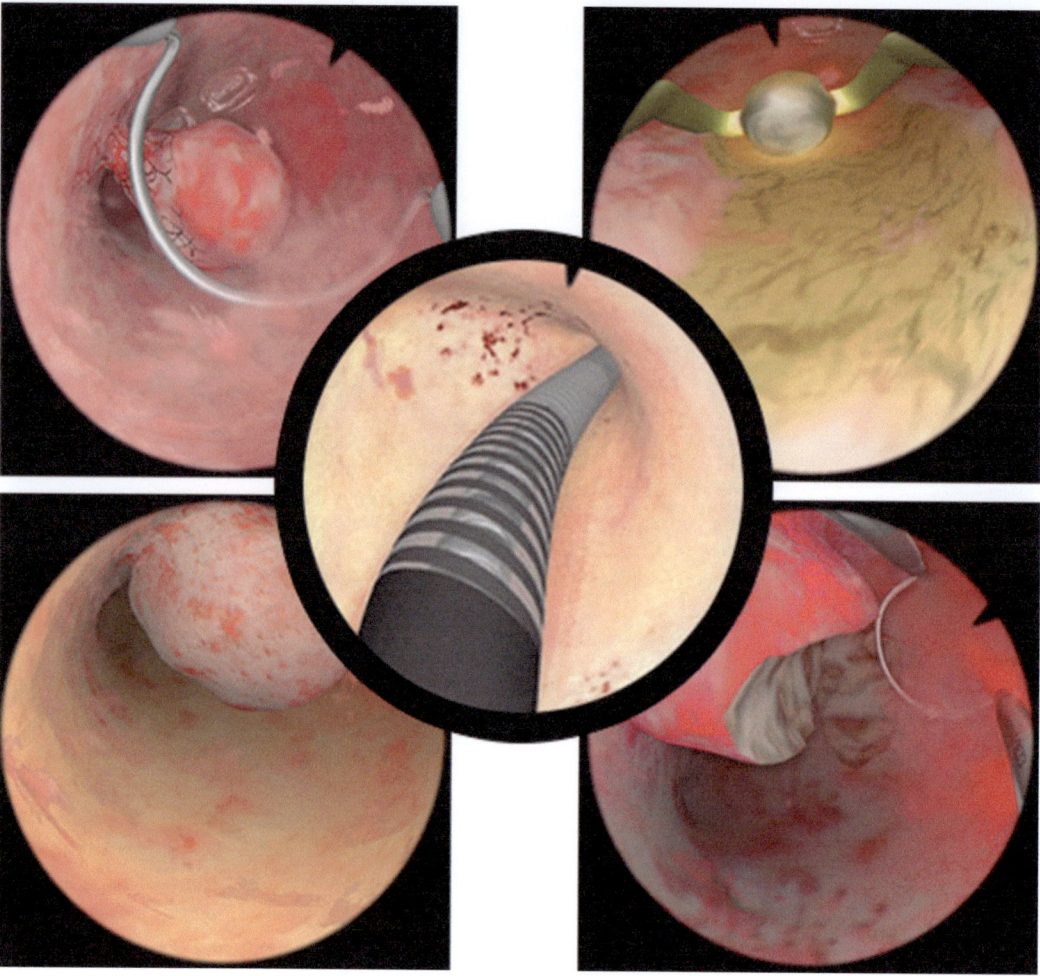

Fig. 17.3 Five examples of varying pathology available in hysteroscopic surgical simulation by 3D Systems™, Cleveland, OH. (Upper left-hand side, polypectomy; upper right-hand side, rollerball endometrial ablation; lower left-hand side, identification of a submucosal myoma; lower right-hand side, myomectomy; center image, sterilization). (Used with permission from 3D Systems™, Cleveland, OH)

Laparoscopic Surgery

Skill Gap Laparoscopic surgery allows for a minimally invasive, cost-effective, and rapid-recovery approach to many common gynecologic procedures. With a natural trend to an ever-changing landscape due to the integration of new technology, this modality of surgery continues to adapt and remain an important skill to be taught in residencies. While laparoscopy remains the gold standard in gynecologic surgery, the learning curve to reach competency is steep. The unique skills employed by laparoscopy must be adapted to a two-dimensional visual field with altered depth perception. This results in challenges with spatial reasoning and obstacles in achieving proficiency with video-eye-hand coordination. This is further compounded by the diminished tactile feedback from the long instruments and the necessary dexterity to complete finer dissections and suturing [17–19].

Solution With the integration of simulation in gynecologic surgery, training in the art of laparoscopy has been fortified and skill acquisition has been markedly improved [17, 18,

20–22]. With the scientifically accepted curriculum established by the Fundamentals of Laparoscopic Surgery (FLS) on box trainers, trainees are taught tasks in PEG transfer, precision cutting, ligating loop placement, and extra- and intra-corporeal knot tying. These tasks focus on obtaining multiple formative assessments in vital skills via a validated low-fidelity model [23–25]. As a result, multiple box trainers have been developed and integrated into didactic sessions in obstetrics and gynecology residencies nationwide. The limitations of these lower-fidelity approaches such as a manual scoring system and large use of consumable equipment are inherent to any box trainer.

With the advent of virtual reality and its application to laparoscopic surgery, the learning potential ceilings are raised to propagate the continued growth of even experienced surgeons— not just novices. The use of a VR simulator allows for the immediate integration of developed curriculum in essential gynecologic procedures. Common procedures from all learning levels from interns to graduating residents are applicable with adnexal surgery modules (i.e., tubal sterilization, treatment of ectopic pregnancy, and oophorectomy) as well as the more advanced total hysterectomy modules and focused didactics with hands-on learning in vaginal cuff closure (Figs. 17.4, 17.5, and 17.6).

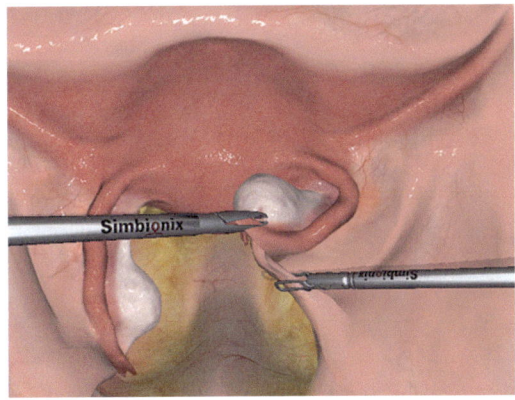

Fig. 17.4 VR simulator of adnexal surgery, 3D Systems™, Cleveland, OH. (Used with permission from 3D Systems™, Cleveland, OH)

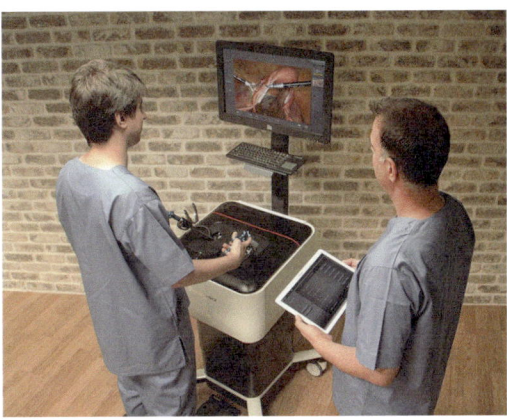

Fig. 17.5 VR simulator of a trainee performing a total laparoscopic hysterectomy with proctor, 3D Systems™, Cleveland, OH. (Used with permission from 3D Systems™, Cleveland, OH)

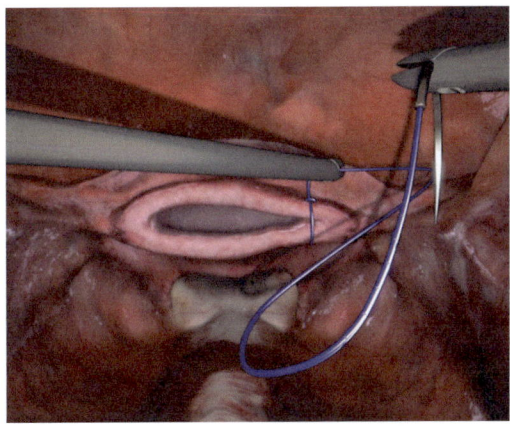

Fig. 17.6 VR simulator of a unidirectional vaginal cuff closure, HYST Mentor 3D Systems™, Littleton, CO. (Used with permission)

The benefits of VR in laparoscopy include education on an interactive 3D pelvis, step-by-step procedural guidance, and a comprehensive return of performance metrics on basic laparoscopic skills such as economy of motion, tissue handling, and instrument safety as well as advanced skills such as laparoscopic suturing, difficult dissections, and lysis of adhesions. Subsequently, with trainee participation in VR simulation, the literature proves superior improvement in technical skill as well as surgical knowledge via the integrated didactic learning programs compared to the conventional

Halstedian approach to surgical education [20–22, 26, 27]. In addition to the accruement of laparoscopic skill, the training via simulation has been validated to translate to the operating room, thus giving the opportunity for improvement in operating time and safety profile as well as compound surgical skill growth [20, 22, 27].

Robotic Surgery

Skill Gap Robotic surgery is on the forefront of gynecologic surgery with an increasing prevalence in obstetrics and gynecology residencies worldwide. While laparoscopic surgery is the gold standard, robotic technology has elevated minimally invasive surgery by allowing gynecologic surgeons to treat significant reproductive pathology inherently limited by the traditional approach. With the combination of the intelligent hardware and structure of the robot, a three-dimensional view of the anatomy is provided while optimizing ergonomics and thus minimizing surgeon fatigue. Human limitations of the "fulcrum effect" are eliminated with the ability to operate with a greater range of motion, visualization is magnified, and tremors are mitigated [28, 29].

Generally, some of the clear shortcomings of the today's current robotic surgical system are an absence of haptic or tactile feedback and cost. With the clear benefits it provides hospitals in several departments of surgery (i.e., gynecology, urology, colorectal, general surgery, vascular, and more), it has proven to be a vital surgical tool that has revolutionized approaches to surgical pathology, and it is here to stay. Given the nature of cost and the challenges with teaching learners when multiple opportunities may not exist, it becomes even more crucial to implement simulation methods to reduce learning time on the equipment and facilitate a more rapid mastery of skill.

Similar to hysteroscopy and laparoscopy as previously described, simulation in robotics has been developed by companies like Intuitive Surgical® and 3D Systems™. Their collaboration has resulted in the creation of a library of modules that are available for repeated practice to not only familiarize oneself with the physical machinery, but master essential skills the use of the robot requires prior to even entering into the operating room. Courses are available in robotic basic skills such as hand-eye coordination, depth perception, bimanual manipulation, camera navigation, and wrist articulation (Fig. 17.7). Often the equipment itself can be challenging to navigate, and not just the procedural features it provides, thus allowing an individual to decrease costly operating room time and even improve patient safety by acquainting themselves ahead of time with its functionality. Once capable of advancement, the learner can then move forward to complete full simulation procedures such as a hysterectomy. The RobotiX Mentor provides the opportunity for practice in all facets of the procedure, from uterine manipulation, ureter identification, bladder mobilization, division of the uterine arteries as well as colpotomy (3D Systems™ and Intuitive Surgical®) (Fig. 17.8). To take it one step further, there are even features such as the LAP Mentor Express (3D Systems™) that allow for the addition of a laparoscopic assistant within the robotic simulator, thereby creating an immersive experience that incorporates team dynamics. This facilitates direct proctorship in addition to training in surgical communication and teamwork. All the modules are on spectrums from basic to advanced thus enabling the learner to start where applicable to them, practice repeat-

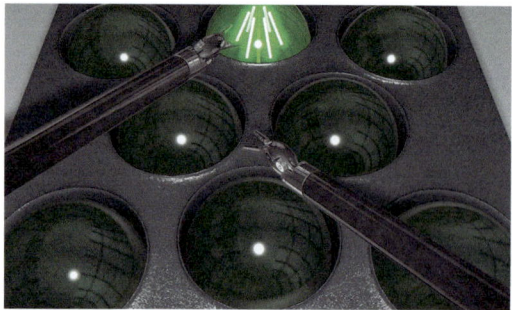

Fig. 17.7 Practicing the clutch feature on the Robotix Mentor, 3D Systems™, Cleveland, OH. (Used with permission from 3D Systems™, Cleveland, OH)

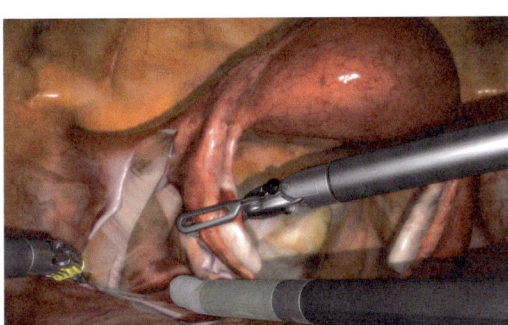

Fig. 17.8 Ureteral dissection on the complete hysterectomy module using the Robotix Mentor and Lap Mentor assist from 3D Systems™. (Used with permission from 3D Systems™, Cleveland, OH)

edly until competency, and ultimately become proficient in multiple training curriculums.

Importantly and similar to the VR simulators in hysteroscopy and laparoscopy described before, upon completion of the tasks, a comprehensive performance report is provided. The immediate feedback on an array of skills provides scores in economy of motion, time, and task-specific metrics.

Unfortunately, but also naturally, not all obstetric and gynecology residencies are created equally. Some programs are distributed unevenly with a heavy weight on, for example, laparoscopy or robotics or vice versa [30, 31]. As a result, this perpetuates skill—or lack thereof—upon graduation, highlighting the areas of potential improvement. In a study published in 2015, only 65% of all the obstetrics and gynecology graduating residents (out of a 95% response rate) felt they had received adequate robotic training [32]. Many studies have also published the demand for creating a standardized curriculum in robotics due to the rising number of complex minimally invasive procedures [30, 33–35]. Now, with the institution of simulation, face, content, construct, and predictive validities of assessment have been proven with robotic simulators, such as the da Vinci Surgical Skill Simulator [36, 37].

In order to continue to improve surgical training for not only obstetrics and gynecology residents but also all fields that use the robot, simulation to bridge gaps in skill is essential.

Summary

We find ourselves in a predicament when we are forced to balance the need to train surgeons with defined objectives and validated measures of competence with the implementation of duty hours in a consistently morphing technological landscape. It has become repeatedly clear that as the gap between our expert surgeons and new trainees widen, a comprehensive education that provides an optimistic safety profile, abides by time constraints, and elevates skill sets will rapidly fall on simulation [21, 22, 38].

Within our surgical heritage, traditional training via apprenticeship models remains ill-defined without structure between the trainee and trainer. Often this results in unequal training across residents individually and training centers nationwide. With this palpable lack of preparedness felt by those graduating, increasing desires for fortified simulation curriculums have become apparent [39–41]. Surgical competence is not simply defined by observation and Halstedian technique, but a combination of cognitive and behavioral abilities as well as perceptual and psychomotor skills. It is unrealistic to expect our current trainees to become proficient in visio-spatial and tactile perception in addition to demonstrate technical competency without supplementation [1, 42–45].

Simulation in hysteroscopy, laparoscopy, and robotics elevates gynecologic surgery to become a tangible arena of mastery. Now, with the advent of comprehensive curriculums and immediate return of objective performance feedback, we can both maintain pace with technologic surgical advancements and continue to evolve with them. Remaining cognizant of the obstacles to incorporation of simulation in gynecologic surgery such as cost will be critical to its success.

References

1. Picarella EA, Simmons JD, Borman KR, Replogle WH, Mitchell ME. "Do one, teach one" the new paradigm in general surgery residency training. J Surg Educ. 2011;68:126–9.

2. Hopkins MR, Dowdy SC. Resident participation in laparoscopic hysterectomy: balancing education with safety. Am J Obstet Gynecol. 2014;211:444–5.

3. Hopkins L, Hampton BS, Abbott JF, et al. To the point: medical education, technology, and the millennial learner. Am J Obstet Gynecol. 2018;218(2):188–92.

4. Lindheim SR, Nouri P, Rabah KA, Yaklic JL. Medical professionalism and enculturation of the millennial physician: meeting of the minds. Fertil Steril. 2016;106:1615–6.

5. Smith ML. Simulation and education in gynecologic surgery. Obstet Gynecol Clin N Am. 2011;38:733–40.

6. Isaacson KB. Complications of hysteroscopy. Obstet Gynecol Clin N Am. 1999;26:39–51.

7. Singhi A. Comparison of complications rates in endoscopic surgery performed by a clinical assistant vs. an experienced endoscopic surgeon. J Gynecol Endosc Surg. 2009;1:40–6.

8. van Dongen H, Kolkman W, Jansen FW. Hysteroscopic surgery: perspectives on skills training. J Minim Invasive Gynecol. 2006;13:121–5.

9. Raymond E, Ternamian A, Leyland N, Tolomiczenko G. Endoscopy teaching in Canada: a survey of obstetrics and gynecology program directors and graduating residents. J Minim Invasive Gynecol. 2006;13:10–6.

10. Goff BA, VanBlaricom A, Mandel L, Chinn M, Nielsen P. Comparison of objective, structured assessment of technical skills with a virtual reality hysteroscopy trainer and standard latex hysteroscopy model. J Reprod Med. 2007;52:407–12.

11. Rackow BW, Solnik MJ, Tu FF, Senapati S, Pozolo KE, Du H. Deliberate practice improves obstetrics and gynecology residents' hysteroscopy skills. J Grad Med Educ. 2012;4:329–34.

12. Savran MM, Sorensen SM, Konge L, Tolsgaard MG, Bjerrum F. Training and assessment of hysteroscopic skills: a systematic review. J Surg Educ. 2016;73:906–18.

13. Kingston A, Abbott J, Lenart M, Vancaillie T. Hysteroscopic training: the butternut pumpkin model. J Am Assoc Gynecol Laparosc. 2004;11:256–61.

14. Clevin L. A training model for hysteroscopy. Ugeskr Laeger. 2004;166:2025–7.

15. Panel P, Bajka M, Le Tohic A, Ghoneimi AE, Chis C, Cotin S. Hysteroscopic placement of tubal sterilization implants: virtual reality simulator training. Surg Endosc. 2012;26:1986–96.

16. Bajka M, Tuchschmid S, Streich M, Fink D, Szekely G, Harders M. Evaluation of a new virtual-reality training simulator for hysteroscopy. Surg Endosc. 2009;23:2026–33.

17. Scott DJ, Bergen PC, Rege RV, et al. Laparoscopic training on bench models: better and more cost effective than operating room experience? J Am Coll Surg. 2000;191:272–83.

18. Scott-Conner CE, Hall TJ, Anglin BL, et al. The integration of laparoscopy into a surgical residency and implications for the training environment. Surg Endosc. 1994;8:1054–7.

19. Melvin WS, Johnson JA, Ellison EC. Laparoscopic skills enhancement. Am J Surg. 1996;172:377–9.

20. Larsen CR, Oestergaard J, Ottesen BS, Soerensen JL. The efficacy of virtual reality simulation training in laparoscopy: a systematic review of randomized trials. Acta Obstet Gynecol Scand. 2012;91:1015–28.

21. Aggarwal R, Ward J, Balasundaram I, Sains P, Athanasiou T, Darzi A. Proving the effectiveness of virtual reality simulation for training in laparoscopic surgery. Ann Surg. 2007;246:771–9.

22. Aggarwal R, Tully A, Grantcharov T, et al. Virtual reality simulation training can improve technical skills during laparoscopic salpingectomy for ectopic pregnancy. BJOG. 2006;113:1382–7.

23. Oropesa I, Sanchez-Gonzalez P, Lamata P, et al. Methods and tools for objective assessment of psychomotor skills in laparoscopic surgery. J Surg Res. 2011;171:e81–95.

24. van Hove PD, Tuijthof GJ, Verdaasdonk EG, Stassen LP, Dankelman J. Objective assessment of technical surgical skills. Br J Surg. 2010;97:972–87.

25. Rooney DM, Brissman IC, Finks JF, Gauger PG. Fundamentals of laparoscopic surgery manual test: is videotaped performance assessment an option? J Surg Educ. 2015;72:90–5.

26. Kotsis SV, Chung KC. Application of the "see one, do one, teach one" concept in surgical training. Plast Reconstr Surg. 2013;131:1194–201.

27. Seymour NE, Gallagher AG, Roman SA, et al. Virtual reality training improves operating room performance: results of a randomized, double-blinded study. Ann Surg. 2002;236:458–63. discussion 63-4

28. Ballantyne GH, Moll F. The da Vinci telerobotic surgical system: the virtual operative field and telepresence surgery. Surg Clin North Am. 2003;83:1293–304. vii

29. Glickson J. Using simulation to train oncology surgeons: gynecologic oncologists practice OR's touch, feel – and pressures. Bull Am Coll Surg. 2011;96:31–8.

30. Moola D, Westermann LB, Pauls R, Eschenbacher M, Crisp C. The impact of robotic-assisted surgery on training gynecology residents. Female Pelvic Med Reconstr Surg. 2016;22:11–5.

31. Berkowitz RL, Minkoff H. A call for change in a changing world. Obstet Gynecol. 2016;127:153–6.

32. Peterson S, Mayer A, Nelson B, Roland P. Robotic surgery training in an OB/GYN residency program: a survey investigating the optimal training and credentialing of OB/GYN residents. Conn Med. 2015;79:395–9.

33. Vogell A, Gujral H, Wright KN, Wright VW, Ruthazer R. Impact of a robotic simulation program on resident surgical performance. Am J Obstet Gynecol. 2015;213:874–5.

34. Jeppson PC, Rahimi S, Gattoc L, et al. Impact of robotic technology on hysterectomy route and associated implications for resident education. Am J Obstet Gynecol. 2015;212:196.e1–6.

35. Vaccaro CM, Crisp CC, Fellner AN, Jackson C, Kleeman SD, Pavelka J. Robotic virtual reality simulation plus standard robotic orientation versus standard robotic orientation alone: a randomized controlled trial. Female Pelvic Med Reconstr Surg. 2013;19:266–70.

36. Alzahrani T, Haddad R, Alkhayal A, et al. Validation of the da Vinci Surgical Skill Simulator across three surgical disciplines: a pilot study. Can Urol Assoc J. 2013;7:E520–9.

37. Culligan P, Gurshumov E, Lewis C, Priestley J, Komar J, Salamon C. Predictive validity of a training protocol using a robotic surgery simulator. Female Pelvic Med Reconstr Surg. 2014;20:48–51.

38. Darzi A, Smith S, Taffinder N. Assessing operative skill. Needs to become more objective. BMJ. 1999;318:887–8.

39. Pellegrini VD Jr. A perspective on the effect of the 80-hour work week: has it changed the graduating orthopaedic resident? J Am Acad Orthop Surg. 2017;25:416–20.

40. O'Sullivan KE, Byrne JS, Walsh TN. Basic surgical training in Ireland: the impact of operative experience, training program allocation and mentorship on trainee satisfaction. Ir J Med Sci. 2013;182:687–92.

41. Kinnear B, Bensman R, Held J, O'Toole J, Schauer D, Warm E. Critical deficiency ratings in milestone assessment: a review and case study. Acad Med. 2017;92:820–6.

42. Moorthy K, Munz Y, Sarker SK, Darzi A. Objective assessment of technical skills in surgery. BMJ. 2003;327:1032–7.

43. Louridas M, Szasz P, de Montbrun S, Harris KA, Grantcharov TP. Can we predict technical aptitude?: a systematic review. Ann Surg. 2016;263:673–91.

44. Grantcharov TP, Bardram L, Funch-Jensen P, Rosenberg J. Assessment of technical surgical skills. Eur J Surg. 2002;168:139–44.

45. Wanzel KR, Hamstra SJ, Caminiti MF, Anastakis DJ, Grober ED, Reznick RK. Visual-spatial ability correlates with efficiency of hand motion and successful surgical performance. Surgery. 2003;134:750–7.

Obstetrics and Gynecology Simulation and Global Health Initiatives

Emily Nicole Bernice Myer
and Chi Chiung Grace Chen

Introduction

Interest in global health care is increasing as more medical schools and residencies develop global health programs, and medical providers choose to practice internationally in some capacity [1, 2]. Simulation can be used prior to international travel in preparing providers and medical trainees for uncommon clinical scenarios, learning how to work in different health-care settings, and developing strategies to manage potential frustrations and unexpected clinical outcomes that may be less commonly encountered in a more familiar environment. Particularly when working in lower resource settings, simulation may also be used to underscore and address potential cultural inequalities and ethical concerns that may arise when working with women and children.

The role of simulation may be even more essential in resource-limited settings where there may be critical shortages of skilled health-care personnel. Medical providers responsible for teaching medical trainees and mid-level practitioners often have more severe time constraints than their counterparts in higher resource settings; therefore, using simulation to augment the teaching of fundamental obstetric and gynecologic skills may be particularly beneficial.

The success of using simulation and sustaining simulation curricula in a global health context depends on three factors: an adequate number of skilled instructors, training materials adapted to the local clinical and cultural setting, and local providers and educators who are trained to teach simulation and committed to incorporating simulation into the educational curricula [3, 4]. Moreover, simulation curricula should ideally include both skills training and clinical scenarios involving all members of the health-care team. This chapter will offer guidance and resources on using simulation both to prepare providers for working in international, specifically lower resource settings, and to teach obstetric and gynecologic skills to providers in those settings. In addition, as high-fidelity simulators are not feasible and may not be well maintained in resource-limited settings, this chapter will focus on low-cost, low-fidelity simulators. Most of the publications on obstetric and gynecologic simulation, including the use of low-fidelity models, have been in higher resource settings; however, many of these models can and should be adapted to fit the specific global health context.

E. N. B. Myer · C. C. G. Chen (✉)
Department of Gynecology and Obstetrics, Division of Female Pelvic Medicine and Reconstructive Surgery, Johns Hopkins University School of Medicine, Baltimore, MD, USA
e-mail: emyer3@jhmi.edu; cchen127@jhmi.edu

Key Learning Points

- Simulation can be used to train domestic providers prior to departure for global health work in obstetrics and gynecology.
- Simulators and simulation curricula can be used in lower resource settings to augment the learning of essential obstetric and gynecologic skills and as a means of introducing comparatively new technology in those settings.
- Simulation should be tailored to the specific global health contexts by taking into account differences in culture, clinical content and health-care systems, and non-customary health-care roles.
- Coordination with local partners in international settings to design simulation curricula both for preparations prior to international travel and for use in those settings is essential to maximize simulation efficacy and sustainability.

General Considerations

In preparing teams for global health experiences and in preparing simulation initiatives for use in global health settings, a needs assessment both of providers planning to travel internationally and of the global health site is essential. The team leader should consider the skill levels and prior global health experiences of team members to help determine the simulation activities needed for preparation. Additionally, the team should consider the governmental structure, cultural characteristics, local health-care infrastructure, and medical needs of the area to which they are planning to travel. It is important to seek permission from the minister of health or colleagues at the planned travel site to discuss the goals of the visit and to obtain permission to practice medicine. Insights into the local culture and health-care infrastructure will help the team better understand patient expectations as well as develop strategies to make sure patients have

access to and are adequately informed regarding treatment options. For example, in many cultures, women may not be able to make their own health-care decisions or decisions for their children. To ensure that women and children have access to and are informed about health-care options, in addition to discussions with the women alone, providers may also need to involve other members in the family such as husbands and/or mothers-in-law [5]. Simulation training in cultural awareness and sensitivity can also be used domestically when caring for refugee populations, which are increasing in more developed countries [6].

Part of the needs assessment also includes working with local providers to better understand the particular needs and challenges of providing care in the specific global setting [5, 7]. Topics to address include availability of medications, operating rooms, and clinical equipment such as speculums and colposcopes. Based on these discussions, pre-departure planning may also require material acquisition. Additionally, the World Health Organization (WHO) international guidelines for management and diagnosis of conditions in maternal, reproductive, and women's health in lower resource settings should be considered to ensure that best practices are being followed [8].

An important aspect of pre-departure preparation includes consideration of ethical challenges that may be particularly pertinent to shorter-term global health trips. The Johns Hopkins Berman Institute of Bioethics has a series of case studies to simulate a variety of common global health ethical scenarios to help prepare medical teams prior to departure (Table 18.1) [9]. In addition, the Working Group on Ethics Guidelines for Global Health Training (WEIGHT) has developed a set of ethical guidelines for institutions, trainees, and global health sponsors [19]. The ethical principles of beneficence, non-maleficence, justice, and autonomy hold true in any health-care setting [20]. Upholding these principles entails assessing the clinical competency of team members and making adequate preparations to ensure that they are qualified to participate in the intended medical and surgical

Table 18.1 Web-based resources for global health

Organization/company	Content	Website source[a]
General preparations		

Johns Hopkins Berman Institute of Bioethics [9]	Case-based scenario for ethical challenges in short-term global health training:
	    Developing cultural understanding
	    Ensuring personal safety
	    Dealing with tasks exceeding level of training
	    Ensuring appropriate benefits
	    Addressing ancillary benefits
	    Recognizing burdens
	    Shifting resources
	    Telling the truth
	    Selecting a research project
	    Understanding informed consent
	Also contains a PDF with a variety of resources for each of these topics
		http://ethicsandglobalhealth.org/
		http://ethicsandglobalhealth.org/Additional-Resources.pdf

Consortium of Universities for Global Health [10]	Global Health Training Modules in a variety of topics related to working in global health:
	    Noncommunicable diseases and injuries
	    Infectious, parasitic, and communicable diseases
	    Priority and vulnerable populations
	    Global child health
	    Health systems, services, resources, and programs
	    Working in low resource countries
	    Global health: priorities, problems, programs, and policies
	Also contains links to a variety of other resources related to these topics
		http://www.cugh.org/resources/educational-modules

Obstetric topics		

Helping Mothers Survive [11]	Hands-on, simulation-based learning modules:
	    Bleeding after birth
	    Preeclampsia and eclampsia
	    Threatened preterm birth care
	    Normal and complicated labor and birth
		http://hms.jhpiego.org/training-materials/

Simulation Use for Global Away Rotations (SUGAR) [12]	Step-by-step instructional simulation development videos:
	    Neonatal resuscitation
	    Bag valve mask ventilation
	    Bubble CPAP
		http://sugarprep.org/pearls/

American College of Obstetricians and Gynecologists [13]	Simulation curricula:
	    Shoulder dystocia
	    Postpartum hemorrhage
	    Breech delivery
	    4th-degree repair
	    Eclampsia
		http://www.acog.org/About-ACOG/ACOG-Departments/Simulations-Consortium/OB-GYN-Simulations-Curricula

Pronto International (Seattle, Washington) [14]	Video simulation:
	    Normal birth
	    Uterine atony management
	    Neonatal resuscitation
	    Shoulder dystocia
	    Preeclampsia and eclampsia
	Birth simulator models:
	    PRONTOPack
	    PARTOPants
		http://prontointernational.org/our-resources/simulation-supplies/about-prontopack/
		http://prontointernational.org/our-resources/video-training-library/

(continued)

Table 18.1 (continued)

Organization/company	Content	Website source[a]

Laerdal Medical (Wappingers Falls, New York) [15]	MamaNatalie simulator:
	  Postpartum hemorrhage
	  Positioning and delivery of the baby
	  Delivery of placenta
	  Fetal heart sounds
	  Cervix landmark
	  Urine bladder catheterization
	  Uterine massage
	  Uterine compression
		http://www.laerdalglobalhealth.com/doc/2545/MamaNatalie

Global Health eLearning Center [16]	Online courses to increase knowledge in global health technical areas:
	  Antenatal and postpartum care
	  Essential newborn care
	  Emergency obstetric and newborn care
	  Malaria in pregnancy
	  Maternal-child HIV
		https://www.globalhealthlearning.org/courses

Practical Obstetric Multi-Professional Training (PROMPT) course [17]	A multi-professional simulation package for training obstetric emergencies	http://www.promptmaternity.org/training/
Gynecologic topics		

Global Health eLearning Center [16]	Online courses to increase knowledge in global health technical areas:
	  Cervical cancer prevention in low resource settings
	  Family planning services
	  IUD
	  Female genital mutilation
	  Youth sexual health
		https://www.globalhealthlearning.org/course/cervical-cancer-prevention-low-resource-settings

Laerdal Medical (Wappingers Falls, New York) [18]	MamaU simulator:
	  Postpartum IUD insertion
	  Uterine balloon tamponade insertions[b]
		http://www.laerdalglobalhealth.com/doc/2580/Mama-U

American College of Obstetricians and Gynecologists [13]	Simulation curricula:
	  Total vaginal hysterectomy
	  Total abdominal hysterectomy
	  Laparoscopic ovarian cystectomy
	  Laparoscopic sterilization
	  Laparoscopic salpingectomy for ectopic pregnancy
	  Bartholin gland marsupialization and placement of Word catheter
	  Cystoscopy
	  Endometrial biopsy
	  Intrauterine device insertion
	  Loop electrosurgical excision procedure
		http://www.acog.org/About-ACOG/ACOG-Departments/Simulations-Consortium/OB-GYN-Simulations-Curricula

[a]All sources last accessed April 2017
[b]Used for postpartum hemorrhage or hemorrhage after gynecologic procedures such as dilation and curettage

tasks prior to departure. Team members should be encouraged to decline tasks for which they feel inadequately trained.

Teams should work with local colleagues to make sure patients will have continued perioperative and postoperative care and necessary medi-cal resources after the expatriate medical team has left [21]. Not only is it essential to work with local colleagues to plan for continued patient care after departure, but if certain specialized follow-up care or resources are not locally avail-able, this should impact one's management decisions. Anticipating and potentially simulating these types of clinically and ethically challenging dilemmas can further prepare the team prior to departure.

Another consideration in preparing for global health work is emotional and personal preparation. In global health settings, providers may encounter conditions with which they are unfamiliar and unprepared to treat. Local resources may be insufficient for curative treatment, patient survival, or improved quality of life that would otherwise not be so in higher resource settings. This may cause providers to be overwhelmed, leading to physical and emotional exhaustion. Making the team aware of these possibilities and discussing, or simulating, challenging clinical scenarios to address coping and management strategies prior to departure are beneficial [22]. While there are no published case scenarios in obstetrics and gyne-

cology for this use, there are several examples to address the feelings of frustration, floundering, failure, and futility in the pediatric literature that can be easily adapted to clinically relevant scenarios in obstetrics and gynecology (Table 18.1) [12]. Understanding the challenges of caring for patients in a planned setting such as during simulation is important to ensure such emotional challenges will not interfere with actual patient care [21].

Pitt and colleagues have reviewed several key points to consider when developing simulation to prepare providers for their international experiences, which are also pertinent in developing simulation and simulation curricula for the international setting (Table 18.2) [4]. Tailoring simulations and simulation curricula to specific global health contexts include widening the differential diagnoses to diseases not commonly encountered in higher resource settings, varying

Table 18.2 Considerations when designing global health simulation clinical scenarios: avoiding common pitfalls

Question to consider	Example of possible difference(s)	Consequence of failing to address
Is the diagnosis seen in this setting?	Certain conditions may be uncommon in low- and middle-income countries (i.e., atopic disease)	Providers may be encouraged to consider diagnoses that are unlikely
Can the diagnosis be made in this setting? If so, is it readily treatable with resources available?	Common diagnostic test (coagulation studies, thyroid hormone levels) may not be available in the setting Access to medication/therapies may be limited	Simulating a scenario that is unable to be diagnosed/treated adds little practical value
Are monitors used in patient care in this setting?	Many settings without monitors would be expected to be track vitals clinically	Scenario may not reflect actual practice
Is the condition diagnosed/treated the same way as it would be at home institution?	WHO guidelines may differ from standard of care in high-resource countries Example: a febrile seizure, which may be treated with reassurance only, would merit evaluation of cerebral malaria in many settings	Providers may be encouraged to follow different practices than regional standard of care
Are the drug names different?	Acetaminophen is most often called paracetamol Trimethoprim-sulfamethoxazole is most often called cotrimoxazole	Unnecessary confusion
Are the units of measurement different?	Glucose is reported in millimole per liter instead of milligram per deciliter (approximately an 18-fold difference) in most of the world	Unnecessary confusion
Are their different expectations of learners than in the home setting?	Nurses may have different roles/expectations Health systems may incorporate community health workers or traditional birth attendants	Scenario may fail to reflect the real-world scenario
Are their cultural differences that may affect the management of the case?	Different goals surrounding end-of-life care Mothers may be expected to defer to fathers or community leaders in decision-making	May lead to an unrealistic scenario or a sense of prescribing one's cultural approach as the "right" way to do something

Reproduced with permission from Pitt et al. [4]

treatments based on available resources, altering the drug names and measurement units, and taking on non-customary health-care roles (e.g., physicians drawing and administering intravenous medications) [4]. Simulation design should strive to be culturally sensitive such as using black rather than white models for simulation in Africa. Adapting training materials to the local environment also means ensuring the simulation is durable and sustainable in that setting. For example, incorporating high-fidelity simulators into the educational curricula in lower resource settings that require routine maintenance and replenishment of materials not readily available are unlikely to be sustainable or effective. Importantly, involving local partners during simulation development, both for preparation before travel and for use in international settings, will help to ensure the relevancy and sustainability of simulation programs.

Obstetric Considerations

Developing countries account for 99% of all maternal and newborn deaths worldwide with approximately 300,000 women dying annually during and following childbirth [23]. This is in part due to a lack of readily available skilled obstetric care and limited access to lifesaving measures to treat common obstetric conditions including hemorrhage, infections, and hypertensive-related disorders [24]. Due to the high burden of maternal morbidity and mortality in lower resource settings, great effort has been put forth to improve global maternal health care including increasing the use of simulation in these settings [23]. Specifically, simulation use has been shown to increase compliance with evidence-based guidelines [25] including active management of the third stage of labor [26]. Additionally, simulation has been shown to reduce the need for cesarean delivery [4], injury associated with shoulder dystocia [27], and overall neonatal morbidity and mortality [28].

When planning simulation curricula either to prepare providers for international work or for use in an international setting, emergency obstetric and newborn care issues to consider are the same as those commonly encountered in any obstetric care context including topics such as management of hemorrhage, assisted vaginal delivery, and neonatal resuscitation. However, what may be different is the availability of specific resources and skilled personnel; therefore, simulations should be modified accordingly.

Although not an exhaustive list and the particular details of various clinical scenarios will vary based on the specific global health context, obstetric emergencies that may be more commonly encountered in lower resource settings include the following:

- Active labor without continuous/intermittent fetal heart rate and/or contraction tracings
- Maternal hemorrhage without available massive transfusion blood products, uterotonic medications, Bakri balloon, readily available operating room, and/or anesthesia
- Maternal severe hypertensive crisis without access to standard intravenous medications and automatic continuous blood pressure monitoring
- Maternal seizure without access to intravenous magnesium or other anti-seizure medications
- Vaginal breech delivery without availability of forceps, nitroglycerin, readily available operating room, and/or anesthesia
- Umbilical cord prolapse without readily available operating room and anesthesia
- Cesarean hysterectomy without availability of additional skilled personnel, such as other obstetricians/gynecologists, gynecologic oncologists, and general surgeon, and massive transfusion blood products
- Assisted vaginal delivery and shoulder dystocia management in patients without regional or local anesthesia
- Cesarean delivery for fetal demise
- Wound infections and/or maternal infection with limited wound care resources including antibiotics, dressings, and local anesthesia for dressing changes
- Maternal and neonatal resuscitation without availability of additional skilled personnel such as neonatologist/pediatrician, code cart, intubation supplies/ventilators, and intensive care unit

– Cultural or family resistance to indicated cesarean delivery due to distrust in Western medical practices
– *List adapted from various resources* [24, 29, 30]

As maternal hemorrhage is one of the most common causes of maternal death worldwide [23], simulation curricula and simulators to teach management of hemorrhage specifically in lower resource settings have been developed. Low-cost simulators include PartoPants (PRONTO International, Seattle, Washington), an adapted pair of scrub pants using simple materials and a baby mannequin to simulate vaginal delivery and postpartum hemorrhage [31], and MamaNatalie (Laerdal Medical, Wappingers Falls, New York),

a low-tech birthing simulator that also simulates vaginal delivery and postpartum hemorrhage after delivery (Table 18.1) [15]. For every purchase of a MamaNatalie (Laerdal Medical, Wappingers Falls, New York) in a higher-income country, one is donated to a lower-income country [15].

Identification and management of perineal lacerations is another obstetric condition with well-described low-fidelity simulators and curricula including beef-tongue and modified kitchen sponge models (Table 18.3) [33, 34]. These simulators have been shown to significantly improve knowledge and confidence of repairs in physician trainees [33, 34]. An instructional DVD has also been used to improve knowledge and skill of perineal repairs in midwives [30]. As unrepaired third- and fourth-degree perineal lacerations have

Table 18.3 Published obstetric and gynecologic low-fidelity simulators

Author	Content
Obstetric simulation	
Deganus 2009 [32]	SYMPTEK (instructions to create models): Episiotomy and repair of perineal lacerations Cervical cerclage Repairing cervical tears Cervical incompetence Controlled cord traction Manual removal of the placenta Bimanual uterine compression (internal and external) Balloon tamponade Repairing cesarean section incisions Uterine artery ligation B-lynch procedure
Illston 2017 [33]	Fourth-degree perineal laceration repair model using beef tongue
Sparks 2006 [34]	Fourth-degree perineal laceration repair model using a modified sponge
Perosky 2011 [35]	Development of a low-cost model made out of rubber, plastic resin, foam, and pressure sensor Light-emitting diodes for use in Africa to simulate bimanual compression for management of postpartum hemorrhage
Mahmud 2013 [30]	Maternity PEARLS: instructional videos for the management of perineal trauma following childbirth
Gynecologic simulation	
Deganus 2009 [32]	SYMPTEK (instructions to create models): Speculum and bimanual examinations Education on vesicovaginal fistula Cervical cancer screening Intrauterine device insertion Manual vacuum aspiration
Tunitsky-Bitton 2014 [36]	Laparoscopic sacrocolpopexy model
Tunitsky-Bitton 2016 [37]	Laparoscopic vaginal cuff closure model
Tunitsky-Bitton 2013 [38]	Ureteral reimplantation model
Hong 2012 [39]	Total abdominal hysterectomy model
Hefler 2012 [40]	LEEP (loop electrosurgical excision procedure) model
Beard 2014 [41]	Laparoscopic skills trainer model

been found to be significantly associated with fecal incontinence, urinary incontinence, and obstetric fistula in resource-limited settings [42], simulation with these models can be used to improve maternal morbidity.

The American College of Obstetricians and Gynecologists Simulations Working Group has also developed low-fidelity obstetric simulators and simulation curricula that can be used for other clinical scenarios in global health settings, including shoulder dystocia, uterine atony, vaginal breech delivery, fourth-degree repair, and eclampsia (Table 18.1) [13]. Ideally, a team-based approach to simulation involving all health-care team members should be considered as a breakdown in team communication has been found to be associated with poor obstetric outcomes, especially if the team does not routinely work together [43, 44].

Gynecologic Considerations

Despite the global burden of gynecologic-related deaths occurring in resource-limited settings, including 97% of unsafe abortions [45] and 85% of all cervical cancer deaths worldwide, most public health attention has been focused on improving obstetric rather than gynecologic outcomes [5]. Barriers to gynecologic care in global settings include cultural factors, resource limitations, and an inadequate number of trained providers [5, 46]. There are limited publications on the impact of gynecologic skills simulation training on clinical outcomes specifically in international settings; therefore, most of the evidence presented in this section is on the use of low-fidelity simulators in higher resource settings that can be adapted for any location.

When planning simulation curricula either to prepare providers for international work or for use in an international setting, key gynecologic care topics to consider include screening of common gynecologic cancers [5], family planning, and urogynecologic conditions [5, 47]. Importantly, surgical simulation training may also include teaching and simulating effective methods to reduce the risk of infection such as

hand washing, surgical site preparation, and administration of perioperative antibiotics [48].

Although not an exhaustive list and the specific details of various clinical scenarios may vary based on the particular global health context, gynecologic scenarios more specific to lower resource settings include the following:

- Dilation and curettage or manual vacuum aspiration for management of septic abortion in patients with severe anemia without availability of ultrasound guidance, uterotonics, and blood products
- Diagnostic and operative laparoscopy with unreliable supply of electricity, carbon dioxide, and limited laparoscopic surgical instruments (e.g., no electrocautery, no surgical clips, etc.)
- Appendectomy, surgical management of bowel obstruction or bowel injury, or incidental finding of malignancy at the time of surgery without availability of additional skilled personnel such as gynecologic oncologists and general surgeons
- Surgical management of a bladder/ureteral injury without availability of additional skilled personnel such as urologists
- Pelvic fistula diagnosis and repair without imaging studies such as CT scans or intraoperative fluoroscopy and without availability to perform cystoscopy and place ureteral stents
- Wound complications including wound debridement and repair of dehiscence without imaging studies such as CT scans, synthetic mesh or biologic graft, and availability of additional skilled personnel including general surgeons and with limited wound care resources including antibiotics, dressings, and local anesthesia for dressing changes
- Management of perioperative hemorrhage- or disease-related complications such as hemorrhage from cervical cancer without massive transfusion blood products, intensive care unit monitoring, and access to radiation or embolization
- Screening for cervical dysplasia without availability of *Papanicolaou* smears

- Postpartum tubal ligation with limited anesthesia availability
- Diagnosis and management of ectopic pregnancy without beta-*human chorionic gonadotropin* levels, ultrasound, and ability to perform diagnostic laparoscopy
- *List adapted from several resources* [8, 29, 49–51]

The WHO provides guidelines on the evaluation and treatment of common gynecologic conditions specific to lower resource settings [8, 48]. For example, in the case of cervical cancer screening, many health-care settings cannot offer Papanicolaou smears as there are no available pathologists to interpret the test. Instead, screening may include human papilloma virus (HPV) testing and/or visual inspection with acetic acid (VIA) using either the naked eye or colposcopy. Any patients with high-risk HPV or area of suspected dysplasia seen on VIA is then treated with loop electrosurgical excision or cold knife conization [8]. A low-cost simulation model using a sausage in a small plastic yogurt cup for teaching these treatments to trainees has been published (Table 18.3) [40].

Few providers are well trained in abortion care internationally [52]; the lack of adequate training has been shown to be a barrier to safe abortion care and contributes to maternal morbidity and mortality [53]. The WHO recommends manual vacuum aspiration (MVA) over dilation and curettage for abortions as it is associated with decreased blood loss, need for anesthesia, and the equipment that can be sterilized for reuse [8]. Low-fidelity simulation models using latex foam blocks wrapped in plastic cling wrap have been developed to teach MVA (Table 18.3) [32]. Providers planning to work in lower resource settings who are less familiar with this technique should consider simulation to reacquire these skills. It is also important to consider the ethical, moral, and cultural barriers concerning performing and teaching abortion care in particular health-care contexts.

Family planning is also an important part of the routine gynecologic care of all reproductive age women. Regardless of the availability of specific types of contraceptive methods, simulation on how to address and educate patients on this potentially culturally sensitive topic [54] and how best to utilize local resources to be consistent with the WHO guidelines [33] should be considered. Additionally, as only certain contraceptive methods may be locally available, this could be an opportunity to work with industry and international partners to use simulation for the introduction of comparatively new and effective technology, such as long-acting reversible contraception (LARC) [51]. Reuseable simulation training devices for many other forms of contraception are also available through the companies manufacturing these devices.

Other gynecologic conditions commonly encountered in any health-care setting include heavy menstrual bleeding, symptomatic uterine fibroids, adnexal masses, pelvic organ prolapse, and pelvic fistulae. What may be more unique to lower resource settings is that women with these conditions may often receive surgical care as first-line therapy as conservative treatment options such as progesterone intrauterine devices for heavy menstrual bleeding or pessaries for pelvic organ prolapse may not be commonly available and the continued follow-up care needed for conservatively managing these conditions may not be feasible. There are several published, low-fidelity models for practicing gynecologic surgical skills including total abdominal hysterectomy model using foam and poster board [39]; cystoscopy model using balloon and rubber ball [55]; laparoscopic hysterectomy vaginal cuff closure model using a laparoscopic box trainer, a neoprene drink sleeve, and vaginal stent/manipulator [37]; laparoscopic sacrocolpopexy model using a laparoscopic box trainer, vaginal stent and a neoprene drink sleeve, and mesh [36]; and ureteral injury repair model using a plastic food container, twine, and pliable gel formed into ureters [38] (Table 18.3).

The American College of Obstetricians and Gynecologists Simulations Working Group has also developed low-fidelity gynecologic simulators and simulation curricula that can be used for the above and other procedures and clinical scenarios in global health settings including total abdominal hysterectomy, total vaginal hysterectomy, colposcopy, cold knife cone biopsy, loop electrosurgical excision procedure, cystoscopy, Bartholin gland marsupialization and word catheter placement, intrauterine device insertion, endometrial biopsy, laparoscopic salpingectomy for ectopic pregnancy, laparoscopic sterilization, and ovarian cystectomy (Table 18.3) [13].

As previously discussed, working with local partners and industry to develop simulation models and curricula may also be useful for introducing and teaching comparatively new surgical technology internationally. For example, although the benefits of laparoscopy in reducing the lengths of hospital stay and risk of perioperative infections may be especially critical in lower resource settings [49], it is still not commonly practiced at international sites. Telesimulation is one tool that has been used to teach basic laparoscopic skills to providers in resource-limited settings, resulting in significant improvements in skill [56]. Telesimulation has also been used to successfully teach other basic surgical skills, such as knot-tying, to interns in lower resource settings [10]. Incorporation of simulation, including use of telesimulation, into the medical training curricula in international settings has the potential to increase the use of laparoscopy and other new technologies in these settings as well as improve basic skills.

preparation before international experiences or for use in international settings, it is important to work with local partners to consider the needs and resources of the particular health-care context as well as take into account differences in health-care infrastructure and culture. The success of using simulation to prepare for international experiences and in developing simulators and simulation curricula for use in international settings depends on an adequate number of skilled instructors, training materials adapted to the local clinical and cultural settings, and commitment from well-trained local providers.

List of Abbreviations

HIV	Human immunodeficiency virus
HPV	Human papilloma virus
LARC	Long-acting reversible contraception
LEEP	Loop electrosurgical excision procedure
MVA	Manual vacuum aspiration
VIA	Visual inspection with acetic acid
WHO	World Health Organization
WEIGHT	Working Group on Ethics Guidelines for Global Health Training

Summary

Simulation training in global health can be used to prepare providers for international experiences as well as for educating international providers, medical trainees, and mid-level practitioners' fundamental obstetrics and gynecologic skills and for the acquisition of comparatively new techniques that may be relevant in those settings. Simulation curricula should ideally include both skills training and clinical scenarios involving all members of the health-care team. Although most obstetrics and gynecology simulation literature, especially pertaining to gynecology, have been developed for and studied in higher resource settings, many of the low-fidelity models presented in this chapter can be readily adapted for lower resource settings. In developing simulation for

References

1. Millar HC, Randle EA, Scott HM, Shaw D, Kent N, Nakajima AK, et al. Global Women's health education in Canadian obstetrics and gynaecology residency programs: a survey of program directors and senior residents. J Obstet Gynaecol Can. 2015;37(10):927–35.
2. Stagg AR, Blanchard MH, Carson SA, Peterson HB, Flynn EB, Ogburn T. Obstetrics and gynecology resident interest and participation in global health. Obstet Gynecol. 2017 Apr 4 [Epub ahead of print].
3. Crofts J, Winter C, Sowter M. Practical simulation training for maternity care—where we are and where next. BJOG. 2011;118(Suppl. 3):11–6.
4. Pitt MB, Eppich WJ, Shane ML, Butteris SM. Using simulation in global health: Considerations for design and implementation. Simul Healthc. 2017;12(3):177–81.
5. Robinson N, Stoffel C, Haider S. Global women's health is more than maternal health: a review of gynecology care needs in low-resource settings. Obstet Gynecol Surv. 2015;70(3):211–22.

6. Ekblad S, Mollica RF, Fors U, Pantziaras I, Lavelle J. Educational potential of a virtual patient system for caring for traumatized patients in primary care. BMC Med Educ. 2013;13(1):110.

7. Nour N, editor. Obstetrics and gynecology in low-resources settings: a practical guide. Cambridge, MA: Harvard University; 2016.

8. World Health Organization. WHO guidelines: maternal, reproductive and women's health [Internet]. [cited 2017 Mar 1]. Available from: http://www.who.int/publications/guidelines/reproductive_health/en/.

9. Johns Hopkins Berman Institute of Bioethics. Ethical Challenges in Short-Term Global Health Training [Internet]. [cited 2017 Feb 3]. Available from: http://ethicsandglobalhealth.org/.

10. Consortium of Universities for Global Health. Global Health Training Modules [Internet]. [cited 2017 Mar 1]. Available from: http://www.cugh.org/resources/educational-modules.

11. Nelissen E, Ersdal H, Østergaard D, Mduma E, Broerse J, Evjen-Olsen B, et al. Helping mothers survive bleeding after birth: an evaluation of simulation-based training in a low-resource setting. Acta Obstet Gynecol Scand. 2014;93(3):287–95.

12. University of Wisconsin System: SUGAR Project. Sugarprep.org [Internet]. [cited 2017 Mar 1]. Available from: sugarprep.org.

13. American College of Obstetricians and Gynecologists. OB-GYN Simulations Curricula [Internet]. [cited 2017 Mar 1]. Available from: http://www.acog.org/Aboug-ACOG/ACOG-Departments/Simulations-Consortium/Ob-GYN-Simulations-Curricula.

14. Pronto International. Pronto International [Internet]. Available from: http://prontointernational.org/our-resources.

15. Laerdal. MamaNatalie Birthing Simulator [Internet]. [cited 2017 Mar 1]. Available from: http://www.laerdal.com/us/products/simulation-training/obstetrics-pediatrics/mamanatalie/.

16. USAID K. Global Health eLearning Center [Internet]. [cited 2017 Mar 1]. Available from: https://www.globalhealthlearning.org/about.

17. PROMPT Maternity Foundation. PROMPT [Internet]. [cited 2017 Mar 1]. Available from: http://www.promptmaternity.org/training/.

18. Laerdal. Mama-U [Internet]. Available from: http://www.laerdalglobalhealth.com/doc/2580/Mama-U.

19. Crump JA, Sugarman J, Barry M, Bhan A, Gardner P, Koplan JP, et al. Ethics and best practice guidelines for training experiences in global health. Am J Trop Med Hyg. 2010;83(6):1178–82.

20. Zaidi MY, Haddad L, Lathrop E. Global health opportunities in obstetrics and gynecology training: examining engagement through an ethical lens. Am J Trop Med Hyg. 2015;93(6):1194–200.

21. American College of Obstetricians and Gynecologists. Ethical considerations for performing gynecologic surgery in low-resource settings abroad. Committee Opinion No. 466. Obstet Gynecol. 2010;116:793–9.

22. Mohamed-Ahmed R, Daniels A, Goodall J, O'Kelly E, Fisher J. "Disaster day": global health simulation teaching. Clin Teach. 2016;13(1):18–22.

23. World Health Organization. Maternal mortality fact sheet [Internet]. 2016 [cited 017 Mar 1]. Available from: https://www.who.int/mediacentre/factsheets/fs348/en/.

24. Ameh CA, Obgyn F, Van Den Broek N. Best practice & research clinical obstetrics and gynaecology making it happen : training health-care providers in emergency obstetric and newborn care. Best Pract Res Clin Obstet Gynaecol. 2015;29:1077–91.

25. Fritz J, Walker DM, Cohen S, Angeles G, Lamadrid-Figueroa H. Can a simulation-based training program impact the use of evidence based routine practices at birth? Results of a hospital-based cluster randomized trial in Mexico. PLoS One. 2017;12(3):e0172623.

26. Walton A, Kestler E, Dettinger JC, Zelek S, Holme F, Walker D. Impact of a low-technology simulation-based obstetric and newborn care training scheme on non-emergency delivery practices in Guatemala. Int J Gynecol Obstet. 2016;132(3):359–64.

27. PROMPT Maternity Foundation. Practical obstetric multi-professional training [Internet]. [cited 2017 Mar 1]. Available from: http://www.promptmaternity.org/

28. Ashish KC, Wrammert J, Clark RB, et al. Reducing perinatal mortality in Nepal using helping babies breathe. Pediatrics. 2016;137(6):e20150117e.

29. Debas HT, Donkon P, Gawande A, Jamison DT, Kruk ME, editors. Essential surgery. 3rd ed. Washington, DC: The International Bank for Reconstruction and Development/The World Bank; 2015.

30. Mahmud A, Kettle C, Bick D, Rowley C, Rathod T, Belcher J, et al. The development and validation of an internet-based training package for the management of perineal trauma following childbirth: MaternityPEARLS. Postgrad Med J. 2013;89(1053):382–9.

31. Cohen SR, Cragin L, Rizk M, Hanberg A, Walker DM. PartoPantsTM: The high-fidelity, low-tech birth simulator. Clin Simul Nurs. 2011;7(1):e11–8.

32. Deganus SA. SYMPTEK homemade foam models for client education and emergency obstetric care skills training in low-resource settings. J Obstet Gynaecol Can. 2009;31(10):930–5.

33. Illston JD, Ballard AC, Ellington DR, Richter HE. Modified beef tongue model for fourth-degree laceration repair simulation. Obstet Gynecol. 2017;129(3):491–6.

34. Sparks RA, Beesley AD, Jones AD. The "sponge perineum:" an innovative method of teaching fourth-degree obstetric perineal laceration repair to family medicine residents. Fam Med. 2006;38(8):542–4.

35. Perosky J, Richter R, Rybak O, Gans-Larty F, Mensah MA, Danquah A, et al. A low-cost simulator for learning to manage postpartum hemorrhage in rural Africa. Simul Healthc. 2011;6(1):42–7.

36. Tunitsky-Bitton E, King CR, Ridgeway B, Barber MD, Lee T, Muffly T, et al. Development and validation of a laparoscopic sacrocolpopexy simula-

tion model for surgical training. J Minim Invasive Gynecol. 2014;21(4):612–8.

37. Tunitsky-Bitton E, Propst K, Muffly T. Development and validation of a laparoscopic hysterectomy cuff closure simulation model for surgical training. Am J Obstet Gynecol. 2016;214(3):392.e1–6.

38. Tunitsky E, Murphy A, Barber MD, Simmons M, Jelovsek JE. Development and validation of a ureteral anastomosis simulation model for surgical training. Female Pelvic Med Reconstr Surg. 2013;19(6):346–51.

39. Hong A, Mullin PM, Al-Marayati L, Peyre SE, Muderspach L, Macdonald H, et al. A low-fidelity total abdominal hysterectomy teaching model for obstetrics and gynecology residents. Simul Healthc. 2012;7(2):123–6.

40. Hefler L, Grimm C, Kueronya V, Tempfer C, Reinthaller A, Polterauer S. A novel training model for the loop electrosurgical excision procedure: An innovative replica helped workshop participants improve their LEEP. Am J Obstet Gynecol. 2012;206(6):535.e1–4.

41. Beard JH, Akoko L, Mwanga A, Mkony C, O'Sullivan P. Manual laparoscopic skills development using a low-cost trainer box in Tanzania. J Surg Educ. 2014;71(1):85–90.

42. Lozo S, Eckardt MJ, Altawil Z, Nelson BD, Ahn R, Khisa W, et al. Prevalence of unrepaired third- and fourth-degree tears among women taken to the operating room for repair of presumed obstetric fistula during two fistula camps in Kenya. Int Urogynecol J Pelvic Floor Dysfunct. 2016;27(3):463–6.

43. Utz B, Kana T, van den Broek N. Practical aspects of setting up obstetric skills laboratories—a literature review and proposed model. Midwifery. 2015;31(4):400–8.

44. Fuchs KM, Miller RS, Berkowitz RL. Optimizing outcomes through protocols, multidisciplinary drills, and simulation. Semin Perinatol. 2009;33(2):104–8.

45. Grimes DA, Benson J, Singh S, Romero M, Ganatra B, Okonofua FE, et al. Unsafe abortion: the preventable pandemic. Lancet. 2006;368(9550):1908–19.

46. Campbell M, Sahin-Hodoglugil NNPM. Barriers to fertility regulation: a review of the literature. Stud Fam Plan. 2006;37(2):87–98.

47. Adler A, Ronsmans C, Calvert C, Filippi V. Estimating the prevalence of obstetric fistula: a systematic review and meta-analysis. BMC Pregnancy Childbirth. 2013;13(1):246.

48. World Health Organization. WHO Guidelines for Safe Surgery 2009. Who [Internet]. 2009;125. Available from: http://whqlibdoc.who.int/publications/2009/9789241598552_eng.pdf.

49. Chao TE, Mandigo M, Opoku-Anane J, Maine R. Systematic review of laparoscopic surgery in low- and middle-income countries: benefits, challenges, and strategies. Surg Endosc Other Interv Tech. 2016;30(1):1–10.

50. 2020 FP. FP2020 Initiative [Internet]. [cited 2017 Mar 1]. Available from: http://www.familyplanning2020.org/.

51. Ngo TD, Nuccio O, Pereira SK, Footman K, Reiss K. Evaluating a LARC expansion program in 14 Sub-Saharan African countries: a service delivery model for meeting FP2020 goals. Matern Child Health J. 2016;1:1–10.

52. Cleeve A, Faxelid E, Nalwadda G, Klingberg-Allvin M. Abortion as agentive action: reproductive agency among young women seeking post-abortion care in Uganda. Cult Health Sex. 2017;1058:1–15.

53. Cook S, de Kok B, Odland ML. "It's a very complicated issue here': understanding the limited and declining use of manual vacuum aspiration for post-abortion care in Malawi: a qualitative study. Health Policy Plan. 2017;32:305–13.

54. Kabagenyi A, Reid A, Ntozi J, Atuyambe L. Sociocultural inhibitors to use of modern contraceptive techniques in rural Uganda: a qualitative study. Pan Afr Med J. 2016;25:1–12.

55. Bowling CB, Gerer WJ, Bryant SA, Gleason JL, Szychowski JM, Varner E, Holley RLRH. Testing and validation of a low cost cystoscopy teaching model. Obstet Gynecol. 2010;116(1):85–91.

56. Okrainec A, Henao O, Azzie G. Telesimulation: an effective method for teaching the fundamentals of laparoscopic surgery in resource-restricted countries. Surg Endosc Other Interv Tech. 2010;24(2):417–22.

Index